Photodynamic Therapy - From Basic Science to Clinical Research

Edited by Natalia Mayumi Inada, Hilde Harb Buzzá, Kate Cristina Blanco and Lucas Danilo Dias

Published in London, United Kingdom

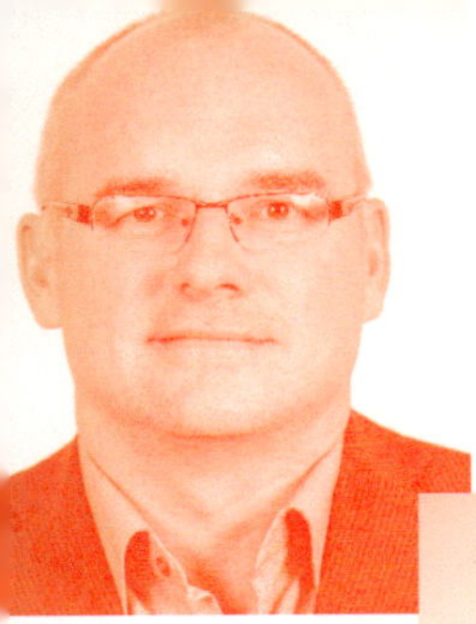
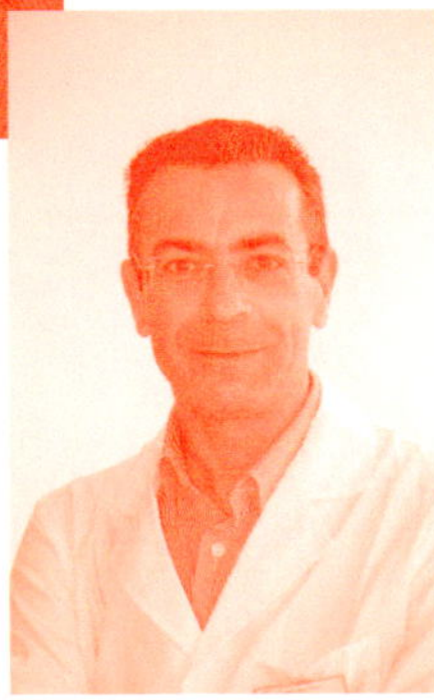
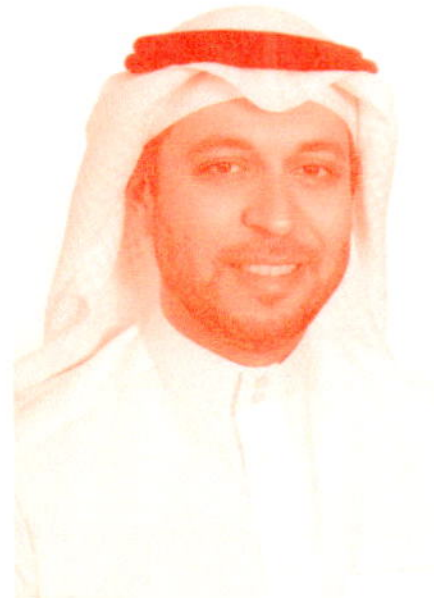
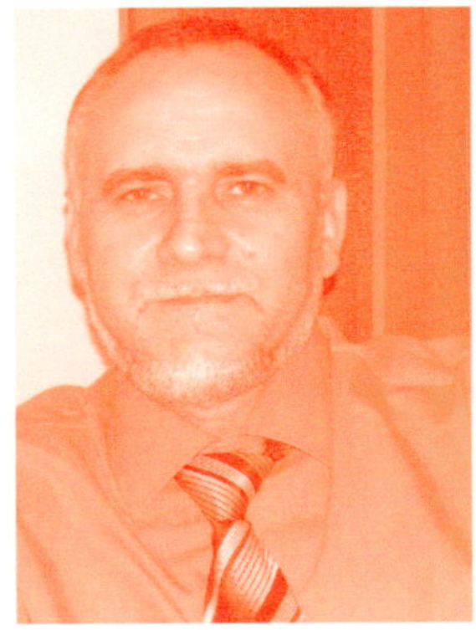
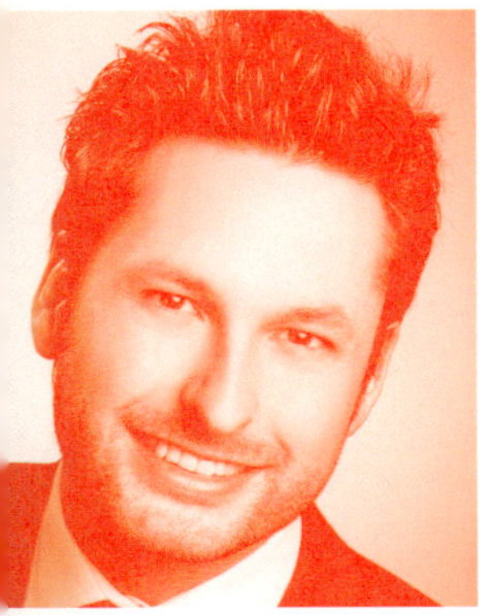
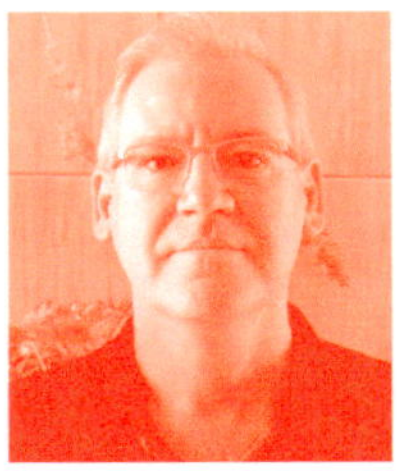
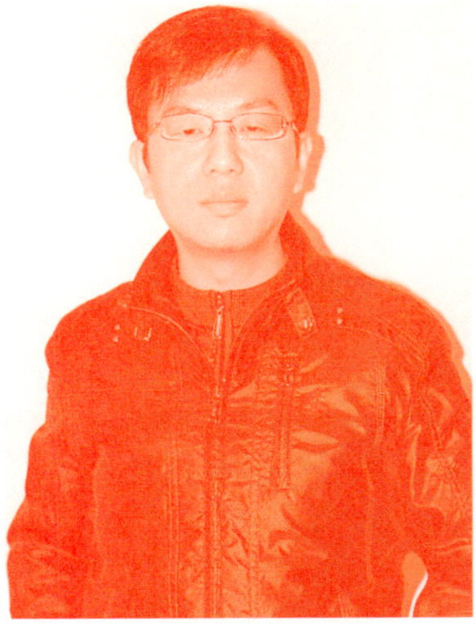

IntechOpen

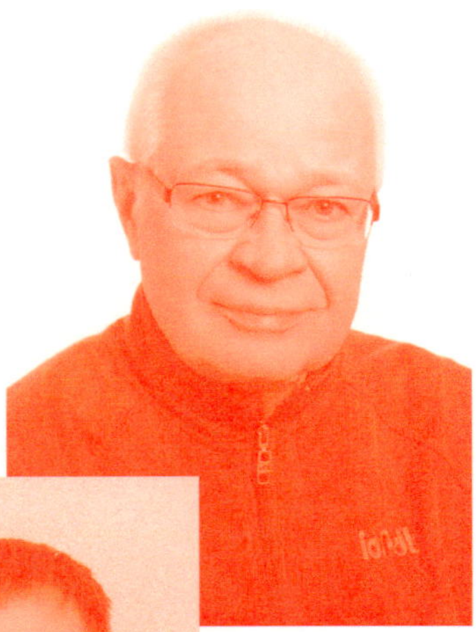
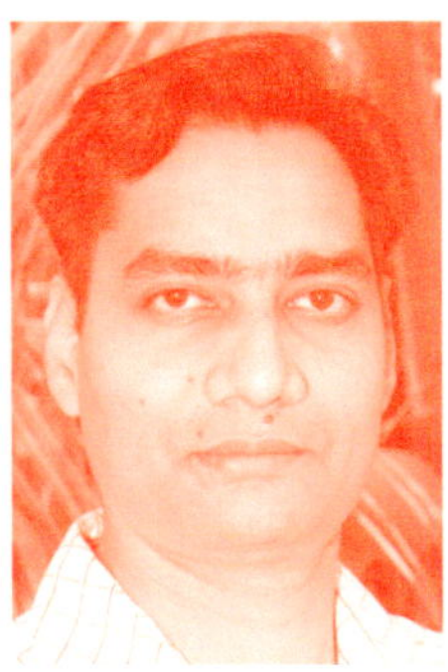
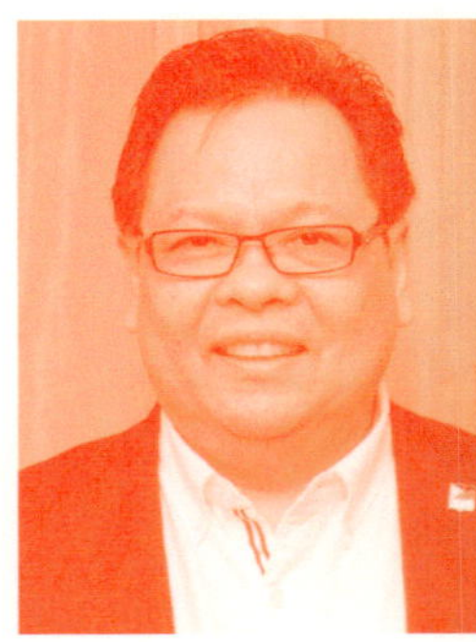
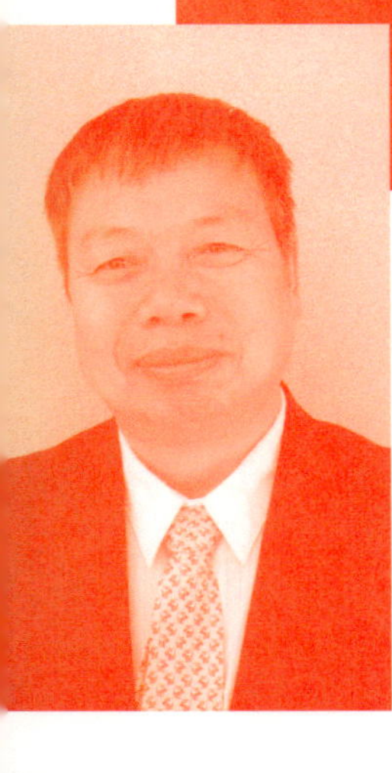
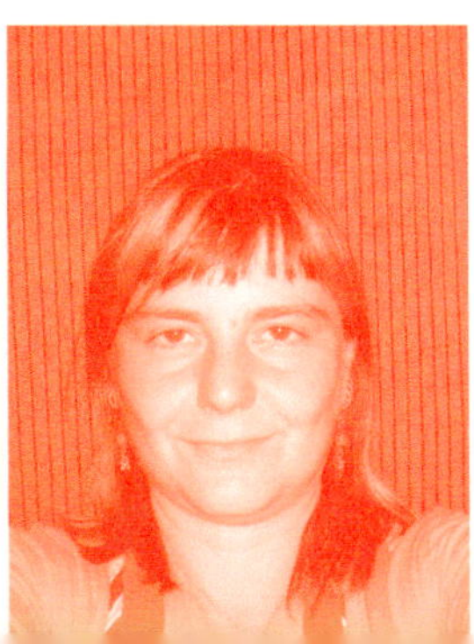
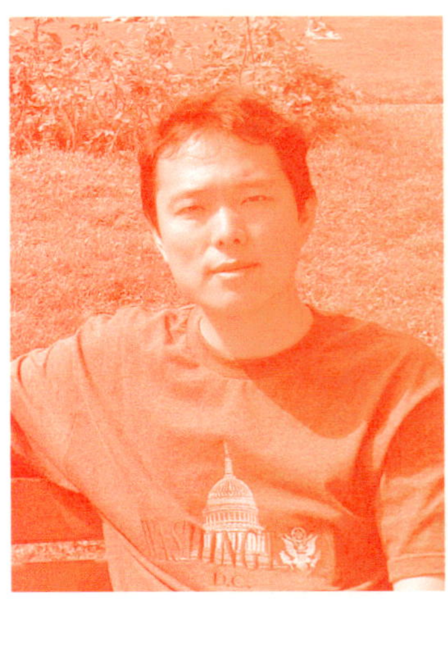

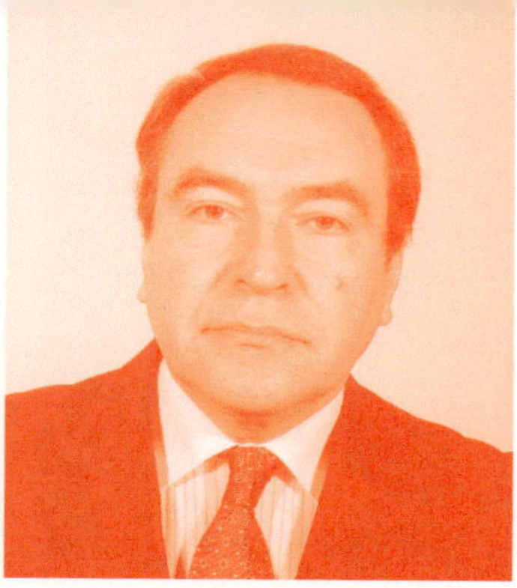
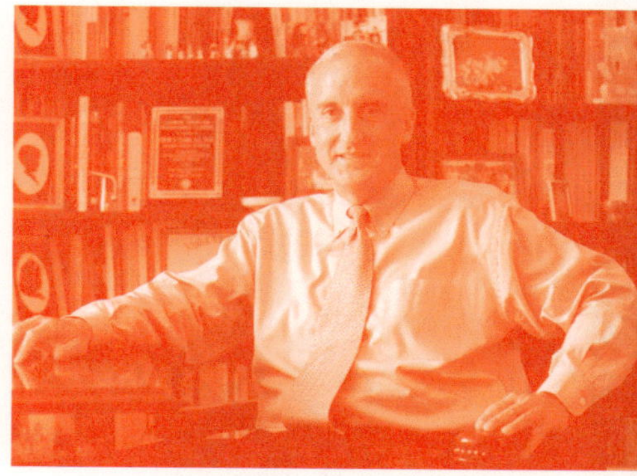
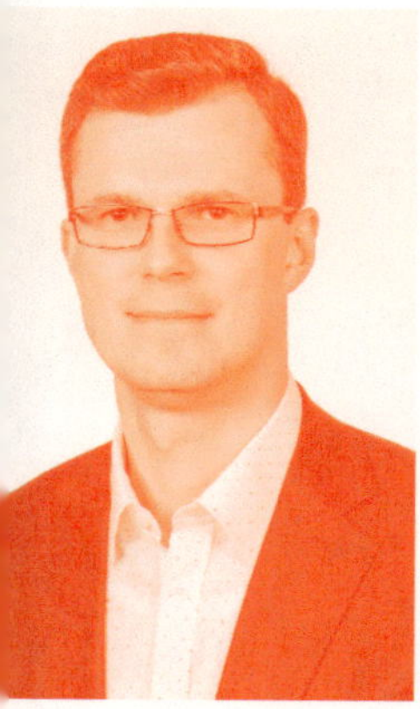
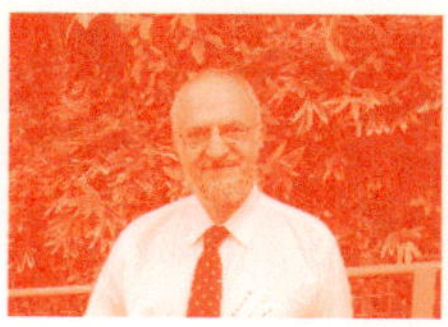
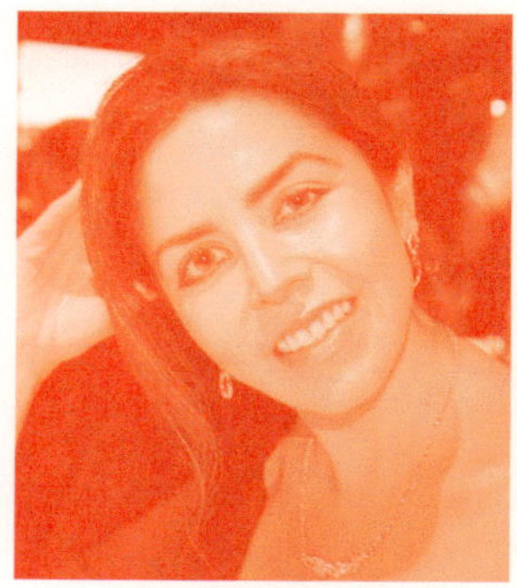

Supporting open minds since 2005

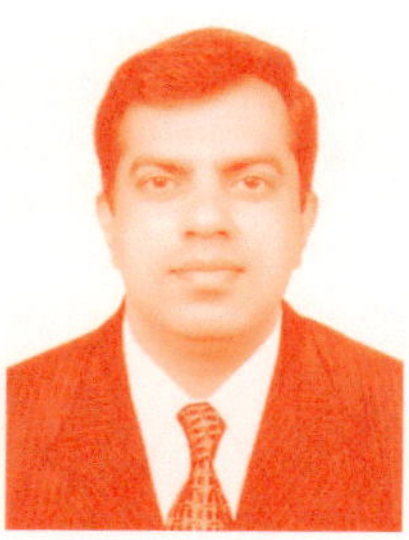
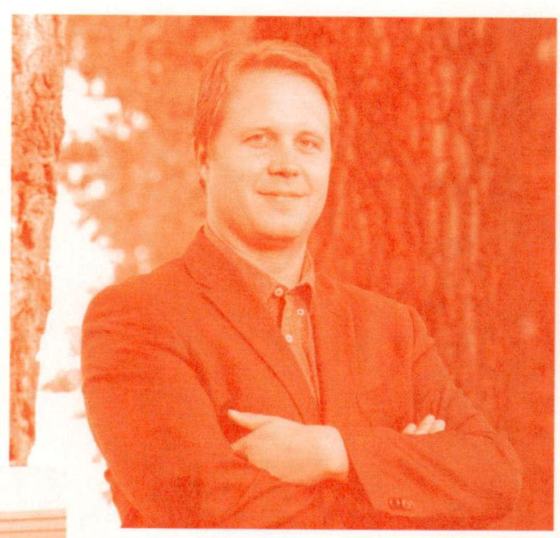
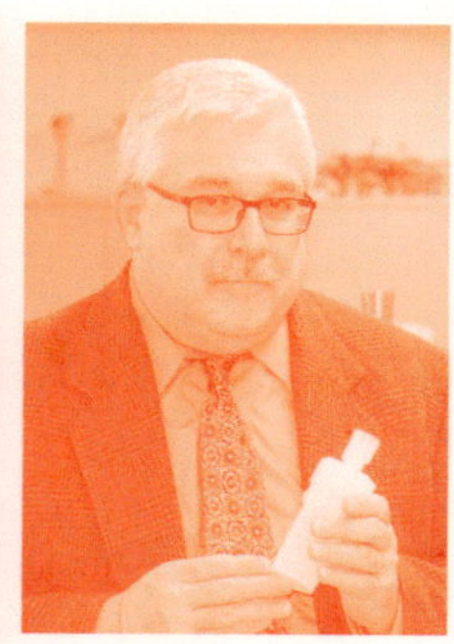
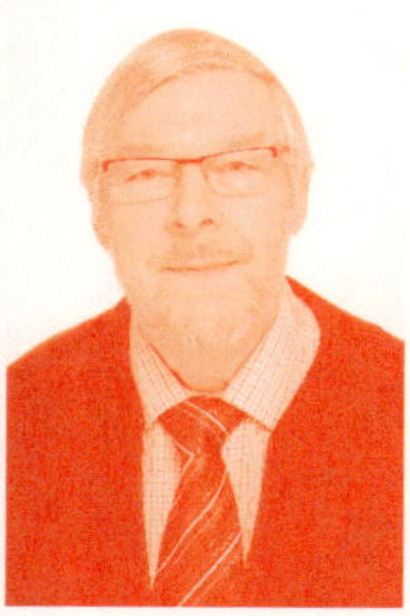
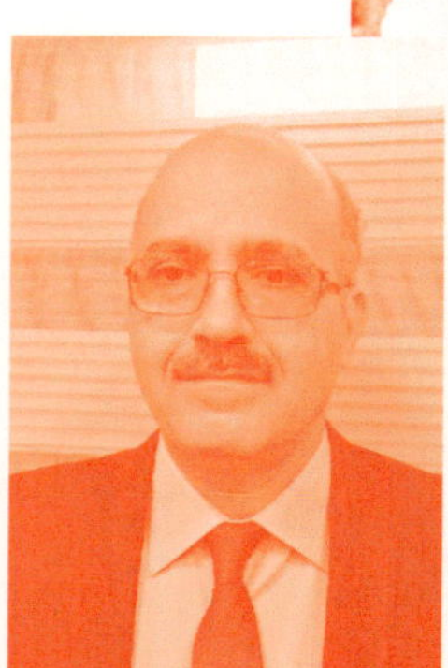
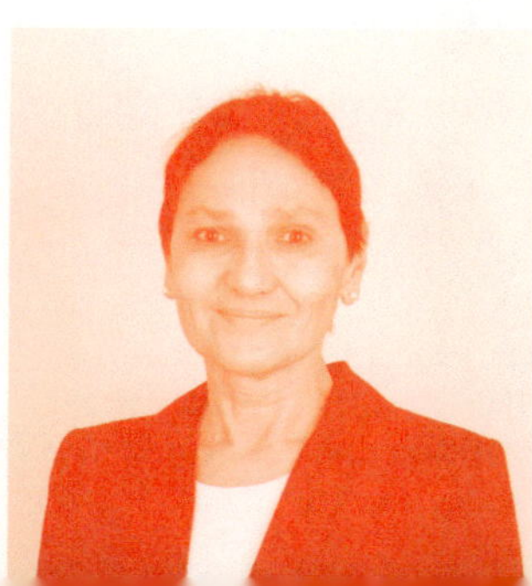
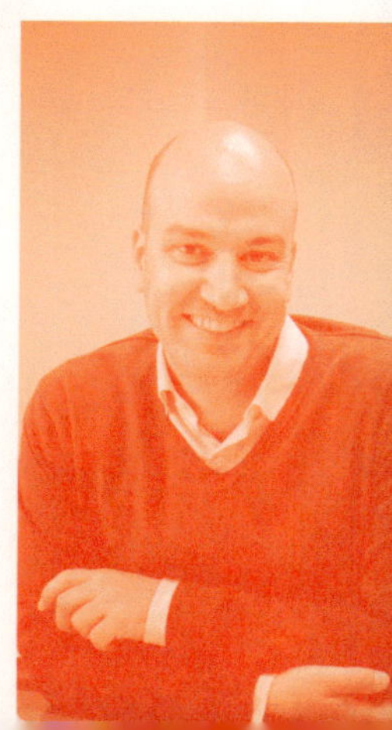

Photodynamic Therapy - From Basic Science to Clinical Research
http://dx.doi.org/10.5772/intechopen.77705
Edited by Natalia Mayumi Inada, Hilde Harb Buzzá, Kate Cristina Blanco and Lucas Danilo Dias

Assistant to the Editors: Giulia Kassab

Contributors
Alessandra Fujita, Daniel Chianfrone, Vinicius Moreira, Anderson Zanchin, Priscila Menezes, Vanderlei Salvador Bagnato, Lucas de Freitas, Cristina Pacheco-Soares, Bruno Henrique Godoi, Juliana Ferreira Strixino, Newton Soares Da Silva, Michelle Barreto Requena, Mirian Denise Stringasci, José Dirceu Vollet-Filho, Natalia Mayumi Inada, Hilde Harb Buzzá, Lucas Danilo Dias, Kate Cristina Blanco, Giulia Kassab, Dragana Gabrić, Bleron Azizi, Ana Budimir, Ivona Bago, Luka Marković, Verica Pavlić, Marko Vuletić, Božana Lončar Brzak, Igor Smojver, Mato Sušić, Kazutaka Hirakawa, André Romero Da Silva, Barbara Silva Silva Figueiredo, Vannyla Viktoria Viana Vasconcelos, Julyana Noval De Souza Ferreira, Priscila Ponate De Souza, Rafaela Vergna De Angeli, Aline Margraf-Ferreira, Carolina W. Galvão, Rafael M. Etto, Christian Palavecino, Camila Perez, Tania Zuñiga, Luiz A. Alves, Evellyn Araujo Dias, Heber Lopes de Mello, Sabrina De Sá Pereira Magalhães, Vinicius Cotta De Almeida, Rodrigo Da Cunha Bisaggio, Niral M. Patel, Ali I. Musani, Vanderlei Salvador Bagnato

First published in London, United Kingdom, 2021 by IntechOpen
IntechOpen is the global imprint of INTECHOPEN LIMITED, registered in England and Wales, registration number: 11086078, 5 Princes Gate Court, London, SW7 2QJ, United Kingdom
Printed in Croatia

British Library Cataloguing-in-Publication Data
A catalogue record for this book is available from the British Library

Additional hard and PDF copies can be obtained from orders@intechopen.com

Photodynamic Therapy - From Basic Science to Clinical Research
Edited by Natalia Mayumi Inada, Hilde Harb Buzzá, Kate Cristina Blanco and Lucas Danilo Dias
p. cm.
Print ISBN 978-1-83968-060-1
Online ISBN 978-1-83968-061-8
eBook (PDF) ISBN 978-1-83968-068-7

For EU product safety concerns:
IN TECH d.o.o., Prolaz Marije Krucifikse Kozulić 3, 51000 Rijeka, Croatia, info@intechopen.com or visit our website at intechopen.com.

Meet the editor

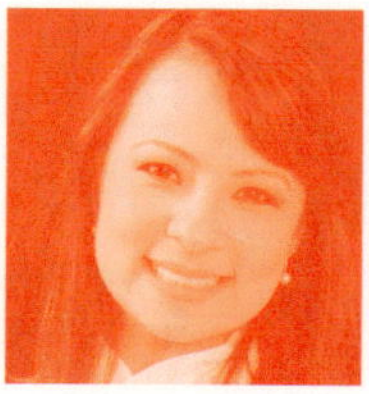

Natalia M. Inada earned a Ph.D. in Medical Pathophysiology from the State University of Campinas (UNICAMP), Brazil, in 2006). She is currently a research scientist at the University of São Paulo (USP), São Carlos Institute of Physics, Brazil, leading the Microbial Control and Cell Culture Labs at the Biophotonics Group. She works in multicenter clinical projects such as the "CerCa Solutions for Diagnosis and Treatment of Cervical Intraepithelial Neoplasia" and "Photodynamic Therapy Brazil for Non-melanoma Skin Cancer." Dr. Inada's research focuses on improving photodynamic therapy with nanodelivery systems, and the treatment of infectious diseases. She has published numerous scientific papers and book chapters, and was awarded for her work many times, including the Mercosur Prize for Science and Technology (2016), the PDT Clinical Trial Excellence (2017), and Poster of Merit (2019) by the International Photodynamic Association.

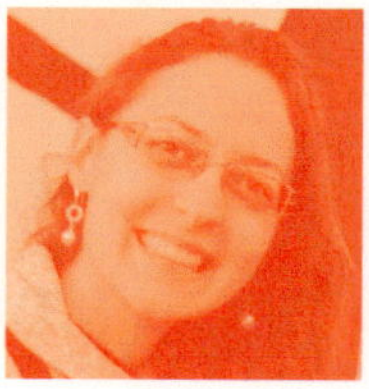

Dr. Hilde Harb Buzza is currently a postdoctoral fellow at the Institute of Physics of São Carlos (IFSC), University of São Paulo (USP), Brazil, studying light application in life science. She graduated with a degree in Physical and Biomolecular Sciences and obtained her Ph.D. in Applied Physics from IFSC. She has experience in the field of photodynamic and photothermal therapies for tumor treatments and infections caused by bacteria and fungi, with studies from the lab to clinical trials. She has worked with the application of nanotechnology in biophotonics and has contributed to teaching and scientific dissemination activities.

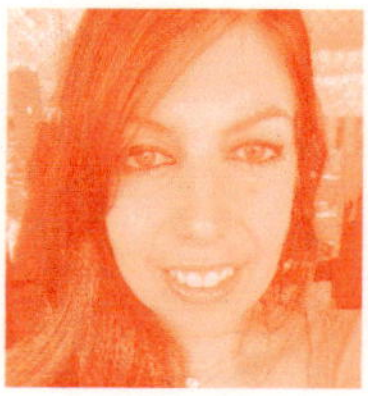

Kate Blanco is a postdoctoral researcher at the São Carlos Institute of Physics, University of São Paulo (USP), Brazil, and has been working at the Optics and Photonics Research Center of the São Paulo Research Foundation (Fapesp). She has a degree in Biomedicine and a doctorate in Microbiology from Universidade Estadual Paulista (Unesp), Brazil. She specializes in industrial fermentation and the production of health products and processes, infections, and microbial control of food using optical techniques.

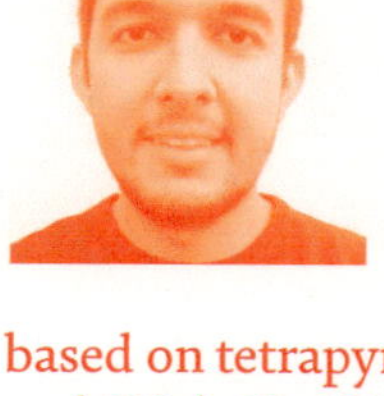

Lucas D. Dias received his Ph.D. in Chemistry at the University of Coimbra, Portugal, and is currently a postdoctoral research fellow at the University of São Paulo (USP), Brazil. His current research interests are in the fields of medicine and catalysis, namely, mechanisms in photodynamic therapy, synthesis of photosensitizers for photodynamic therapy, design and synthesis of photocatalysts, and synthesis of homogeneous and immobilized catalysts based on tetrapyrrolic macrocycles for the activation of small molecules (O_2, CO and CO_2). Dr. Dias has published thirty-two peer-reviewed papers in national/international journals, authored more than forty communications (oral and posters) in national/international scientific meetings, and is the inventor of one patent.

Contents

Preface

Photodynamic Therapy - From Basic Science to Clinical Research features chapters written by experienced and renowned authors in the field. This book brings together chapters that cover the basic principles of photodynamic therapy as well as clinical studies of its use in treating oncologic and other diseases. It also presents innovative strategies in photodynamic therapy, including information on polymer nanoparticles.

I would like to acknowledge Dr. Lucas Danilo Dias, Dr. Kate Cristina Blanco, Dr. Hilde Harb Buzzá and MSc. Giulia Kassab for their exceptional contributions to the editorial process. This book was prepared with great care and by many valuable hands so that we can expand the dissemination of photodynamic therapy as well as inspire new research.

Natalia Mayumi Inada
São Carlos Institute of Physics,
University of São Paulo,
São Carlos-SP, Brazil

Hilde Harb Buzzá, Kate Cristina Blanco and Lucas Danilo Dias
University of Sao Paulo,
Brazil

Chapter 1

Electron Transfer-Supported Photodynamic Therapy

Kazutaka Hirakawa

Abstract

Photodynamic therapy (PDT) is a less-invasive treatment of cancer and precancerous lesions. Porphyrin derivatives have been used and studied as the photosensitizers for PDT. In general, the biomacromolecules oxidation by singlet oxygen, which is produced through energy transfer from the photoexcited photosensitizers to oxygen molecules, is an important mechanism of PDT. However, the traditional PDT effect may be restricted, because tumors are in a hypoxic condition and in certain cases, PDT enhances hypoxia via vascular damage. To solve this problem, the electron transfer-mediated oxidation of biomolecules has been proposed as the PDT mechanism. Specifically, porphyrin phosphorus(V) complexes demonstrate relatively strong photooxidative activity in protein damage through electron transfer. Furthermore, other photosensitizers, *e.g.*, cationic free-base porphyrins, can oxidize biomolecules through electron transfer. The electron transfer-supported PDT may play the important roles in hypoxia cancer therapy. Furthermore, the electron transfer-supported mechanism may contribute to antimicrobial PDT. In this chapter, recent topics about the biomolecules photooxidation by electron transfer-supported mechanism are reviewed.

Keywords: Photoinduced electron transfer, porphyrin phosphorus(V) complex, protein oxidation, cationic porphyrin, phenothiazine dyes

1. Introduction

Photodynamic therapy (PDT) is a less-invasive treatment of cancer and other nonmalignant conditions [1–3]. This treatment is a medicinal application of photochemistry. Antimicrobial treatment, called as antimicrobial photodynamic therapy (aPDT) or photodynamic antimicrobial chemotherapy (PACT), is also important application [4–7]. In the case of cancer treatment, less-toxic PDT reagents, photosensitizers, cause oxidative damage to biomolecules, including protein, nucleic acids, and/or other compounds, under visible-light irradiation. This photosensitized reaction results in necrosis or apoptosis of cancer cells [1–3]. As the PDT photosensitizers, porphyrins have been extensively studied and used [8–11]. For example, porfimer sodium [12, 13] and talaporfin sodium [13], an oligomer and a monomer of a free-base anionic porphyrin, respectively, are well-known photosensitizers in clinical use. In general, the porphyrin photosensitizer (*e.g.*, almost 60 mg/body for talaporfin sodium) is given for the target tissue, followed by irradiation of the visible light (e.g., 664 nm, 150 mW cm^{-2}, and 10 J cm^{-2}). To reduce the risk of adverse side effects, the development of efficient photosensitizers that work with harmless weak light is important. Furthermore, consideration of PDT mechanism is also important to develop effective photosensitizer. Most of porphyrins have relatively large quantum yield (Φ_Δ) for singlet oxygen ($^1O_2$), a reactive oxygen species (ROS), generation [14]. $^1O_2$ can be easily generated by relatively small energy photon of long wavelength visible light and/or near infrared radiation (wavelength $\gtrsim$ 770 nm) through energy transfer from photoexcited photosensitizer to oxygen molecule [15–17]. Radiation in the long wavelength region called "optical window", 600 ~ 1300 nm, can penetrate human tissue deeply [18]. Therefore, $^1O_2$ is the important reactive species of porphyrin-based PDT. However, the phototoxic effect of $^1O_2$ on PDT is restricted because of the hypoxic condition of tumors [19–22]. Furthermore, in certain cases, PDT itself enhances hypoxia [23] via vascular damage [24]. This "hypoxia problem" of tumor is very important to improve the PDT effect.

Oxidation is defined as the oxygenation, hydrogen extraction, and electron extraction. Electron extraction from biomolecules to photoexcited photosensitizer is also the mechanism of oxidative biomolecule damage. This electron transfer oxidation may be an important mechanism to resolve the "hypoxia problem" and to develop the effective PDT photosensitizers. Phosphorus(V) porphyrins [25, 26] and cationic free-base porphyrins [27] have relatively strong oxidative activity through electron transfer [28]. Furthermore, electron transfer process can be control by surroundings condition, for example pH of medium [29, 30].

In this chapter, recent studies about the electron transfer-supported photosensitizer for PDT are reviewed. The examples of activity control of photosensitizer for the cancer-selective PDT are also introduced. In the last section, the role of electron transfer mechanism in aPDT is discussed.

2. Electron transfer oxidation as a mechanism of photosensitized biomolecule damage

In general, photosensitized biomolecule damage can be explained by oxygen-independent mechanism (Type I mechanism) and oxygen-mediated mechanism (Type II mechanism) (**Figure 1**) [31–33]. Because the electron transfer-mediated biomolecule oxidation does not absolutely require oxygen, this mechanism is categorized as Type I mechanism. On the other hand, biomolecule oxidation through $^1O_2$ generation is defined as Type II mechanism (Type II, major). Another ROS-mediated process, superoxide ($O_2^{\bullet-}$)-mediated biomolecule oxidation is also categorized as the Type II mechanism (Type II, minor). Although $O_2^{\bullet-}$ is produced through electron transfer from photoexcited photosensitizer, it's not categorized as the Type I mechanism. The initial process of electron transfer-mediated biomolecule oxidation is an electron extraction from the targeting biomolecule, such as protein, to the photoexcited photosensitizer.

2.1 Driving force dependence of electron transfer

The driving force of electron transfer, Gibbs energy (ΔG), is determined by the excitation energy of photosensitizer (photon energy) and the redox potential of photosensitizer and targeting biomolecule. The electron transfer is a relaxation process of photoexcited photosensitizer. Fast electron transfer is advantageous for an efficient electron transfer. Due to the Marcus theory [34, 35], the rate constant of electron transfer (k_{ET}) is expressed using ΔG as follows:

$$k_{ET} = \sqrt{\frac{4\pi^3}{h^2 \lambda K_B T}} V_{DA}{}^2 \exp\frac{-\left(\Delta G^* + \lambda\right)^2}{4\lambda K_B T}, \tag{1}$$

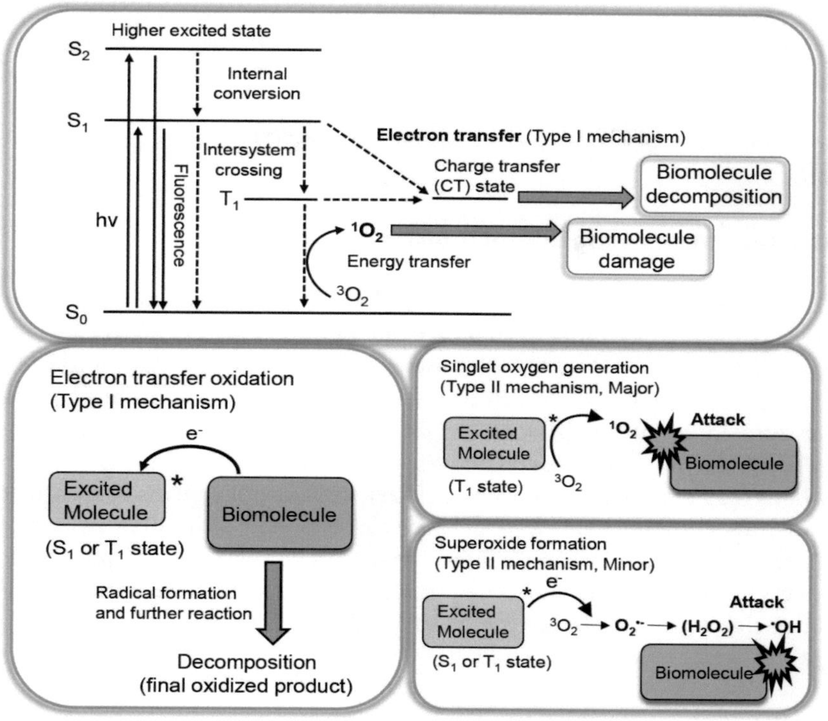

Figure 1.
Relaxation process of photoexcited state of photosensitizer and the typical photosensitized biomolecule damaging mechanisms.

where h is Plank constant, λ is the reorganization energy, K_B is the Boltzmann constant, and V_{DA} is the effective electronic Hamiltonian matrix element. The λ can be calculated from the following equation:

$$\lambda = \frac{e^2}{4\pi\varepsilon_0}\left(\frac{1}{2r_D}+\frac{1}{2r_A}+\frac{2}{d}\right)\left(\frac{1}{n^2}-\frac{1}{\varepsilon}\right), \tag{2}$$

where e is the elementary charge, ε_0 is the vacuum permeability (8.854×10^{-12} F m^{-1}), r_D and r_A are the radius of the electron donor and that of acceptor, respectively, d is the distance between electron donor and acceptor, n is the refractive index, and ε is the static dielectric constant of surrounding material. Since the V_{DA} is determined by the overlap between wavefunctions of electron donor and acceptor, the electron transfer rate strongly depends on the d, and decreased exponentially with an increase in d. Therefore, association between photosensitizer and targeting biomolecule is very important. The ΔG, driving force of electron transfer, is expressed as follows:

$$\Delta G = e\left(E_{red} - E_{ox}\right) - E_{0-0}, \tag{3}$$

where E_{red} is the redox potential of a one-electron reduction of photosensitizer, E_{ox} is the redox potential of a one-electron oxidation of targeting biomolecule, and E_{0-0} is the 0–0 energy (singlet excited (S_1) energy) of photosensitizer. The Eq. (1) indicates that k_{ET} becomes maximum at $\Delta G = \lambda$. However, in general, large -ΔG is advantageous for fast electron transfer. Therefore, small (small absolute value) E_{red} and/or large (large absolute value) E_{ox} is appropriate for effective electron transfer. To evaluate the electron transfer in the triplet excited (T_1) state, the "E_{0-0}" term in Eq. (3) is replaced with the T_1 state energy. Because T_1 state energy is smaller than E_{0-0}, in general, electron transfer oxidation by T_1 state photosensitizer becomes difficult.

2.2 Excitation energy and electron transfer

Excitation energy (photon energy) strongly affects the electron transfer rate and efficiency as the Eq. (3). Indeed, an ultraviolet photosensitizer can oxidize DNA, which is relatively resistant to the electron extraction, through photoinduced electron transfer [32, 33]. However, ultraviolet radiation is harmful for human tissue. Furthermore, long wavelength visible light or near infrared radiation can penetrate human tissue deeply as mentioned above as the optical window [18]. Therefore, visible light (or near infrared) photosensitizer, such as porphyrins and phthalocyanines, are important for PDT. To realize the electron transfer photosensitizer, which can be excited by long wavelength light, the design and synthesis of photosensitizer molecules with small E_{red} value are required. However, a molecule with small E_{red} has tend to decay through reduction by surrounding molecules, and small E_{red} is not appropriate for stability of molecule.

2.3 Kinetics of electron transfer

In general, electron transfer can be demonstrated by a transient absorption spectrum measurement [36, 37] and a time-resolved electron paramagnetic resonance measurement [38, 39]. The k_{ET} values can be determined by the analysis of transient absorption spectra. Fluorescence lifetime measurement is also an important method [40]. Although fluorescence lifetime is affected by various factors other than electron transfer, it is sensitive and convenient method. If other factors can be excluded, this method is advantageous for the kinetic evaluation of electron transfer. The k_{ET} value can be obtained using fluorescence lifetime by the following equation:

$$k_{ET} = \frac{1}{\tau_f} - \frac{1}{\tau_f^0}, \tag{4}$$

where τ_f is the observed fluorescence lifetime of photosensitizer with electron donor (targeting biomolecule) and τ_f^0 is that without electron donor. In general, k_{ET} becomes larger than $10^8 \sim 10^9$ s^{-1} in the case of electron transfer in the S_1 state, because lifetime of most of porphyrin S_1 state is order of several nanosecond. In the case of T_1 state, the lifetime is order of microsecond and the rate constant becomes relatively small. As mentioned above, the T_1 state is not appropriate for electron transfer oxidation from the thermodynamic point of view.

3. Phosphorus(V) porphyrin photosensitizer

Porphyrin derivatives have been used as clinical photosensitizer for PDT [8–11]. Porfimer sodium [12, 13] and Talaporfin sodium [13] are famous examples of clinically used photosensitizers. The PDT mechanism of these porphyrins is $^1O_2$ generation. The photochemical property of porphyrin can be changed by the replacement of the central atom and substitution. It has been reported that phosphorus(V) porphyrin can oxidize biomolecules, such as nucleobase [41], protein [42–48], and other biomolecules [49, 50] through electron transfer.

3.1 General property of phosphorus(V) porphyrin

General procedure of synthesis method of phosphorus(V) porphyrin is a reflux of free base porphyrin with phosphoryl chloride in dry pyridine [51]. The photochemical property of phosphorus(V) porphyrin can be improved by the substitution of the *meso*- or *β*-positions and the axial ligand (**Figure 2**) [42–53]. An example of phosphorus(V) porphyrin, diethoxyP(V)tetrakis(4-methoxyphenyl) porphyrin chloride, is shown in **Figure 3**. The calculation with density functional theory (DFT) at ωB97X-D/6-31G* level shows the distorted structure of phosphorus(V) porphyrin. Their distorted structures have been reported from the results of X-ray crystal analysis [54]. Phosphorus(V) porphyrins introduced in this chapter are listed in **Table 1**. Because phosphorus(V) porphyrin is a cationic

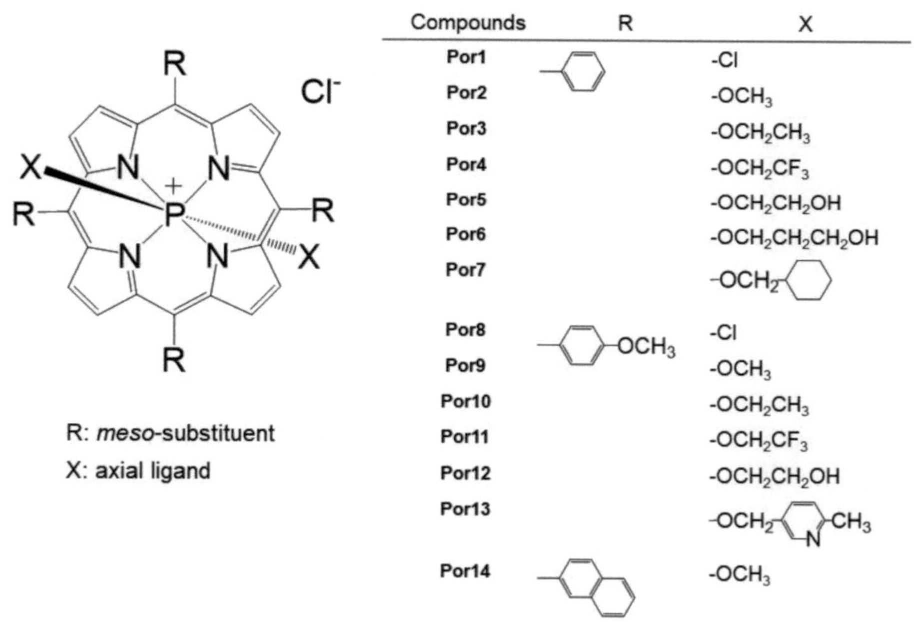

Figure 2.
Structures of phosphorus(V) porphyrins.

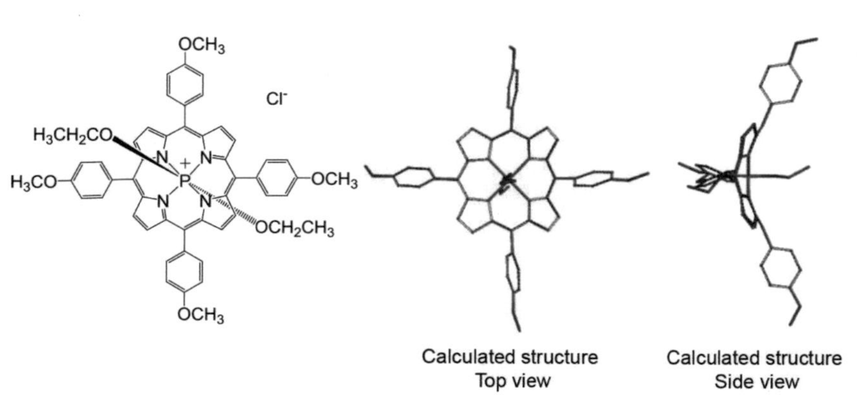

Figure 3.
Optimized structure of **Por10** *by the DFT calculation at ωB97X-D/6-31G* level.*

porphyrin, its water solubility is relatively large. Furthermore, hydrophilic substitution markedly increases the water solubility [55]. One of the most important characteristics of phosphorus(V) porphyrin is relatively small E_{red} value due to the positive charge of the central phosphorus atom, resulting in the strong oxidative activity in the photoexcited state. This character is very important as electron transfer-supported photosensitizer for PDT. Furthermore, in general, phosphorus(V) porphyrin has relatively large quantum yield of photosensitized $^1O_2$ generation in an aqueous solution (Φ_Δ is more than 0.5, **Table 1**) due to the effective intersystem crossing [42–47]. In the presence of enough oxygen molecules, phosphorus(V) porphyrin can oxidize biomolecule through $^1O_2$ generation, a traditional PDT mechanism.

3.2 Photosensitized protein damage by phosphorus(V) porphyrin through electron transfer

Isolated amino acids, a water-soluble protein, and enzymes have been used as the targeting biomacromolecules to examine photosensitizer activity of phosphorus(V) porphyrins [42]. For example, human serum albumin (HSA), a water-soluble protein, is a convenient target. The crystal structure and amino acid sequence of HSA have been clarified [56]. In addition, HSA has major drug specific binding sites identified as Sudlow's site I and site II [57]. The mono-cationic phosphorus(V) porphyrins listed in **Table 1** are well-soluble in organic solvents (*e.g.*, alcohol) rather than water, indicating the hydrophobic character beside the hydrophilicity. Therefore, binding interaction between HSA and phosphorus(V)

Compounds	E_{red} / V	E_{0-0} / eV	Φ_f	Φ_Δ	Ref.
Por1	−0.30	2.04, $PBS_{1.25EtOH}$		0.96, EtOH	[42]
Por2	−0.50[a]	2.03, $PBS_{1.25EtOH}$[a] 2.03, PBS[b]	0.017, $PBS_{2.5EtOH}$[c] 0.023, EtOH[c]	0.64, PBS[b] 0.93, $PBS_{2.5EtOH}$[c]	[42][a], [43][b], [52][c]
Por3	−0.54[e]	2.04, PBS[e]		0.59, PBS[d]	[44][d], [50][e]
Por4	−0.40[e]	2.03, PBS[e]		0.68, PBS[d]	[44][d], [50][e]
Por5	−0.51	2.03, PBS	0.048, PBS	0.88, PBS	[45]
Por6	−0.51	2.03, PBS	0.043, PBS	0.80, PBS	[45]
Por7	−0.54	2.02, $PBS_{1.25EtOH}$		0.94, EtOH	[42]
Por8	−0.33		0.029, PBS	0.97, PBS	[46]
Por9	−0.58		0.024, PBS	0.86, PBS	[46]
Por10	−0.58	1.96, $PBS_{1.0EtOH}$	0.067, EtOH	0.84, EtOH	[47]
Por11	−0.43	1.98, $PBS_{1.0EtOH}$	0.086, EtOH	0.82, EtOH	[47]
Por12	−0.57		0.029, PBS	0.83, PBS	[46]
Por13	−0.55	2.01, $PBS_{1.0EtOH}$	pH-dependent	pH-dependent	[48]
Por14		2.00, $PBS_{2.5EtOH}$	0.034, EtOH	ND, $PBS_{2.5EtOH}$	[52]

E_{red}: measured in acetonitrile (vs. saturated calomel electrode; SCE), PBS: 10 mM sodium phosphate buffer (pH 7.6) solution, EtOH: ethanol, $PBS_{ETOH2.5}$: PBS containing 2.5% ethanol, $PBS_{ETOH1.25}$: PBS containing 1.25% ethanol, $PBS_{ETOH1.0}$: PBS containing 1.0% ethanol, Φ_f: Fluorescence quantum yield. ND: not detected.

Table 1.
Examples of phosphorus(V) porphyrin photosensitizers and their photochemical properties.

porphyrins is expected and their binding site can be speculated. Because the electron transfer-mediated oxidation strongly depends on the distance between photosensitizer and the target molecule, a binding interaction is very important. HSA has one tryptophan, which is easily oxidized by oxidative stress, including $^1O_2$ and electron transfer reaction [42–47, 58]. Tryptophan can emit relatively strong fluorescence and its damage can be detected by fluorescence measurement [45, 58]. Using these characteristics of HSA, the oxidative damage of tryptophan residue by photosensitized reaction can be easily examined by a fluorometry [45–47, 58].

Qualitative study of HSA photodamage by phosphorus(V) porphyrins was reported using **Por2** [43]. **Por2** oxidized the tryptophan of HSA through $^1O_2$ generation and electron transfer. It has been considered that damaged tryptophan is changed to *N*-formylkynurenine and other decomposed products [59, 60]. $^1O_2$ can oxidize the tryptophan residue of HSA [61]. Using isolated amino acids, it has been demonstrated that tyrosine and tryptophan can be oxidized by photoexcited **Por2** [42].

Photosensitized HSA damage by **Por5** and **Por6** was quantitatively clarified [45]. **Por5** and **Por6** bound to HSA and damaged its tryptophan residue during photoirradiation. **Por5** and **Por6** photosensitized $^1O_2$ generation, and the contribution of $^1O_2$ was confirmed by the inhibitory effect of a $^1O_2$ quencher, sodium azide (NaN_3, [62]). From the kinetic analysis, the contribution of electron transfer mechanism to HSA damage was demonstrated [45]. Fluorescence lifetime measurement and the calculation of ΔG supported the electron transfer mechanism.

To realize the effective PDT photosensitizer, response of photosensitizers to long wavelength visible light or near infrared region is important. To improve the abovementioned phosphorus(V) porphyrins, **Por5** and **Por6**, *meso*-phenyl substituted derivatives were designed and synthesized [46]. **Por8**, **Por9**, and **Por12** can be excited under the irradiation of long-wavelength visible light (> 630 nm). These phosphorus(V) porphyrins induced tryptophan oxidation in HSA under illumination with light-emitting diode (central wavelength: 659 nm), and this protein photodamage was barely inhibited by NaN_3 [46]. Fluorescence lifetimes of phosphorus(V) porphyrins was decreased by HSA, suggesting the electron transfer quenching. The ΔG value of electron transfer from tryptophan to the S_1 state of these porphyrins calculated from their redox potentials also supported the electron transfer-mediated oxidation.

3.3 Cancer selective photodynamic action of phosphorus(V) porphyrin photosensitizers

Above mentioned phosphorus(V) porphyrins, **Por8**, **Por9**, and **Por12**, exhibited the cancer cell selective toxicity under visible light irradiation [46].

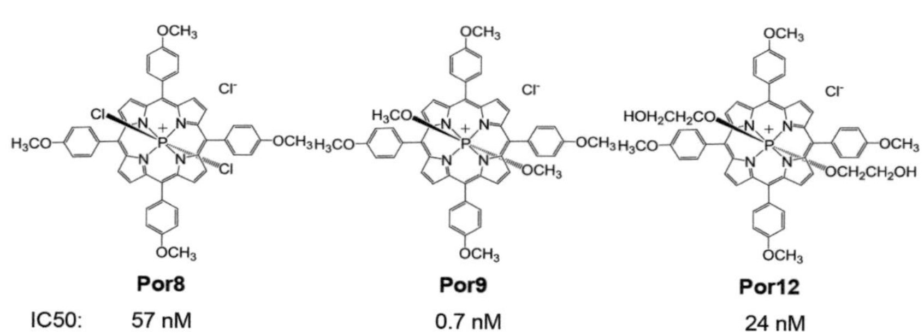

Figure 4.
*Structures of **Por8, Por9,** and **Por12,** and their IC50 values for HeLa cells under photoirradiation [46].*

Photocytotoxicity to HeLa cells by these porphyrins are the following order: **Por9** > **Por12** > **Por8** in the condition of previous report (**Figure 4**) [46]. Although the half maximal inhibitory concentration (IC50) value for **Por8** is largest (least phototoxicity) in the three phosphorus(V) porphyrins, its photocytotoxicity to cancer cells is sufficiently high. Furthermore, **Por8** did not exhibit photocytotoxicity to HaCaT cells, cultured human skin cells (normal cell model). **Por9** and **Por12** exhibited phototoxicity to HaCaT cells, however, these IC50 value were significantly larger than those for HeLa cells and cellular DNA damage in HaCat cells were not observed. These three phosphorus(V) porphyrins demonstrated significant PDT effects on mice tumor models [46]. The observed PDT effects by these porphyrins are almost the same, and are comparable with that of talaporfin sodium. These results suggest the cancer selectivity of **Por8**, **Por9**, and **Por12**, and lower carcinogenic risk to normal cells. Specifically, **Por8**, of which the redox potential is most advantageous for the electron transfer-mediated biomolecule oxidation, demonstrated the highest cancer-selectivity and significant PDT effect under irradiation with long-wavelength visible light.

3.4 Photoinduced electron transfer by phosphorus(V) porphyrin triggers the chain reaction for NADH decomposition

The electron transfer mechanism can contribute to oxidation other various biomolecules. For example, nicotinamide adenine dinucleotide (NADH), an important endogenous reductant, becomes an important targeting molecule [50]. The S_1 states of **Por3** and **Por4** easily extract electron from NADH, resulting in the formation of

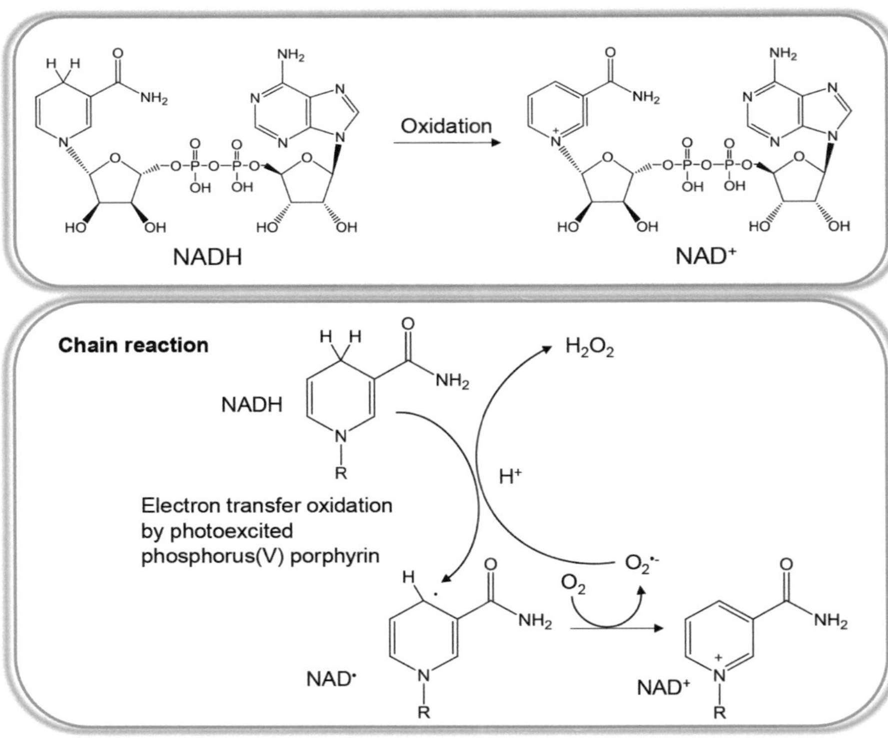

Figure 5.
Structures of NADH and its oxidized form, and the electron transfer-triggered chain reaction of NADH decomposition.

$NAD^{\bullet}$, a radical. Further oxidation leads to the irreversible decomposition of NADH to NAD^+ (**Figure 5**). The total quantum yield of NADH decomposition (Φ_D) is expressed as follows:

$$\Phi_D = \Phi_{ET} \times \Phi_{FR}, \tag{5}$$

where Φ_{ET} is the quantum yield of the initial process (electron transfer) and Φ_{FR} is that of the further reaction to form NAD^+. Analysis of the quantum yields, obtained values of Φ_{FR} became much larger than unity. These findings suggest that the electron accepting by the photoexcited **Por3** and **Por4** triggers a chain reaction of NADH oxidation (**Figure 5**). The initial electron transfer to photoexcited **Por3** or **Por4** produces $NAD^{\bullet}$. The $NAD^{\bullet}$ immediately reacts with molecular oxygen to produce $O_2^{\bullet-}$:

$$NAD^{\bullet} + O_2 \rightarrow NAD^+ + O_2^{\bullet-}. \tag{6}$$

In the following process, $O_2^{\bullet-}$ oxidizes NADH and hydrogen peroxide (H_2O_2) is produced [63]:

$$NADH + O_2^{\bullet-} + H^+ \rightarrow NAD^{\bullet} + H_2O_2. \tag{7}$$

The electron transfer-mediated reaction induces the chain reaction, resulting in the acceleration of NADH decomposition and secondary generation of reactive oxygen species. In the case of direct photosensitized reaction, ultraviolet photon is required to produce H_2O_2 [28]. The secondary formed H_2O_2 may produce hydroxyl radicals ($^{\bullet}OH$), very strong ROS. These results suggest that electron transfer reaction with visible light irradiation induces a severe toxic effect through a chain reaction and the formation of H_2O_2, similarly to the ultraviolet radiation.

3.5 Photosensitized oxidation of folic acid by phosphorus(V) porphyrin through electron transfer

Folic acid, a vitamin, is also oxidized through photoinduced electron transfer [64]. Because the fluorescence intensity of folic acid is significantly increased by the decomposition, a fluorometry of folic acid can be used as a convenient indicator to evaluate the photosensitizer activities [65, 66]. For example, photosensitized decomposition of folic acid by **Por2** through electron transfer was reported [49]. Photoexcited porphyrin can produce $^1O_2$, and folic acid is also oxidized by $^1O_2$. The contribution of $^1O_2$-mediated decomposition can be excluded by the effect of $^1O_2$ quencher and the effect of electron transfer reaction can be evaluated.

4. Contribution of the electron transfer mechanism in photosensitized reaction by cationic porphyrins

Photooxidation activity through electron transfer depends on the redox potential. It has been demonstrated that photoexcited hematoporphyrin, a free base porphyrin, induces the oxidative electron transfer from the tryptophan residue of bovine serum albumin [67, 68]. Cationic porphyrins show relatively small E_{red} values due to their positive charge. In this section, several examples of electron transfer-mediated oxidation of biomolecules by cationic porphyrins.

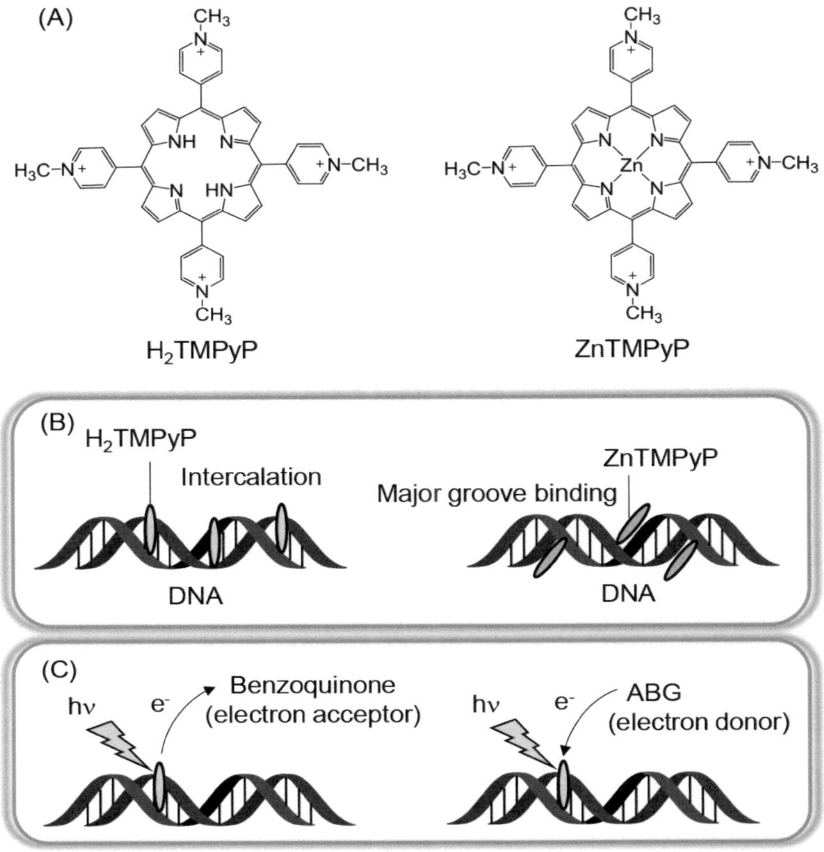

Figure 6.
Structures of H_2TMPyP and ZnTMPyP (A), their binding interaction with DNA (B), and the electron transfer reactions (C). ABG: Amino benzoyl-L-glutamic acid.

4.1 Protein photooxidation through electron transfer by cationic porphyrins

The photosensitized protein damage by tetrakis(*N*-methyl-*p*-pyridinio) porphyrin (H_2TMPyP, **Figure 6**) and its zinc complex (ZnTMPyP, **Figure 6**) was reported [69]. Photosensitized reaction of H_2TMPyP has been extensively studied [14, 70]. Water-solubility of H_2TMPyP and its analogues is appropriate for biological study. Furthermore, electrostatic interaction between these cationic porphyrins and biomacromolecules is considered to enhance the electron transfer reaction with targeting biomolecules. The Φ_Δ value of H_2TMPyP is relatively large [14, 69, 71], and photosensitized biomolecule damage caused by H_2TMPyP through $^1O_2$ generation is generally accepted [70, 72]. However, E_{red} of H_2TMPyP is relatively small [27], and negative ΔG values for photosensitized oxidation of several amino acids through electron transfer are estimated. Therefore, electron transfer-mediated photooxidation of biomolecules is expected.

H_2TMPyP and ZnTMPyP bound to HSA and caused photosensitized oxidation of the tryptophan residue [69]. Three amino acids–tryptophan, phenylalanine, and tyrosine–were also used as target biomolecules, and tryptophan and tyrosine were photodamaged by these cationic porphyrins. However, H_2TMPyP and ZnTMPyP could not photosensitize the damage of phenylalanine. The protein damage (oxidation of the tryptophan residue) was enhanced in deuterium oxide and inhibited by NaN_3. Analysis of the scavenger effect showed that the absolute quantum yields of electron transfer-mediated oxidation are 5.3×10^{-3} and 4.0×10^{-3} for H_2TMPyP

and ZnTMPyP, respectively. The E_{red} of H_2TMPyP (−0.23 V vs. SCE) [27] is lower than that of ZnTMPyP (−0.85 V) [73]. The values of -ΔG for electron transfer from tryptophan to their S_1 states suggest that H_2TMPyP (−1.03 eV) is more oxidative than ZnTMPyP (−0.53 eV). The estimated value of k_{ET} estimated from the fluorescence lifetime for H_2TMPyP was 1.0×10^8 s^{-1}. On the other hand, the fluorescence lifetime of ZnTMPyP was not affected by the interaction with HSA in the presented experimental condition. Because of the relatively shorter fluorescence lifetime of ZnTMPyP (1.3 ns), the estimation of k_{ET} may be difficult by the fluorescence lifetime measurement. Furthermore, protein photodamage by the T_1 states of H_2TMPyP and ZnTMPyP were also discussed [69]. The lifetimes of their T_1 states are relatively long: H_2TMPyP (2.1 μs) and ZnTMPyP (2.7 μs), suggesting that the electron transfer in the T_1 state is kinetically advantageous. The estimated -ΔG of the electron transfer from tryptophan to their T_1 states (−0.65 eV for H_2TMPyP and − 0.15 eV for ZnTMPyP) suggests that this electron transfer is also possible in terms of energy.

4.2 Electron transfer from DNA to photoexcited cationic porphyrins and microenvironmental effect of DNA on photoinduced electron transfer

Photoinduced electron transfer between DNA and the cationic porphyrins, H_2TMPyP and ZnTMPyP, was analyzed by the fluorescence measurements (**Figure 6**) [74]. Absorption spectrum and circular dichroism measurements showed that H_2TMPyP mainly intercalates to calf thymus DNA, whereas ZnTMPyP binds into a DNA groove. An electrostatic interaction with DNA raises their redox potentials of the binding cationic porphyrins. In the presence of DNA, the fluorescence intensity of these porphyrins was almost the same as that without DNA. The E_{ox} of H_2TMPyP (>1.30 V vs. SCE in water) [27], ZnTMPyP (1.18 V vs. SCE in water) [73], and guanine (1.24 V vs. SCE in acetonitrile) [75, 76] suggested that electron transfer by the S_1 state of H_2TMPyP is possible in terms of energy. Furthermore, the electron donating character of guanines increased in the double-stranded structure [77–79]. However, the fluorescence measurements indicated that the S_1 states of these porphyrins are barely quenched by DNA. These results could be explained by that an electrostatic interaction between cationic porphyrins and an anionic DNA strand should increase the redox potential of porphyrins, leading to the inhibition of the electron transfer. In the cases of their higher excited states, secondary excited singlet (S_2) states, the electron transfer from DNA was observed. The lifetime of S_2 state is significantly short (a few picoseconds). However, the E_{red} value of their S_2 states are large (larger E_{red} value of the excited state indicates stronger oxidative activity); >2.14 V vs. SCE for H_2TMPyP and 1.94 V vs. SCE for ZnTMPyP. Therefore, the S_2 states of porphyrins are thermodynamically strong oxidants through electron transfer mechanism.

Photoinduced electron transfer from these porphyrins to benzoquinones, electron acceptors, and that from *N*-(4-aminobenzoyl)-L-glutamic acid (ABG), an electron donor, to these porphyrins were also studied [74]. As mentioned above, the electrostatic interaction with DNA raises the redox potential of cationic porphyrins (*i.e.* decreases the oxidative property of cationic porphyrins). Therefore, the DNA microenvironment inhibited the electron transfer from ABG, an electron-donating quencher, to the binding porphyrins. On the other hand, the electron transfer from the binding porphyrins to benzoquinones, an electron-accepting quencher, was enhanced. A steric effect by the DNA strand was also important. A hydrophobic bulky electron acceptors forms stacking complex with porphyrins, resulting in the strong fluorescence quenching. The interaction with DNA strand cleaves this stacking interaction and inhibit the electron transfer to the benzoquinone. In summary, the DNA microenvironment significantly affects the electron transfer property of the binding cationic porphyrins through an electrostatic interaction and the steric effect.

5. Activity control based on the electron transfer

Electron transfer can be controlled by the surrounding environment. For example, pH is an important factor to control the photoinduced electron transfer [29, 30, 48, 80, 81]. Since it has been reported that cancer cells are slightly acidic (pH 6 ~ 7) against normal tissues (pH 7 ~ 7.4) [82–85], control of the electron transfer of the photosensitizer by pH can be applied for the development of cancer-selective PDT. In the cases of pH-dependent $^1O_2$ photosensitizers, the redox control [30, 86–88], the structure change [89], and the control of intersystem crossing [90] by pH have been reported as the important concepts. Several types of pH-activatable-porphyrin photosensitizers [30, 88], including a phosphorus(V) porphyrin [48, 81], have been reported. In addition, a self-quenching of the photoexcited molecules can be also used to control the activity [47]. In this section, several examples about the activity control of electron transfer-photosensitizers are introduced.

5.1 Electron transfer control by pH

The biomolecule oxidation activity of photosensitizer through electron transfer can be controlled by using changeable electron donor. **Por13** was designed and synthesized to control the photodynamic activity of phosphorus(V) porphyrin photosensitizer (**Figure 7**) [48]. As an electron-donor, 6-methylpyridine was used. The photoexcited **Por13** is quenched through intramolecular electron transfer and this quenching is suppressed by protonation of the methylpyridine moiety, an electron donor. The pK_a of protonated methylpyridine moiety was about 7, and fluorescence lifetime of **Por13** was lengthened under an acidic condition by

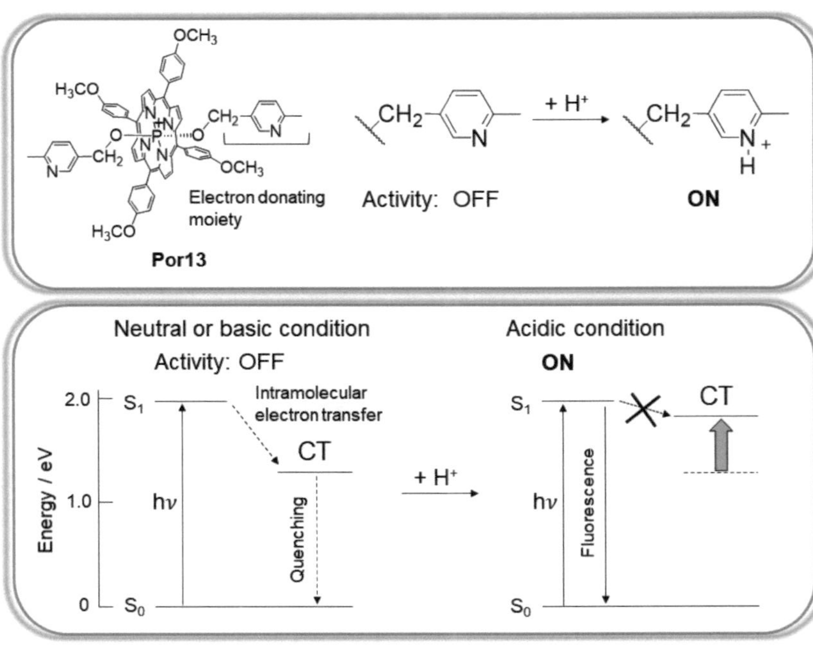

Figure 7.
Scheme of the activity control of photosensitizer, Por13, by pH and the relaxation processes of photoexcited state.

suppression of the quenching through intramolecular electron transfer by methylpyridine. The quantum yields of photosensitized $^1O_2$ generation and biomolecule oxidation through electron transfer mechanism were also increased under acidic condition. NADH oxidation by **Por13** through photoinduced electron transfer was successfully enhanced under acidic conditions. However, photosensitized protein damage (oxidative damage of HSA) through electron transfer was decreased under an acidic condition, and relatively strong protein damage was observed under a neutral condition. It is explained by the fact that a relatively weak association between protein and **Por13** under an acidic condition due to electrostatic repulsion. Protonated protein under acidic condition decreases the association with cationic porphyrin, resulting in the suppression of the electron transfer from the amino acids. Furthermore, the hydrophobic environment of protein inhibits the electron transfer-quenching of **Por13**. This study shows the difficulty of activity control of photosensitizers by pH, because other factors significantly affect the photoinduced electron transfer.

5.2 Activity control through the self-quenching of photosensitizers

DiethoxyP(V)tetrakis(*p*-methoxyphenyl)porphyrins, **Por10** and **Por11**, analogues of above mentioned **Por9**, were synthesized [47]. Their water-solubilities were smaller than that of **Por9**, and these porphyrins form self-aggregation complexes (**Figure 8**). Photoexcited states of **Por10** and **Por11** were effectively quenched through this aggregation (concentration quenching). These phosphorus(V) porphyrins can bind to the hydrophobic pocket of HSA, resulting in dissociation of their self-aggregation states (**Figure 8**). Calculating simulation showed the distance between the tryptophan residue and the porphyrin molecules as follows: 24.4 Å (**Por10**) and 23.5 Å (**Por11**). Fluorescence lifetime of these porphyrins were recovered by the dissociation of self-aggregation. Photoirradiation to these porphyrins binding to HSA induced the oxidation of tryptophan through $^1O_2$ generation and electron transfer. The axial fluorination of ethoxy chain of central phosphorus atom reduced the E_{red} of porphyrin ring. The electron transfer

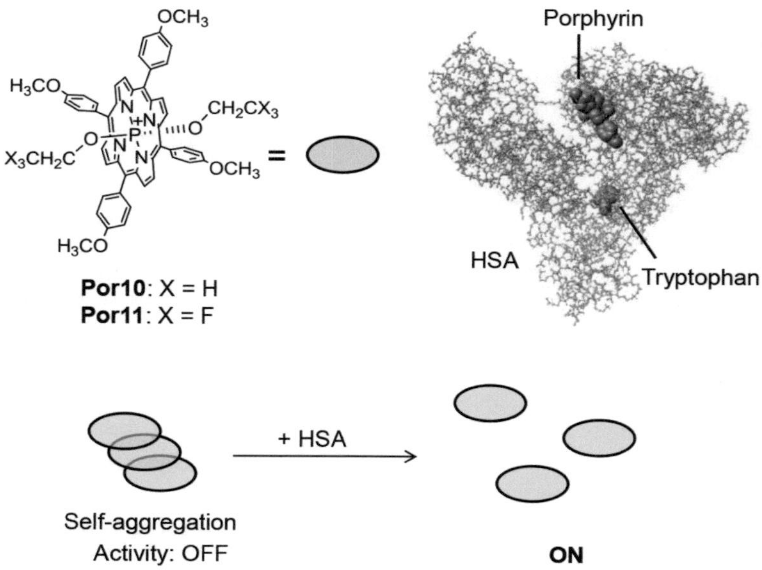

Figure 8.
Scheme of the activity control of photosensitizers, **Por10** *and* **Por11***, through the self-aggregation and interaction with HSA.*

rate constant from the tryptophan residue of HSA to **Por11** is larger than that of **Por10**, due to the effect of axial fluorination. The substitution by fluorine, the highest electronegative element, showed the improving effect on photooxidation of protein through electron transfer. However, the fluorination decreased the binding interaction with HSA. In the presence of same concentration of porphyrins, **Por10** exhibits higher damaging activity to HSA under photoirradiation. These results suggest that selective interaction is important for electron transfer-mediated photodamage of biomolecules. These porphyrins demonstrated the photocytotoxicity to HaCaT cells. The IC50 value of **Por11** was lower (stronger cytotoxicity) that **Por10**. Photooxidative activity of **Por11** through electron transfer and enhanced cellular uptake by the fluorination may play the important role in this photocytotoxic effect. Furthermore, **Por10** and **Por11** barely induce cellular DNA damage to HaCaT cells, similarly to **Por8**, **Por9**, and **Por12**. Therefore, their carcinogenic risks are also small. The self-aggregation of photosensitizers can be used to suppress their photosensitizing activity. These results suggest that the PDT activity of self-aggregation photosensitizers can be reversed using association with targeting biomacromolecules, such as protein.

6. Electron transfer mechanism and antimicrobial photodynamic therapy

PDT can be applied for disinfection and sterilization [4–7]. Microbial, including bacterium and viruses can be removed by photosensitized reaction. The physical treatment, such as PDT, is advantageous against antibiotic-resistant bacteria [91, 92]. PDT for microbial treatment is called as aPDT and/or PACT. Red light (relatively long wavelength visible light) is used for aPDT. Because $^1O_2$ can be easily produced by relatively small energy photons, it is considered as the important reactive species for aPDT process. Phenothiazine dyes, such as Methylene Blue is used as the photosensitizer for aPDT [93], because Methylene Blue can absorb relatively long-wavelength visible light and its Φ_Δ value is relatively large [94]. However, the aPDT mechanism has not been well-understand. Biological environments are under a hypoxic condition [95], the mechanism mediated by $^1O_2$ generation mechanism may be restricted. Therefore, the electron transfer mechanism may play an important role in the aPDT mechanism.

6.1 Photosensitized DNA damage through electron transfer

DNA is a potentially important targeting biomacromolecules for PDT and aPDT [1–3, 28]. In the cases of DNA damage, the generation of reactive oxygen species, such as $^1O_2$ (Type II mechanism), and the direct oxidation of nucleobases through photoinduced electron transfer (Type I mechanism) are important. In general, $O_2^{\bullet-}$ formation and following H_2O_2 and/or $^\bullet OH$ production (Type II mechanism, minor) require relatively shorter wavelength radiation, such as ultraviolet ray [28, 32, 33]. Therefore, the contribution of the $O_2^{\bullet-}$ generation (Type II minor) mechanism is considered to be small in the aPDT mechanism. As mentioned above, photosensitized $^1O_2$ generation is the important mechanism of aPDT. Guanine is the selective target of $^1O_2$, and every guanine is oxidized by $^1O_2$ in a DNA sequence [28, 33]. Similar to the $^1O_2$ generation mechanism, guanine is also damaged through electron transfer selectively [28, 32, 33]. However, single guanines in double-stranded DNA and guanine residue in single-stranded DNA are resistant to electron transfer mechanism, in the contrary to the $^1O_2$ mechanism [28, 33]. Since π-π interaction between consecutive guanines decrease the E_{ox} of guanine, the consecutive guanines, such as GG and GGG, are selectively oxidized through electron transfer mechanism [77–79]. Similar compounds are produced of guanine oxidation through the both mechanisms of $^1O_2$ generation and electron transfer [72].

The mechanism of DNA damage photosensitized by Nile Blue (**Figure 9**) has been studied as a potential photosensitizing reaction [96]. The reported value of Φ_Δ by Nile Blue is very small (0.005) [66, 97]. Therefore, Nile Blue is an appropriate model to examine the oxygen-independent mechanism. Nile Blue bound to DNA strand through an electrostatic interaction and the fluorescence lifetime was decreased, supporting the electron transfer quenching. Using ^{32}P-5′-end-labeled DNA fragments, DNA damaging mechanism of Nile Blue was examined and consecutive guanine damage was observed. From the analysis of DNA damaging pattern, the contribution of DNA damage through electron transfer mechanism was estimated to be 72% (the contribution of $^1O_2$ mechanism is 28%). The ΔG of electron transfer from guanine to the S_1 state of Nile Blue is negative (−0.15 eV) [96], and this value is considered to become smaller in the case of consecutive guanine, as mentioned above [77–79]. The estimated k_{ET} value is relatively large (1.0×10^{10} s^{-1}). These values supported the electron transfer-mediated DNA oxidation. The mechanism of DNA damage photosensitized by Nile Blue is shown in **Figure 9**. Relevantly, rhodamine-6G, a fluorescence dye, induces the electron transfer-mediated oxidation of DNA [98] and folic acid [64] with photoirradiation. In general, fluorescence dyes hardly photosensitize $^1O_2$ generation. On the other hand, photooxidative activity through electron transfer depends on the redox potential of molecules. These results suggest that the electron transfer-oxidation becomes important PDT mechanism for non-$^1O_2$ generating dyes.

6.2 Photosensitized protein damage through electron transfer

Photosensitized protein damage by Methylene Blue and its analogues (**Figure 10**) were studied [99]. Similar to the cases of phosphorus(V) porphyrin photosensitizers, HSA was used as the targeting biomacromolecules. DNA binding through electrostatic force of these cationic compounds are well-known [40, 71, 74, 96, 100]. However, the interaction between these cationic dyes and HSA is small and a hydrophobic

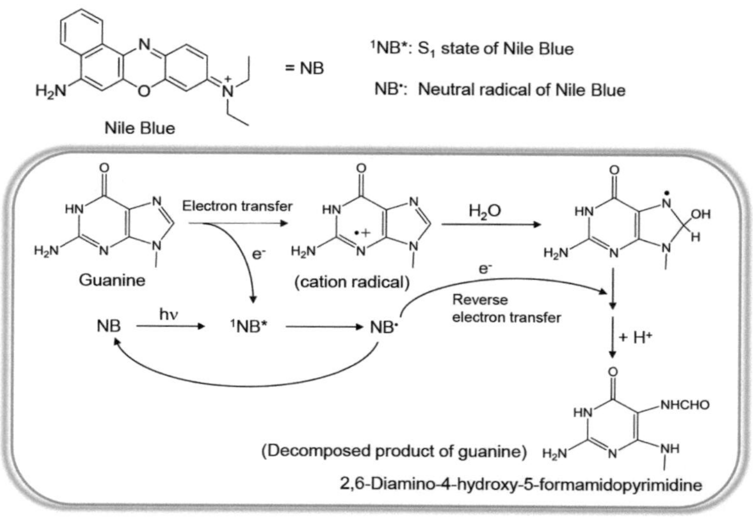

Figure 9.
Structure of Nile Blue and the proposed mechanism of guanine decomposition through photoinduced electron transfer.

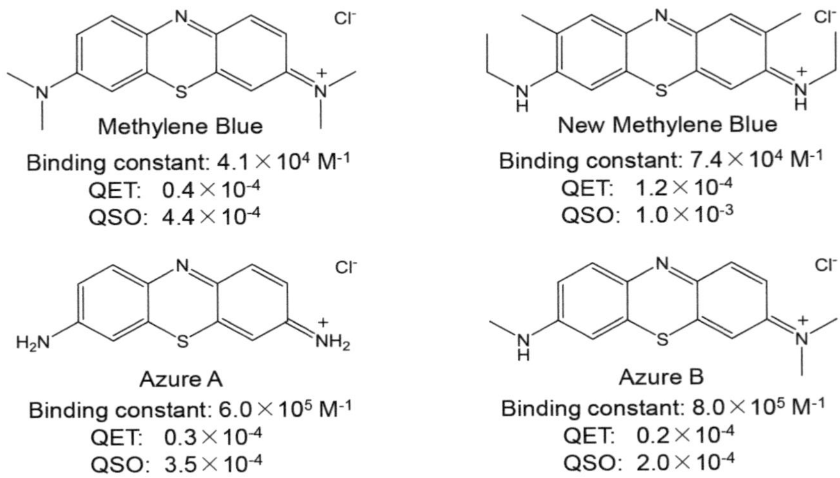

Figure 10.
Structures of Methylene Blue and its analogues. Binding constants with HSA were examined in a 10 mM sodium phosphate buffer (pH 7.6). QET: The quantum yield of HSA oxidation through electron transfer mechanism. QSO: The quantum yield of HSA oxidation through $^1O_2$ *generation.*

interaction (not electrostatic interaction) may be a driving force of the association with HSA [58]. The reported binding constant, which were estimated by the Benesi-Hildebrand Equation [101] are shown in **Figure 10**. Fluorometry of HSA tryptophan residue demonstrated the photosensitized oxidation through both mechanisms, electron transfer and $^1O_2$ generation [99]. The analyzed quantum yields through these mechanisms are shown in **Figure 10**. Fluorescence decay of these dyes was complex. From the analysis of their observed fluorescence decay, the estimated k_{ET} values were order of 10^9 s^{-1}, supporting the electron transfer mechanism. Furthermore, this result suggests the existence of markedly fast electron transfer species, much faster than the detection limit of this study (within ~50 ps) [99]. DFT calculation also supported the electron transfer mechanism. The energy gap between the highest occupied molecular orbital (HOMO) of amino acids and that of photosensitizers are important for the electron transfer mechanism. The plot between the HOMO values of these cationic dyes and the protein damaging quantum yield through electron transfer demonstrated a relatively good relationship. Furthermore, the relationship between the Φ_Δ and the damaging quantum yield through $^1O_2$ generation is also observed. These results shown that the electron transfer mechanism is also important for photosensitized protein oxidation by Methylene Blue and its analogues, as $^1O_2$ generation mechanism does. The electron transfer mechanism is not completely independent of oxygen molecule, because oxygen support the electron transfer by removing the excess electron from the reduced photosensitizer. However, other endogenous oxidative agents, such as metal ions, may support the electron transfer mechanism, in *vivo*, the electron transfer mechanism may play an important role in the aPDT under hypoxic condition.

7. Conclusions

This chapter reviewed the several topics about the photosensitizers, which play electron transfer-supported mechanism. $^1O_2$ is the important reactive species in PDT and aPDT. However, hypoxic condition in biological environment is not appropriate for reactive oxygen-dependent mechanism. Electron transfer is not completely independent of oxygen; however, this mechanism does not absolutely require oxygen. Endogenous oxidative substances other than oxygen can support the electron transfer mechanism. In the study of PDT photosensitizer for cancer, phosphorus(V) porphyrins showed the selectivity for cancer cell and relatively strong PDT effects. Most important property of these photosensitizers is strong photooxidative activity through electron transfer under long-wavelength visible light irradiation. Furthermore, the photosensitizing activity of phosphorus(V) porphyrins through electron transfer mechanism can be controlled by surroundings, such as pH. In the processes of aPDT, the electron transfer mechanism may be important. For developing the effective drugs for aPDT, molecular design based on the electron transfer is also useful as well as that based on the $^1O_2$ generating activity. The activity of electron transfer oxidation depends on the redox potential, and a long lifetime of photoexcited state is advantageous. For PDT photosensitizers, relatively strong response to long-wavelength radiation is required. In the molecular design of PDT photosensitizers including phosphorus(V) porphyrins, the calculations of HOMO energy level and the excitation energy are important as the initial steps.

Acknowledgements

This work was supported in part by Grants-in-Aid for Scientific Research (B) from Japan Society for the Promotion of Science (JSPS KAKENHI 17H03086) and Futaba Electronics Memorial Foundation (10407).

Conflict of interest

The author declares no conflict of interest.

Author details

Kazutaka Hirakawa[1,2]

1 Department of Engineering, Applied Chemistry and Biochemical Engineering Course, Graduate School of Integrated Science and Technology, Shizuoka University, Hamamatsu, Japan

2 Department of Optoelectronics and Nanostructure Science, Graduate School of Science and Technology, Shizuoka University, Hamamatsu, Japan

*Address all correspondence to: hirakawa.kazutaka@shizuoka.ac.jp

References

[1] Dolmans DEJGJ, Fukumura D, Jain RK. Photodynamic therapy for cancer. Nature Reviews Cancer. 2003;3:380-387. DOI:10.1038/nrc1071

[2] Castano AP, Mroz P, Hamblin MR. Photodynamic therapy and anti-tumour immunity. Nature Reviews Cancer. 2006;6:535-545. DOI:10.1038/nrc1894

[3] Abrahamse H, Hamblin MR. New photosensitizers for photodynamic therapy. Biochemical Journal. 2016;473:347-364. DOI: 10.1042/BJ20150942

[4] Sperandio FF, Huang YY, Hamblin MR. Antimicrobial photodynamic therapy to kill Gram-negative bacteria. Recent Patents on Anti-Infective Drug Discovery. 2013;8:108-120. DOI: 10.2174/1574891x113089990012

[5] Amos-Tautua BM, Songca SP, Oluwafemi OS. Application of porphyrins in antibacterial photodynamic therapy. Molecules. 2019;24:2456. DOI: 10.3390/molecules24132456

[6] Shen JJ, Jemec GBE, Arendrup MC, Saunte DML. Photodynamic therapy treatment of superficial fungal infections: a systematic review. Photodiagnosis and Photodynamic Therapy. 2020:101774. DOI: 10.1016/j.pdpdt.2020.101774

[7] Souza EQM, da Rocha TE, Toro LF, Guiati IZ, Ervolino E, Garcia VG, Wainwright M, Theodoro LH. Antimicrobial photodynamic therapy compared to systemic antibiotic therapy in non-surgical treatment of periodontitis: Systematic review and meta-analysis. Photodiagnosis and Photodynamic Therapy. 2020:101808. DOI: 10.1016/j.pdpdt.2020.101808

[8] Tsolekile N, Nelana S, Oluwafemi OS. Porphyrin as diagnostic and therapeutic agent. Molecules. 2019;24:2669. DOI: 10.3390/molecules24142669

[9] Xue X, Lindstrom A, Li Y. Porphyrin-based nanomedicines for cancer treatment. Bioconjugate Chemistry. 2019;30:1585-1603. DOI: 10.1021/acs.bioconjchem.9b00231

[10] Lin Y, Zhou T, Bai R, Xie Y. Chemical approaches for the enhancement of porphyrin skeleton-based photodynamic therapy. The Journal of Enzyme Inhibition and Medicinal Chemistry. 2020;35:1080-1099. DOI: 10.1080/14756366.2020.1755669

[11] Yu W, Zhen W, Zhang Q, Li Y, Luo H, He J, Liu Y. Porphyrin-based metal-organic framework compounds as promising nanomedicines in photodynamic therapy. ChemMedChem. DOI: 10.1002/cmdc.202000353

[12] Lu J, Roy B, Anderson M, Leggett CL, Levy MJ, Pogue B, Hasan T, Wang KK. Verteporfin- and sodium porfimer-mediated photodynamic therapy enhances pancreatic cancer cell death without activating stromal cells in the microenvironment. The Journal of Biomedical Optics. 2019;24:1-11. DOI: 10.1117/1.JBO.24.11.118001

[13] Ohmori S, Arai T. In vitro behavior of Porfimer sodium and Talaporfin sodium with high intensity pulsed irradiation. Lasers in Medical Science. 2006;21:213-223. DOI: 10.1007/s10103-006-0403-0

[14] Lang K, Mosinger J, Wagnerová DM. Photophysical properties of porphyrinoid sensitizers non-covalently bound to host molecules; models for photodynamic therapy. Coordination Chemistry Reviews. 2004;248:321-350. DOI: 10.1016/j.ccr.2004.02.004

[15] DeRosa MC, Crutchley RJ. Photosensitized singlet oxygen and its applications. Coordination Chemistry Reviews. 2002;233-234:351-371. DOI: 10.1016/S0010-8545(02)00034-6

[16] Schweitzer C, Schmidt R. Physical mechanisms of generation and deactivation of singlet oxygen. Chemical Reviews. 2003;103:1685-1758. DOI: 10.1021/cr010371d

[17] Mascio PD, Martinez GR, Miyamoto S, Ronsein GE, Medeiros MHG, Cadet J. Singlet molecular oxygen reactions with nucleic acids, lipids, and proteins. Chemical Review. 2019;119:2043-2086. DOI: 10.1021/acs.chemrev.8b00554

[18] Anderson RR, Parrish JA. The optics of human skin. Journal of Investigative Dermatology. 1981;77:13-19. DOI: 10.1111/1523-1747.ep12479191

[19] Choudhry H, Albukhari A, Morotti M, Haider S, Moralli D, Smythies J, Schödel J, Green CM, Camps C, Buffa F, Ratcliffe P, Ragoussis J, Harris AL, Mole DR. Tumor hypoxia induces nuclear paraspeckle formation through HIF-2α dependent transcriptional activation of NEAT1 leading to cancer cell survival. Oncogene. 2015;34:4482-4490. DOI: 10.1038/onc.2014.378

[20] Cabral P, Cerecetto H. Radiopharmaceuticals in tumor hypoxia imaging: a review focused on medicinal chemistry aspects. Anti-Cancer Agents in Medicinal Chemistry. 2017;17:318-332. DOI: 10.2174/187152061666616030 7142514

[21] Stieb S, Eleftheriou A, Warnock G, Guckenberger M, Riesterer O. Longitudinal PET imaging of tumor hypoxia during the course of radiotherapy. European Journal of Nuclear Medicine and Molecular Imaging. 2018;45:2201-2217. DOI: 10.1007/s00259-018-4116-y

[22] Kumari R, Sunil D, Ningthoujam RS. Naphthalimides in fluorescent imaging of tumor hypoxia - An up-to-date review. Bioorganic Chemistry. 2019;88:102979. DOI: 10.1016/j.bioorg.2019.102979

[23] Liu Y, Liu Y, Bu W, Cheng C, Zuo C, Xiao Q, Sun Y, Ni D, Zhang C, Liu J, Shi J. Hypoxia induced by upconversion-based photodynamic therapy: towards highly effective synergistic bioreductive therapy in tumors. Angewandte Chemie International Edition. 2015;54:8105-8109. DOI: 10.1002/anie.201500478

[24] Victor HF, Wieman TJ, Wiehle SA, Cerrito PB. The role of microvascular damage in photodynamic therapy: the effect of treatment on vessel constriction, permeability, and leukocyte adhesion. Cancer Research. 1992;52:4914-4921.

[25] Marrese CA, Carrano CJ. The synthesis, characterization and electrochemistry of 5,10,15,20-tetrap henylporphinatodichlorophosphoru s(V) chloride. Inorganic Chemistry. 1983;22:1858-1862. DOI: 10.1021/ic00192a024

[26] Takeuchi Y, Hirakawa K, Susumu K, Segawa H. Electrochemical determination of charge transfer direction of "center-to-edge" phosphorus(V) porphyrin arrays. Electrochemistry. 2004;72:449-451. DOI: 10.5796/electrochemistry.72.449

[27] Kalyanasundaram K, Neumann-Spallart M. Photophysical and redox properties of water-soluble porphyrins in aqueous media. The Journal of Physical Chemistry. 1982;86:5163-5169. DOI: 10.1021/j100223a022

[28] Hirakawa K. DNA damage through photo-induced electron transfer and photosensitized generation of reactive oxygen species. In: Kimura H, Suzuki A, editors. New Research on DNA Damage. New York: Nova Science Publishers; 2008. p. 197-219. ISBN: 978-1-60456-581-2

[29] Hirakawa K, Segawa H. Acid dissociation of the axial hydroxylgroup of hydroxy(1-pyrenebutoxy) phosphorus(v) porphyrin controls the intramolecular excitation energy transfer. Photochemical and Photobiological Sciences. 2010;9:704-709. DOI: 10.1039/B9PP00204A

[30] Horiuchi H, Kuribara R, Hirabara A, Okutsu T. pH-Response optimization of amino-substituted tetraphenylporphyrin derivatives as pH-activatable photosensitizers. The Journal of Physical Chemistry A. 2016;120:5554-5561. DOI: 10.1021/acs.jpca.6b05019

[31] Foote CS. Definition of type I and type II photosensitized oxidation. Photochemistry and Photobiology. 1991;54:659. DOI: 10.1111/j.1751-1097.1991.tb02071.x

[32] Ito K, Kawanishi S. Site-specific DNA damage induced by UVA radiation in the presence of endogenous photosensitizer. Biological Chemistry. 1997;378:1307-1312.

[33] Hiraku Y, Ito K, Hirakawa K, Kawanishi S. Photosensitized DNA damage and its protection via a novel mechanism. Photochemistry and Photobiology. 2007;83:205-512. DOI: 10.1562/2006-03-09-IR-840

[34] Marcus RA. On the theory of oxidation-reduction reactions involving electron transfer. I. The Journal of Chemical Physics. 1956;24:966-978. DOI: 10.1063/1.1742723

[35] Marcus RA, Sutin N. Electron transfers in chemistry and biology. Biochimica et Biophysica Acta. 1985;811:265-322. DOI: 10.1016/0304-4173(85)90014-X

[36] Keane PM, Kelly JM. Transient absorption and time-resolved vibrational studies of photophysical and photochemical processes in DNA-intercalating polypyridyl metal complexes or cationic porphyrins. Coordination Chemistry Reviews. 2018;364:137-154. DOI: 10.1016/j.ccr.2018.02.018

[37] Fujitsuka M, Kim SS, Lu C, Tojo S, Majima T. Intermolecular and intramolecular electron transfer processes from excited naphthalene diimide radical anions. The Journal of Physical Chemistry B. 2015;119:7275-7282. DOI: 10.1021/jp510850z

[38] Higashino T, Yamada T, Yamamoto M, Furube A, Tkachenko NV, Miura T, Kobori Y, Jono R, Yamashita K, Imahori H. Remarkable dependence of the final charge separation efficiency on the donor-acceptor interaction in photoinduced electron transfer. Angewandte Chemie International Edition. 2016;55:629-633. DOI: 10.1002/anie.201509067

[39] Hasegawa M, Nagashima H, Minobe R, Tachikawa T, Mino H, Kobori Y. Regulated electron tunneling of photoinduced primary charge-separated state in the photosystem II reaction center. The Journal of Physical Chemistry Letters. 2017;8:1179-1184. DOI: 10.1021/acs.jpclett.7b00044

[40] Hirakawa K, Nishimura Y, Arai T, Okazaki S. Singlet oxygen generating activity of an electron donor-connecting porphyrin photosensitizer can be controlled by DNA. The Journal of the Physical Chemistry B. 2013;117:13490-13496. DOI: 10.1021/jp4072444

[41] Hirakawa K, Kawanishi S, Hirano T, Segawa H. Guanine-specific DNA oxidation photosensitized by the tetraphenylporphyrin phosphorus(V) complex via singlet oxygen generation and electron transfer. Journal of Photochemistry and Photobiology B: Biology. 2007;87:209-217. DOI: 10.1016/j.jphotobiol.2007.04.001

[42] Ouyang D, Hirakawa K. Photosensitized enzyme deactivation

and protein oxidation by axialsubstituted phosphorus(V) tetraphenylporphyrins. Journal of Photochemistry and Photobiology B: Biology. 2017;175:125-131. DOI: 10.1016/j.jphotobiol.2017.08.036

[43] Hirakawa K, Fukunaga N, Nishimura Y, Arai T, Okazaki S. Photosensitized protein damage by dimethoxyphosphorus(V) tetraphenylporphyrin. Bioorganic and Medicinal Chemistry Letters. 2013;23:2704-2707. DOI: 10.1016/j.bmcl.2013.02.081

[44] Hirakawa K, Azumi K, Nishimura Y, Arai T, Nosaka Y, Okazaki S. Photosensitized damage of protein by fluorinated diethoxyphosphorus(V)porphyrin. Journal of Porphyrins and Phthalocyanines. 2013;17:56-62. DOI: 10.1142/S1088424612501258

[45] Hirakawa K, Umemoto H, Kikuchi R, Yamaguchi H, Nishimura Y, Arai T, Okazaki S, Segawa H. Determination of singlet oxygen and electron transfer mediated mechanisms of photosensitized protein damage by phosphorus(V)porphyrins. Chemical Research in Toxicology. 2015;28:262-267. DOI: 10.1021/tx500492w

[46] Hirakawa K, Ouyang D, Ibuki Y, Hirohara S, Okazaki S, Kono E, Kanayama N, Nakazaki J, Segawa H. Photosensitized protein-damaging activity, cytotoxicity, and antitumor effects of P(V)porphyrins using long-wavelength visible light through electron transfer. Chemical Research in Toxicology. 2018;31:371-379. DOI: 10.1021/acs.chemrestox.8b00059

[47] Hirakawa K, Suzuki A, Ouyang D, Okazaki S, Ibuki Y, Nakazaki J, Segawa H. Controlled photodynamic action of axial fluorinated diethoxyP(V)tetrakis(p-methoxyphenyl)porphyrin through self-aggregation. Chemical Research in Toxicology. 2019;32:1638-1645. DOI: 10.1021/acs.chemrestox.9b00172

[48] Hirakawa K, Ohnishi, Y, Ouyang D, Horiuchi H, Okazaki S. pH-Dependent photodynamic activity of bis(6-methyl-3-pyridylmethoxy)P(V)tetrakis(p-methoxyphenyl)porphyrin. Chemical Physics Letters. 2020;746:137315. DOI: 10.1016/j.cplett.2020.137315

[49] Hirakawa K, Morimoto S. Electron transfer mediated decomposition of folic acid by photoexcited dimethoxophosphorus(V)porphyrin. Journal of Photochemistry and Photobiology A: Chemistry. 2016;318:1-6. DOI: 10.1016/j.jphotochem.2015.11.028

[50] Hirakawa K, Murata A. Photosensitized oxidation of nicotinamide adenine dinucleotide by diethoxyphosphorus(V) tetraphenylporphyrin and its fluorinated derivative: Possibility of chain reaction. Spectrochimica Acta Part A: Molecular and Biomolecular Spectroscopy. 2018;188:640-646. DOI: 10.1016/j.saa.2017.07.055

[51] Susumu K, Segawa H, Shimidzu T. Synthesis and photochemical properties of the orthogonal porphyrin triad composed of free-base and phosphorus(V) porphyrins. Chemistry Letters. 1995;24:929-930. DOI: 10.1246/cl.1995.929

[52] Hirakawa K, Aoki S, Ueda Y, Ouyang D, Okazaki S. Photochemical property and photodynamic activity of tetrakis(2-naphthyl)porphyrin phosphorus(V) complex. Rapid Communication in Photoscience. 2015;4:37-40. DOI: 10.5857/RCP.2015.4.2.37

[53] Meshkov I, Bulach V, Gorbunova YG, GostevFE,NadtochenkoVA,TsivadzebAU, Hosseini MW. Tuning photochemical properties of phosphorus(V) porphyrin photosensitizers. Chemical

Communications. 2017;53:9918-9921. DOI: 10.1039/c7cc06052a

[54] Barbour T, Belcher WJ, Brothers PJ, Rickard CEF, Ware DC. Preparation of group 15 (phosphorus, antimony, and bismuth) complexes of meso-tetra-p-tolylporphyrin (TTP) and x-ray crystal structure of [Sb(TTP)(OCH(CH_3)$_2$)$_2$] Cl. Inorganic Chemistry. 1992;31:746-754. DOI: 10.1021/ic00031a011

[55] Matsumoto J, Shiragami T, Hirakawa K, Yasuda M. Water-solubilization of P(V) and Sb(V) porphyrins and their photobiological application. International Journal of Photoenergy. 2015:148964. DOI: 10.1155/2015/148964

[56] He XM, Carter DC. Atomic structure and chemistry of human serum albumin. Nature. 1992;358:209-215. DOI: 10.1038/358209a0

[57] Sudlow G, Birkett DJ, Wade DN. The characterization of two specific drug binding sites on human serum albumin. Molecular Pharmacology. 1975;11:824-832.

[58] Hirakawa K. Evaluation of photodynamic agent activity using human serum albumin. In: Cohen D, editor. Human Serum Albumin: Structure, Binding and Activity. New York: Nova Science Publishers; 2019. p. 1-33 (Chapter 3). ISBN: 978-1-53614-787-2

[59] Thomas AH, Serrano MP, Rahal V, Vicendo P, Claparols C, Oliveros E, Lorente C. Tryptophan oxidation photosensitized by pterin. Free Radical Biology and Medicine. 2013;63:467-475. DOI: 10.1016/j.freeradbiomed.2013.05.044

[60] Reid LO, Roman EA, Thomas AH, Dántola ML. Photooxidation of tryptophan and tyrosine residues in human serum albumin sensitized by pterin: a model for globular protein photodamage in skin. Biochemistry. 2016;55:4777-4786. DOI: 10.1021/acs.biochem.6b00420

[61] Jensen RL, Arnbjerg J, Ogilby PR. Reaction of singlet oxygen with tryptophan in proteins: a pronounced effect of the local environment on the reaction rate. Journal of the American Chemical Society. 2012;134:9820-9826. DOI: 10.1021/ja303710m

[62] Li MY, Cline CS, Koker EB, Carmichael HH, Chignell CF, Bilski P. Quenching of singlet molecular oxygen ($^1O_2$) by azide anion in solvent mixtures. Photochemistry and Photobiology. 2001;74:760-764. DOI: 10.1562/0031-8655(2001)074<0760:qosmoo>2.0.co;2

[63] Goldstein S, Czapski G. Reactivity of peroxynitrite versus simultaneous generation of $^{\bullet}$NO and $O_2^{\bullet-}$ toward NADH, Chemical Research in Toxicology. 2000;13:736-741. DOI: 10.1021/tx000099n

[64] Hirakawa K, Ito H. Rhodamine-6G can photosensitize folic acid decomposition through electron transfer. Chemical Physics Letters. 2015;627:26-29. DOI: 10.1016/j.cplett.2015.03.030

[65] Hirakawa K. Using folic acids to detect reactive oxygen species. In: Taylor JC, editor. Advances in Chemistry Research. Volume 26. New York: Nova Science Publishers; 2015. p. 111-126. ISBN: 978-1-63463-630-8

[66] Hirakawa K. Fluorometry of singlet oxygen generated via a photosensitized reaction using folic acid and methotrexate. Analytical and Bioanalytical Chemistry. 2009;393:999-1005. DOI: 10.1007/s00216-008-2522-x

[67] Silvester JA, Timmins GS, Davies MJ. Protein hydroperoxides and carbonyl groups generated by

porphyrin-induced photo-oxidation of bovine serum albumin. Archives of Biochemistry and Biophysics. 1998;350:249-258. DOI: 10.1006/abbi.1997.0495

[68] Silvester JA, Timmins GS, Davies MJ. Photodynamically generated bovine serum albumin radicals: evidence for damage transfer and oxidation at cysteine and tryptophan residues. Free Radical Biology and Medicine. 1998;24:754-766. DOI: 10.1016/s0891-5849(97)00327-4

[69] Ouyang D, Inoue S, Okazaki S, Hirakawa K. Tetrakis(N-methyl-p-pyridinio)porphyrin and its zinc complex can photosensitize damage of human serum albumin through electron transfer and singlet oxygen generation. Journal of Porphyrins and Phthalocyanines. 2016;20:813-821. DOI: 10.1142/S1088424616500991

[70] Tada-Oikawa S, Oikawa S, Hirayama J, Hirakawa K, Kawanishi S. DNA damage and apoptosis induced by photosensitization of 5,10,15,20-tetrakis (N-methyl-4-pyridyl)-21H,23H-porphyrin via singlet oxygen generation. Photochemistry and Photobiology. 2009;85:1391-1399. DOI: 10.1111/j.1751-1097.2009.00600.x

[71] Hirakawa K, Taguchi M, Okazaki S. Relaxation process of photoexcited meso-naphthylporphyrins while interacting with DNA and singlet oxygen generation. The Journal of Physical Chemistry B. 2015;119:13071-13078. DOI: 10.1021/acs.jpcb.5b08025

[72] Burrows CJ, Muller JG. Oxidative nucleobase modifications leading to strand scission. Chemical Reviews 1998;98:1109-1151. DOI: 10.1021/cr960421s

[73] Neumann-Spallart M, Kalyanasundaram KZ. On the one and two-electron oxidations of water-soluble zinc porphyrins in aqueous media. Z. Naturforsch. 1981;36b:596-600.

[74] Hirakawa K, Nakajima S. Effect of DNA microenvironment on photosensitized reaction of water-soluble cationic porphyrins. Recent Advances in DNA and Gene Sequences. 2014;8:35-43. DOI: 10.2174/2352092208666141013231434

[75] Lewis FD, Wu Y. Dynamics of superexchange photoinduced electron transfer in duplex DNA. Journal of the Photochemistry and Photobiology C: Photochemistry Reviews. 2001;2:1-16. DOI: 10.1016/S1389-5567(01)00008-9

[76] Seidel CAM, Schulz A, Sauer MHM. Nucleobase-specific quenching of fluorescent dyes. 1. nucleobase one-electron redox potentials and their correlation with static and dynamic quenching efficiencies. The Journal of Physical Chemistry. 1996;100: 5541-5553. DOI: 10.1021/jp951507c

[77] Sugiyama H, Saito I. Theoretical studies of GG-specific photocleavage of DNA via electron transfer: significant lowering of ionization potential and 5′-localization of HOMO of stacked GG bases in B-form DNA. Journal of the American Chemical Society. 1996;118:7063-7068. DOI: 10.1021/ja9609821

[78] Yoshioka Y, Kitagawa Y, Takano Y, Yamaguchi K, Nakamura T, Saito I. Experimental and theoretical studies on the selectivity of GGG triplets toward one-electron oxidation in B-form DNA. Journal of the American Chemical Society. 1999;121:8712-8719. DOI: 10.1021/ja991032t

[79] Yoshioka Y, Kawai H, Sato T, Yamaguchi K, Saito I. Ab initio molecular orbital study on the G-selectivity of GGG triplet in copper(I)-mediated one-electron oxidation. Journal of the American Chemical Society. 2003;125:1968-1974. DOI: 10.1021/ja028039m

[80] Aigner D, Freunberger SA, Wilkening M, Saf R, Borisov SM, Klimant I. Enhancing photoinduced electron transfer efficiency of fluorescent pH-probes with halogenated phenols, Analytical Chemistry. 2014;86:9293-9300. DOI: 10.1021/ac502513g

[81] Horiuchi H, Isogai M, Hirakawa K, Okutsu T. Improvement of the ON/OFF switching performance of a pH-activatable porphyrin derivative by the introduction of phosphorus(V), ChemPhotoChem. 2019;3:138-144. DOI: 10.1002/cptc.201800248

[82] Vaupel P, Kallinowski F, Okunieff P. Blood flow, oxygen and nutrient supply, and metabolic microenvironment of human tumors: a review, Cancer Research. 1989;49:6449-6465.

[83] Estrella V, Chen T, Lloyd M, Wojtkowiak J, Cornnell HH, Ibrahim-Hashim A, Bailey K, Balagurunathan Y, Rothberg JM, Sloane BF, Johnson J, Gatenby RA, Gillies RJ. Acidity generated by the tumor microenvironment drives local invasion. Cancer Research. 2013;73:1524-1535. DOI: 10.1158/0008-5472.CAN-12-2796

[84] Korenchan DE, Bok R, Sriram R, Liu K, Santos RD, Qin H, Lobach I, Korn N, Wilson DM, Kurhanewicz J, Flavell RR. Hyperpolarized in vivo pH imaging reveals grade-dependent acidification in prostate cancer. Oncotarget. 2019;10:6096-6110. DOI: 10.18632/oncotarget.27225

[85] Vasquez-Montes V, Gerhart J, Thévenin D, Ladokhin AS. Divalent cations and lipid composition modulate membrane insertion and cancer-targeting action of pHLIP, Journal of Molecular Biology. 2019;431:5004-5018. DOI: 10.1016/j.jmb.2019.10.016

[86] Zhu X, Lu W, Zhang Y, Reed A, Newton B, Fan Z, Yu H, Ray PC, Gao R. Imidazole-modified porphyrin as a pH-responsive sensitizer for cancer photodynamic therapy, Chemical Communications. 2011;47:10311-10313. DOI: 10.1039/c1cc13328d

[87] Tian J, Zhou J, Shen Z, Ding L, Yu JS, Ju H. A pH-activatable and anilinesubstituted photosensitizer for near-infrared cancer theranostics. Chemical Science. 2015;6:5969-5977. DOI: 10.1039/c5sc01721a

[88] Horiuchi H, Hirabara A, Okutsu T. Importance of the orthogonal structure between porphyrin and aniline moieties on the pH-activatable porphyrin derivative for photodynamic therapy, Journal of the Photochemistry and Photobiology A: Chemistry. 2018;365:60-66. DOI: 10.1016/j.jphotochem.2018.07.034

[89] Tørring T, Toftegaard R, Arnbjerg J, Ogilby PR, Gothelf KV. Reversible pH regulated control of photosensitized singlet oxygen production using a DNA i-motif. Angewandte Chemie International Edition. 2010;49:7923-7925. DOI: 10.1002/anie.201003612

[90] Wang C, Qian Y. A novel BODIPY-based photosensitizer with pH-active singlet oxygen generation for photodynamic therapy in lysosomes. Organic and Biomolecular Chemistry. 2019;17:8001-8007. DOI: 10.1039/c9ob01242g

[91] Tim M. Strategies to optimize photosensitizers for photodynamic inactivation of bacteria. Journal of the Photochemistry and Photobiology B: Biology. 2015;150:2-10. DOI: 10.1016/j.jphotobiol.2015.05.010

[92] Ma W, Liu C, Li J, Hao M, Ji Y, Zeng X. The effects of aloe emodin-mediated antimicrobial photodynamic therapy on drug-sensitive and resistant *Candida albicans*. Photochemical and Photobiological

Sciences. 2020;19:485-494. DOI: 10.1039/c9pp00352e

[93] Tardivo JP, Del Giglio A, de Oliveira CS, Gabrielli DS, Junqueira HC, Tada DB, Severino D, de Fátima TR, Baptista MS. Methylene blue in photodynamic therapy: From basic mechanisms to clinical applications. Photodiagnosis and Photodynamic Therapy. 2005;2:175-191. DOI: 10.1016/S1572-1000(05)00097-9

[94] Usui Y, Kamogawa K. A standard system to determine the quantum yield of singlet oxygen formation in aqueous solution. Photochemistry and Photobiology. 1974;19:245-247. DOI: /10.1111/j.1751-1097.1974.tb06506.x

[95] Jørgensen E, Bay L, Bjarnsholt T, Bundgaard L, Sørensen MA, Jacobsen S. The occurrence of biofilm in an equine experimental wound model of healing by secondary intention. Veterinary Microbiology. 2017;204:90-95. DOI: 10.1016/j.vetmic.2017.03.011

[96] Hirakawa K, Ota K, Hirayama J, Oikawa S, Kawanishi S. Nile blue can photosensitize DNA damage through electron transfer. Chemical Research in Toxicology. 2014;27:649-655. DOI: 10.1021/tx400475c

[97] Wainwright M, Mohr H, Walker W.H. Phenothiazinium derivatives for pathogen inactivation in blood products. Journal of the Photochemistry and Photobiology B: Biology. 2007;86:45-58. DOI: 10.1016/j.jphotobiol.2006.07.005

[98] Hirakawa K, Ochiai S, Oikawa S, Kawanishi S. Oxygen-independent DNA damage photosensitized by rhodamine-6G. Trends in Photochemistry and Photobiology. 2011;13:29-35.

[99] Hirakawa K, Ishikawa T. Phenothiazine dyes photosensitize protein damage through electron transfer and singlet oxygen generation. Dyes and Pigments. 2017;142:183-188. DOI: 10.1016/j.dyepig.2017.03.035

[100] Vardevanyan PO, Antonyan AP, Parsadanyan MA, Torosyan MA, Karapetian AT. Joint interaction of ethidium bromide and methylene blue with DNA. The effect of ionic strength on binding thermodynamic parameters. Journal of Biomolecular Structure and Dynamics. 2016;34:1377-1382. DOI: 10.1080/07391102.2015.1079557

[101] Benesi HA, Hildebrand JH. A spectrophotometric investigation of the interaction of iodine with aromatic hydrocarbons. Journal of the American Chemical Society. 1949;71:2703-2707. DOI: 10.1021/ja01176a030

Chapter 2

Can PDT Alter the Glycosylation of the Tumor Cell Membrane?

Bruno Henrique Godoi, Juliana Ferreira Strixino, Newton Soares da Silva and Cristina Pacheco Soares

Abstract

Photodynamic Therapy (PDT) is a cancer treatment that used the interaction of a photosensitizing drug and a light source. PDT can lead to changes in the expression of various cellular elements, compromising cell adhesion, and cytoskeleton integrity in cells undergoing treatment. However, the pathways of cellular alterations caused by this treatment are little known. Alterations in expression in surface glycoproteins and glycolipids are significant features in malignant tumor transformation and are strongly associated with tumor cell adhesion, invasion, and metastasis. This study evaluated photodynamic therapy effects on indirect distribution surface glycoproteins in human laryngeal carcinoma HEp-2 cell line surface, using Click-iT™ Metabolic Glycoprotein Labeling Reagent. Aluminum Phthalocyanine Tetrasulfonate (AlPcS4) was administrated at 5 μM/mL, followed by one hour of the incubation period for its accumulation in the tumor cells. After this time, cultures were irradiated with LED (light-emitting diode) dispositive (BioPdi/IRRAD-LED) λ = 660 nm. Evaluation of glycoproteins was performed by flow cytometry. Knowledge of the cellular alterations caused by the treatment will allow obtaining tools for the potentiation or optimization and personalization of the anticancer treatment. This therapy has a low cost and better efficacy, when applied early, about radiotherapy chemotherapy.

Keywords: glycosylation, flow cytometry, cell culture, aluminum phthalocyanine tetrasulfonate

1. Introduction

Photodynamic therapy (PDT) is an oncology treatment based on photochemical reactions involved photosensitizer (PS) and light irradiation of an appropriate wavelength. The interaction of PS and light, producing reactive oxygen species (ROS), can directly induce cellular damage to organelles and cell membranes. PDT's action on cellular organelles, mainly in the endoplasmic reticulum (ER) and Golgi, interferes with several metabolic pathways [1]. The glycosylation process is a post-translational modification that occurs in the ER [2]. It results in the addition of carbohydrate motifs—glycans to proteins that are, in most cases, destined for the cell surface. The resultant glycoprotein structures at the cell surface form a carbohydrate-rich layer, which presents an essential role in the cell's interaction with its surrounding environment. Glycosylation of a given protein is a process catalyzed by glycosyltransferases, localized in the Golgi, leading to the formation of protein-bound glycans with specific and diverse biological functions [3]. These carbohydrate side chains can modulate the protein's interaction with its environment, influencing key factors such as protein half-life, solubility, binding activity, and specificity. Two significant types of glycosylation occur on proteins. (1) O-linked glycosylation refers to the addition of N-acetyl-galactosamine to serine or threonine residues by the enzyme UDP-N-acetyl-D-galactosamine transferase, followed by the addition of other carbohydrates, such as galactose, N-acetyl-D-glucosamine, or sialic acid; (2) N-linked glycosylation occurs in the ER [4, 5]. It refers to the insertion of an oligosaccharide chain enzymatically attached to the amide group of asparagine in the consensus sequence Asn-X-Ser/Thr (where X represents any residue except proline). Alterations in glycosylation of malignant cells can take a variety of forms, including changes in the amount, linkage, and acetylation of sialic acids; changes in the branching of N-glycans mediated by glycosyltransferases; alterations in the expression of glycosaminoglycans such as heparan sulfate; and altered glycosylation of mucins, which are heavily glycosylated epithelial-derived proteins known to be implicated in certain cancers [5, 6].

Changes in glycoprotein glycans are significant in malignant tumor transformation and are closely associated with tumor cell adhesion, invasion, and metastasis [7]. Christiansen et al., 2014 [8] demonstrated changes in cell surface glycosylation in five different types of cancer: breast, colon, liver, skin (melanoma), and ovarian, and how these changes may be associated with carcinogenesis. Synthesis and expression of cell-surface carbohydrates is a highly regulated process that affects several cell-cell interactions. The presence of specific oligosaccharides in highly malignant cells is essential for expressing the metastatic phenotype [9]. Elevation of glycoproteins above normal levels reflects local tissue destruction processes with the release of preformed tissue proteins or becomes a local synthesis and releases glycoproteins through tumor cells [10].

Waiting for glycans and glycoconjugates to play a relevant role in various tumor progression stages, biosynthetic cell machinery involved in glycan biosynthesis and modification is a promising target for cancer treatment. Treatments that act on such targets should be researched to act or stimulate specific glycosylation inhibitors that may target a pro-metastatic biological product or interfere with the immune response's modulation.

2. Methods

2.1 Cell culture

The HEp-2 cell line (human laryngeal carcinoma) and MCF7 cell line (human mammary carcinoma) were obtained from the Bank of Cells of Rio de Janeiro (BCRJ). Cells were cultured in 25 cm^2 culture flask (Greiner), routinely maintained in Dulbecco's Modified Eagles Medium (DMEM) supplemented with 10% fetal bovine serum (FBS), 1% antibiotic-antimycotic (Gibco-Life-Technology), at 37°C, an atmosphere containing 5% CO2 (Forma Scientific CO2, MODEL 3110).

2.2 Photosensitizer

Aluminum phthalocyanine tetrasulfonate (AlPcS4-Frontier Scientific) at a 5 μM/mL concentration is diluted in phosphate-buffered saline (PBS).

Experimental groups HEp-2 cells were divided into four groups: control, a photosensitizer (cells incubated with AlPcS4), laser (irradiated cells only), and photodynamic therapy (PDT) (cells incubated with AlPcS4 and irradiated).

2.3 Photodynamic therapy

Cells were cultivated in 6-well plates at a density of 1 × 10^6 cells/well, at 37°C in a 5% CO_2 atmosphere, and incubated for 18 hours for cell adhesion. After plating, cells were incubated with AlPcS4 for 1 hour at 37°C in an atmosphere containing 5% CO2. Then, they were washed with PBS to remove the photosensitizer not absorbed by the cells. Irradiation was performed by using a LED dispositive (Biopdi/IRRAD-LED) λ = 660 nm. Each well was exposed to 25 mW, an energy density of 5 J/cm2. Immediately after treatment, all groups were incubated with 25 μM Click-iT™ Metabolic Glycoprotein Labeling (according to the manufacturer's instructions, Thermo Fisher Scientific™- **Table 1**) for 24 and 48 hours to evaluate the changes in the protein glycosylation process by the Golgi complex (**Figure 1**). At the end of the incubation periods, the cells were scraped, added into 5 ml tubes, and centrifuged at 5259 g at 4°C for 5 minutes for cell sedimentation. After this, cells were resuspended and washed in PBS 2 times, fixed with 4% paraformaldehyde in PBS for 15 minutes, washed two more times with PBS, and permeabilized with 0.25% Triton x-100 in PBS for 15 minutes, washed with 3% BSA in PBS twice, and then incubated with an FTIC-conjugated antibody for one hour while diluted 1: 1000 in a Click-iT reaction buffer for one hour. At the end of the incubation period, it was washed

Markers	Target	Incubation time
Click-iT® GalNAz	O-linked glycans	24–72 hours
Click-iT® ManNAz	Sialic acid-modified glycoproteins	24–72 hours
Click-iT® GlcNAz	O-GLcNAz-modified glycoproteins	24–72 hours

Table 1.
The markers used to evaluate glycoproteins.

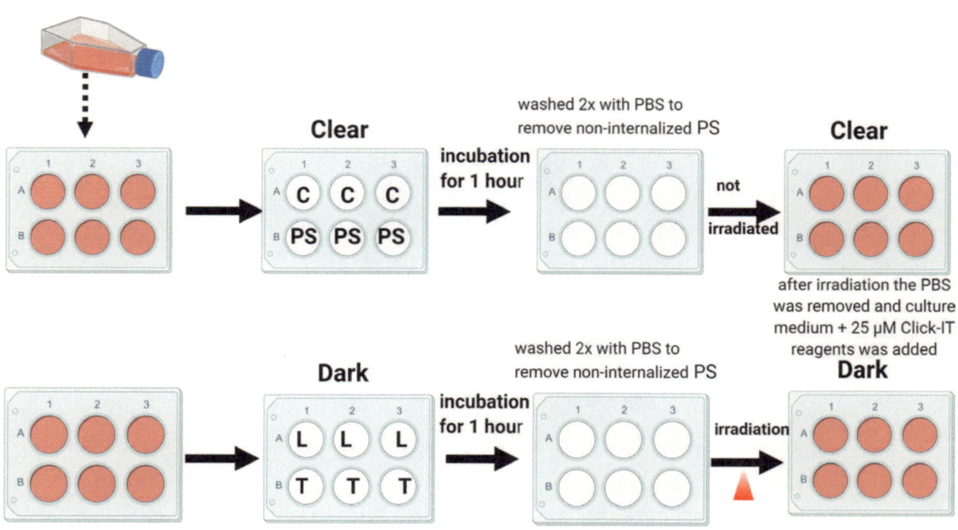

Figure 1.
Scheme of the experimental procedure. C – Control; PS – Photosensitizer; L – Led only; T – Treatment = PS + Led. Created with BioRender.com.

with PBS, resuspended in the Click-iT reaction buffer, and read by BD AccuriC6 Plus flow cytometer. All experiments were performed in duplicate (n = 6).

2.4 Statistical analysis

The data presented are in the form of mean and standard deviation, compared by the two-way ANOVA test and confirmed by the Tukey test. Statistical significance was admitted with $P < 0.05$ with $^{*}P < 0.05$; $^{**}P < 0.01$; $^{***}P < 0.001$; $^{****}P < 0.0001$ being considered significant. Experiments were performed in three independent replications with n = 8. GraphPad Prism 6® software was used to per-form statistical and graphical analyses.

3. Results

The evaluation of the glycoprotein synthesis by Flow Cytometry demonstrates that the modified sialic acid glycoproteins (Click-iT® ManNAz - **Figure 2**) in the treatment group present a higher fluorescence intensity in 24 hours, concerning the O-GLcNAz-modified glycoproteins and the O- glycans linked. The HEp-2 strain presents the synthesis of sialic acid-modified glycoproteins and O-GlcNAz-modified effectively in the first 24 hours; after 48 hours, a decrease in the synthesis of these glycoproteins is observed (**Figures 3** and **4**). They were probably modified due to the action of glycosidases and glycosyltransferases, changing their structures. O-linked glycans are less fluorescent in the first 24 hours; however, in the group treated within 48 hours, an increase in the synthesis of these glycoproteins is observed, which can be considered a possible target for photodynamic treatment.

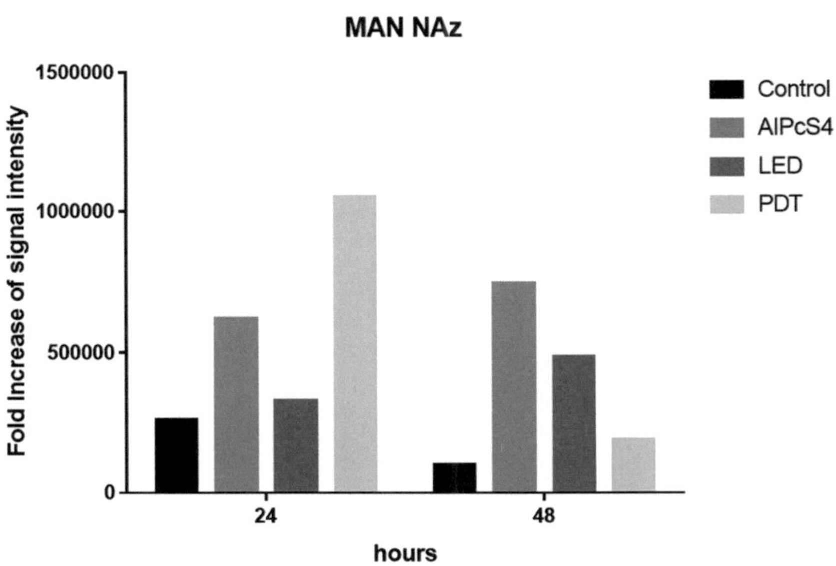

Figure 2.
Analysis of cells treated with Click-iT®-ManNAz, the graph shows the fluorescence intensity of the cells of the control, LED, and treatment groups in the periods of 24 and 48 hours. The treatment group showed a high fluorescence intensity within 24 hours, with a severe fluorescence reduction occurring in all groups within 48 hours.

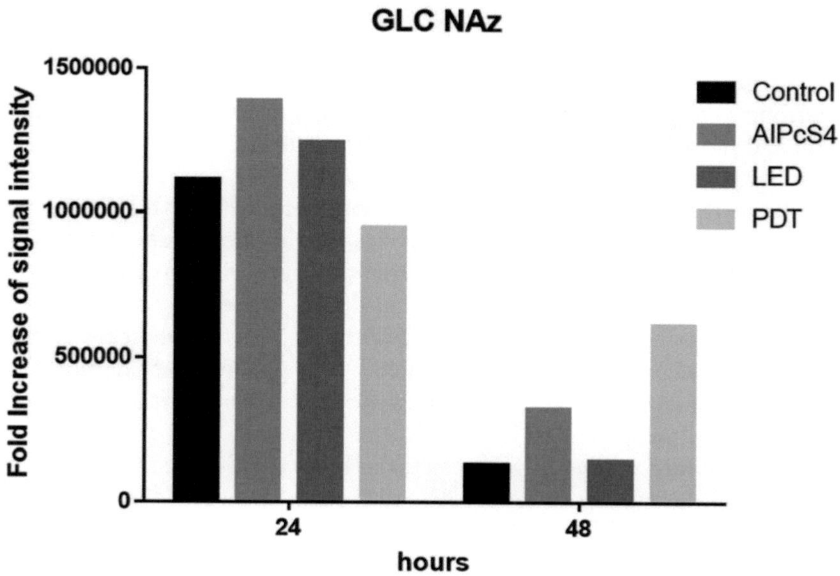

Figure 3.
Analysis of cells treated with Click-iT®-GlcNAz, the graph shows the fluorescence intensity of the cells of the control, led, and treatment groups in the periods of 24 and 48 hours. The fluorescence intensity in all groups in the 24 hours is the same for all. Within 48 hours it is possible to observe an increase in fluorescence intensity in the treatment group compared the control and LED groups.

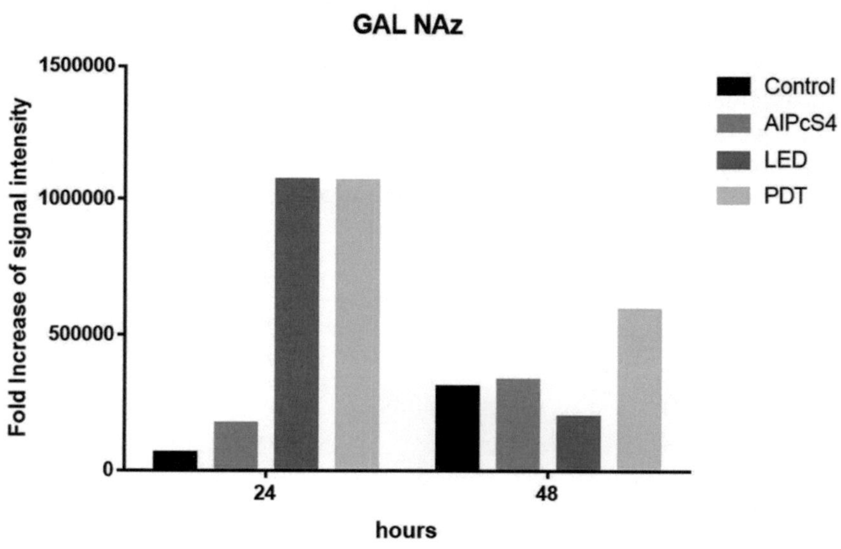

Figure 4.
Analysis of cells treated with Click-iT®-GalNAz, the graph shows the fluorescence intensity of the cells of the control, LED, and treatment groups in the periods of 24 and 48 hours. The treatment group, compared to the other groups, has a high fluorescence intensity.

4. Discussion

The use of the technique called metabolic oligosaccharide engineering (metabolic oligosaccharide engineering) allows for the labeling of glycans with probes for visualization in cells by enriching specific types of glycoconjugates for proteomic analysis. This methodology promotes the metabolic labeling of glycans with a specific reactive functional group, the azide. Azide-labeled carbohydrates are endocytosed by cells and integrated with glycan biosynthesis in various glycoconjugates. The cells are incubated for periods of 24 to 72 hours to allow the synthesis of surface glycoproteins to be monitored [11, 12].

According to prior research [13, 14], glycosylation markers can assist in cancer detection and monitoring since the malignant transformation of cancer cells associated with changes in cell glycosylation are associated with tumor progression and, finally, metastasis. The schemes shown above demonstrate the biosynthesis of glycoproteins in a normal cell (**Figure 5**). The results obtained demonstrate indirectly that the photodynamic treatment altered the glycosylation of proteins in the lattice, consequently compromising the glycosylation in the Golgi and the insertion of glycoproteins in the plasma membrane (**Figure 6**). The statement concerning the reticule is based on previous data obtained by our group, which demonstrated changes in the reticular tubular network and the presence of surface glycoproteins N-acetyl glucosamine terminals [15, 16].

The glycoproteins, when sent via vesicle traffic to the Golgi complex, change with the removal of mannose residues, the addition of N-acetyl glucosamine, galactose, and sialic acid. The addition of carbohydrates is associated with the function that the glycoprotein will play on the cell surface.

The glycosylation markers can be used for cancer detection and monitoring, since changes in cell glycosylation are associated with the transformation of cancer cells into glycosylation, tumor progression, and, finally, metastasis [13, 14]. The schemes shown above demonstrate the biosynthesis of glycoproteins in a normal cell (**Figures** 7 and **8**). The results obtained indirectly demonstrate that the photodynamic treatment altered the glycosylation of proteins in the lattice, consequently compromising the glycosylation in the Golgi and the insertion of glycoproteins in the plasma membrane. The reticule statement is based on previous data obtained by our group [15], which demonstrated changes in the reticular tubular network.

The photodynamic treatment action on surface glycans has a significant impact on cell signaling and the regulation of cell-tumor cell adhesion and cell-matrix

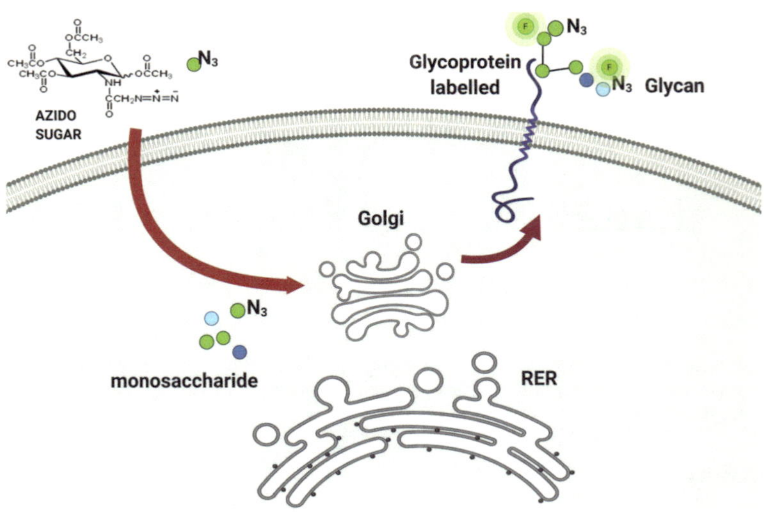

Figure 5.
Membrane glycoprotein biosynthesis scheme. The monosaccharide complexed with azide (Click-iT™ Metabolic Glycoprotein Labeling Reagent), crosses the plasma membrane, becoming available in the cytoplasm. Golgi, responsible for the glycosylation process, captures the monosaccharide, which will be used in the processing of membrane protein, coming from the rough endoplasmic reticulum. After the incorporation of the labeled monosaccharide into the protein, the vesicle is released and fused to the plasma membrane, exposing the glycoprotein, allowing its detection by microscopy or cytometry. Created with BioRender.com.

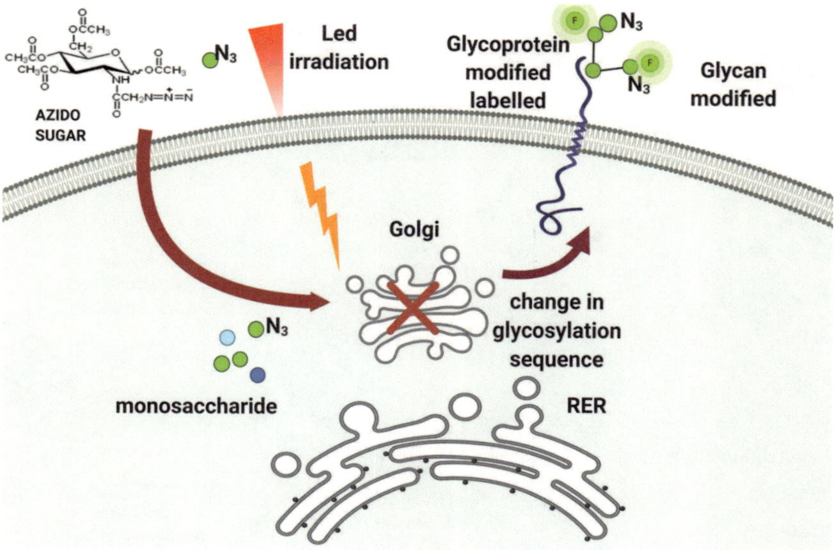

Figure 6.
Membrane glycoprotein biosynthesis scheme after PDT. The monosaccharide complexed with azide (Click-iT™ metabolic glycoprotein labeling reagent), crosses the plasma membrane, becoming available in the cytoplasm. Golgi, responsible for the glycosylation process, captures the monosaccharide, which will be used in the processing of membrane protein, coming from the rough endoplasmic reticulum, but after PDT changes the sequence of monosaccharides, modifies the glycan modifying the glycoprotein. After the incorporation of the labeled monosaccharide into the protein, the vesicle is released and fused to the plasma membrane, exposing the glycoprotein, allowing its detection by microscopy or cytometry. Created with BioRender.com.

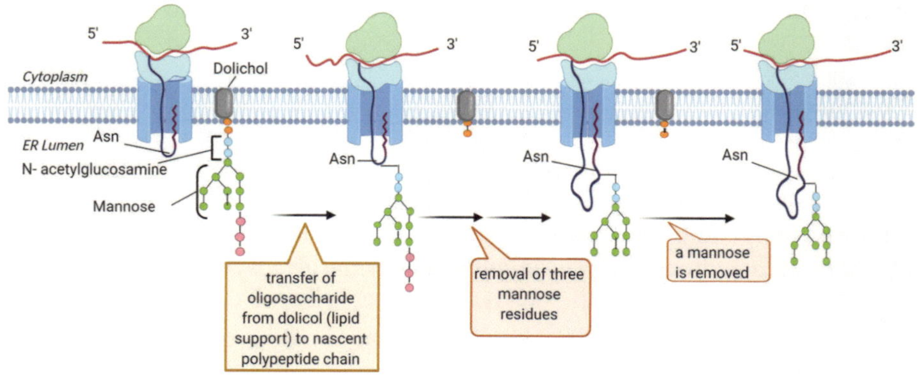

Figure 7.
Glycosylation scheme in the rough endoplasmic reticulum. Created with BioRender.com.

interaction, compromising the interaction between cancer cells and the tumor microenvironment.

An exciting result refers to the $AlPcS_4$ group, with reduced glycosylation of proteins with mannose and galactose terminal monosaccharides, when compared to the control group. This data suggests that phthalocyanine endocytosed by the tumor cell requires more lysosomes to be degraded, a demand supplied by Golgi, which releases transport vesicles with acid hydrolases to the lysosomes via the mannose −6-phosphate receptor. For the substitution of mannose by galactose, mannosidase action must occur; however, as there is a need for more hydrolases and more transporters, the final carbohydrate does not change.

In the 48 hours, the $AlPcS_4$ and LED groups show similar behavior to the control group, indicating that, after the period of interaction with the photosensitizer and

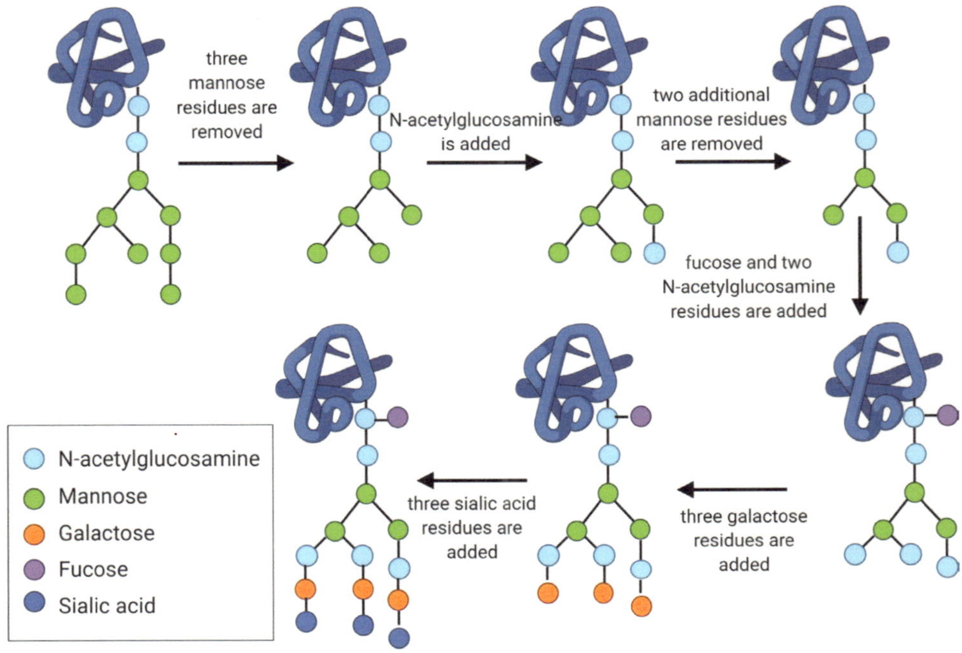

Figure 8.
Glycosylation scheme in the Golgi apparatus. Created with BioRender.com.

the action of light, the cell restores its synthesis process. Reinforcing the information that light and separate photosensitizers cannot cause damage to cells.

5. Conclusion

The action of photodynamic treatment on surface glycans has a significant impact on cell signaling and the regulation of cell-tumor, cell-adhesion, and cell-matrix interactions, compromising the interaction between cancer cells and the tumor microenvironment. The involvement of the glycosylation process in the Golgi apparatus prejudice the survival of tumor cells and can be exploited to develop strategies for immune system activation.

Acknowledgements

The authors acknowledge support from FAPESP (São Paulo Research Foundation, Contract grant number 2016/17984-1), CNPq - National Council for Scientific and Technological Development grant 305920/2017-0 and FINEP (Financier of Studies and Projects) n° 01.18.0053.00.

Conflict of interest

The authors declare no conflict of interest.

Author details

Bruno Henrique Godoi[1], Juliana Ferreira Strixino[2], Newton Soares da Silva[3] and Cristina Pacheco Soares[1*]

1 Laboratory of Dynamics of Cellular Compartments, Institute of Research and Development, Universidade do Vale do Paraíba, São José dos Campos, São Paulo, Brazil

2 Laboratory of Photobiology Applied to Health, Institute of Research and Development, Universidade do Vale do Paraíba, São José dos Campos, São Paulo, Brazil

3 Laboratory of Cellular and Tissue Biology, Institute of Research and Development, Universidade do Vale do Paraíba, São José dos Campos, São Paulo, Brazil

*Address all correspondence to: cpsoares@univap.br

References

[1] Zhang, X., & Wang, Y. Glycosylation Quality Control by the Golgi Structure. Journal of molecular biology, 428(16), 3183-3193. 2016 doi:10.1016/j.jmb.2016.02.030

[2] Maftoum-Costa Naves M, KT, Oliveira AL, Tedesco AC, Pacheco-Soares, C. Mitochondria, endoplasmic reticulum and actin filament behavior after PDT with chloroaluminum phthalocyanine liposomal in HeLa cells. Cell Biology International, 2008. 32, 1024-1028.

[3] Aebi M, N-linked protein glycosylation in the ER, Biochimica et Biophysica Acta (BBA) - Molecular Cell Research, Volume 1833, Issue 11, 2013. 2430-2437, ISSN 0167-4889, https://doi.org/10.1016/j.bbamcr.2013.04.001.

[4] Lodish H, Berk A, Zipursky SL, et al. Molecular Cell Biology. 4th edition. New York: W. H. Freeman; Section 17.7, Protein Glycosylation in the ER and Golgi Complex. 2000. Available from: https://www.ncbi.nlm.nih.gov/books/NBK21744/,

[5] Peixoto, A., Relvas-Santos, M., Azevedo, R., Santos, L. L., & Ferreira, J. A. Protein Glycosylation and Tumor Microenvironment Alterations Driving Cancer Hallmarks. Frontiers in oncology, 9, 380. 2019. doi:10.3389/fonc.2019.00380.

[6] Joy M. Burchell, Richard Beatson, Rosalind Graham, Joyce Taylor-Papadimitriou, Virginia Tajadura-Ortega. O-linked mucin-type glycosylation in breast cancer. Biochem Soc Tran. 2018. 46 (4): 779-788. doi: https://doi.org/10.1042/BST20170483

[7] Gruszewska E, Chrostek L. The alterations of glycosylation in malignant diseases. Pol Merkur Lekarski. 2013. 34(199):58-61.

[8] Christiansen M.N, Chik J.H.L, Lee L et al. Cell surface protein glycosylation in cancer. Proteomics. 2014. 14, 4-5. DOI: 10.1002/pmic.201300387

[9] Dennis JW, Laferte S, Waghorne C, Breitman Ml, Kerbel RS Beta 1-6 branching of Asn-linked oligosaccharides is directly associated with metastasis. Science. 1987. 01 MAY, 582-585.

[10] Shetty RK, Bhandary SK, Kali A. Significance of serum l-fucose glycoprotein as cancer biomarker in head and neck malignancies without distant metastasis. J Clin Diagn Res. 2013. 7:2818-20.

[11] Dube, D. H., & Williams, D. A. Metabolic Glycan Engineering in Live Animals: Using Bio-orthogonal Chemistry to Alter Cell Surface Glycans. Handbook of In Vivo Chemistry in Mice, 2019. 209-248. doi:10.1002/9783527344406.ch8

[12] Almaraz, R. T., Aich, U., Khanna, H. S., Tan, E., Bhattacharya, R., Shah, S., & Yarema, K. J. Metabolic oligosaccharide engineering with N-Acyl functionalized ManNAc analogs: Cytotoxicity, metabolic flux, and glycan-display considerations. Biotechnology and Bioengineering. 2011. 109(4), 992-1006. doi:10.1002/bit.24363

[13] Rodrigues JG, Balmaña M, Macedo JA, Poças J, Fernandes Â, de-Freitas-JuniorJCM, PinhoSS, GomesJ, Magalhães A, Gomes C, Mereiter S, ReisCA. Glycosylationincancer: Selected roles in tumour progression, immune modulation and metastasis. Cell Immunol. 2018. 333:46-57. doi: 10.1016/j.cellimm.2018.03.007. Epub Mar 20.

[14] Silsirivanit A (2019) Glycosylation markers in cancer Adv Clin Chem.

2019. 89:189-213. doi: 10.1016/bs.acc.2018.12.005. Epub Jan 17.

[15] Ferreira, S.D.R.M., Tedesco, A.C., Sousa, G. et al. Analysis of mitochondria, endoplasmic reticulum and actin filaments after PDT with $AlPcS_4$. Lasers Med Sci 2004. 18, 207-212. doi:10.1007/s10103-003-0282-6.

[16] Pinto, G.P., Lopes, K.A.R., Salles, N.G. et al. N-acetyl Glucosamine Distribution and Mitochondrial Activity of Tumor Cell Exposed to Photodynamic Therapy. J Fluoresc. 2016. 26, 1923-1926 doi:10.1007/s10895-016-1914-0.

Chapter 3

Sonodynamic and Photodynamics Used as a Combined Therapy in the Treatment of Malignant Neoplasms: Facts and Open Questions

Heber Lopes de Mello, Luiz Anastacio Alves,
Evellyn Araujo Dias, Sabrina de Sá Pereira Magalhães,
Vinicius Cotta-de-Almeida and Rodrigo da Cunha Bisaggio

Abstract

Photodynamic therapy (PDT) used in combination with sonodynamic therapy (SDT) is a new approach that aims to increase the effectiveness of tumor treatment when compared to the effect of each independent therapy. PDT is based on stimulating sensitizers with photons, while the most accepted theory for SDT is that sensitizers are stimulated by the sonoluminescence phenomenon. However, after the excitation of the sensitizer, both therapies follow a common path, leading to the generation of free radicals and inducing cell death. One of the positive aspects of this combination is the augmentation of anti-tumor activity with fewer side effects, since cell death may be induced using lower sensitizer concentrations or less exposure to ultrasound or light. Another benefit of combining PDT and SDT, especially with the use of low-frequency ultrasound is the induction of sonophoresis. For instance, on the skin, it may facilitate the absorption of the sensitizer. However, research involving both PDT and SDT exhibit many variants, including differences in irradiation sources and their intensities, among others. These aspects contribute to a lack of standardization, leading to result variations, hindering assessment on the real contribution that these combined therapies can offer in tumor treatment. Thus, further research in the pre-clinical and clinical areas are crucial.

Keywords: cancer therapy, ultrasound, sonodynamic therapy, sonophotodynamic therapy, sonophoresis

1. Introduction

Currently, medicine has gone through great advances due to basic and applied research, as well as the implantation and discovery of new technologies. However, the treatment of malignant neoplasms (cancers) requires improvement. According to the WHO, malignant neoplasms were the second leading cause of death worldwide in 2018 [1], and CDC estimates indicate that malignant neoplasms will be the main cause of death in the USA by 2030 [2].

Malignant neoplasms are a group of diseases exhibiting the common characteristic of invasion of adjacent tissues by proximity or migration to other tissues and organs by lymphatic, blood circulation or body cavities, in a process known as metastasis. Malignant neoplasms exhibit six basic characteristics defined by Hannah and Weingberg in 2000: they are able to resist cell death, induce angiogenesis, exhibit replicative immortality, evade growth suppression, activate invasion (metastasis) and sustain proliferative signaling [3]. The origin of malignant neoplasms is still unknown, and several theories have been postulated in this regard, including Somatic Mutation theory, Evolutionary theory and Cancer Stem cell theory [4, 5]. Environmental factors, such as ultraviolet radiation, ionizing radiation and carcinogens, may alter the genetic structure of cells and explain a portion of cancer cases. To illustrate oncogenesis complexity, smoking is known to increase the risk for cancer up to 100-fold. However, when comparing the mutation numbers of lung cell carcinomas in smokers and non-smokers, this increase is only 1.15-fold [4]. Today, it is clear that the tumoral microenvironment is also part of the oncogenesis process.

Traditional cancer treatments, such as chemotherapy, radiotherapy and surgery, in spite of being effective for several types of tumors, saving millions of lives, are often aggressive, expensive and not always efficient. Chemotherapy is based on the use of drugs in order to reach and destroy tumor cells and radiotherapy applies ionizing radiation to destroy and prevent tumor growth. These therapies are the most common in cancer treatments, but they affect not only tumor cells but also healthy ones, which can lead to side effects, such as nausea and hair loss. Surgery can be used in several cases in which the tumor can be removed either partially or completely, although it can be very invasive and expensive [6]. These treatments are often combined to enhance results, increasing the possibility of longer remission times and, in some cases, cures. Other treatment modalities have begun to be recently applied, such as Immunotherapy, Hormone Therapy and Stem Cell Transplant, alongside, or not, traditional treatments.

Photodynamic therapy (PDT) and sonodynamic therapy (SDT) emerge as alternative or adjuvant treatments for cancer cases, exhibiting a minimally invasive approach. These therapies are based on the administration (either systemic or topical) of a photosensitizer (PS) or a sonosensitizer (SS), generally non-toxic when used in the appropriate concentrations, resulting in cell death when irradiated with light or ultrasound [7].

2. Ultrasound applied to medicine

2.1 Ultrasound in biological systems

Ultrasound is a mechanical wave exhibiting frequencies above 20 kHz, out of the human hearing range [8]. Historical evidence indicates that ultrasounds were first applied in humans to examine a brain tumor by Karl Dussik, in 1942 [9], who reported that, when ultrasound is focused, its biological effects are more localized [10]. Ultrasound applied to therapeutic purposes can be used at low intensities (0.125–3 W/cm^2) to stimulate normal physiological responses to injury and facilitate the transport of substances across the skin (sonophoresis), or it can be used at high intensities (>5 W/cm^2) to selectively destroy target tissues [11].

Acoustic cavitation occurs when ultrasound waves pass through an aqueous medium and it is an important ultrasound interaction with biological tissues. The disturbance caused by ultrasound causes oscillations in the ambient pressure that can lead to gases present in the solution to form small "bubbles". With the maintenance of the ultrasound waves, these bubbles may continue to increase in size and, eventually,

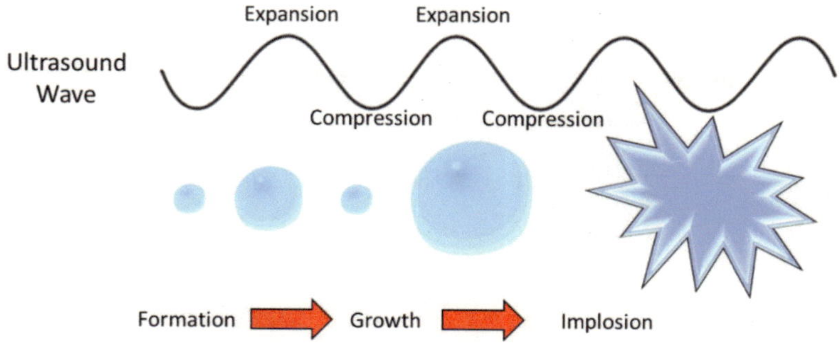

Figure 1.
Scheme depicturing the development of cavitation bubbles. The ultrasound waves cause the cavitation bubble to increase and decrease in size in sustained cycles, until the bubbles reach an unstable and critical size. When the bubbles implode, high temperatures and the release of energy in the form of light (Sonoluminescence) can occur.

collapse (**Figure 1**), releasing energy [12]. Another ultrasound effect is thermal; where the mechanical waves cause frictional heat in tissues by molecule vibration and, depending on the temperature, lead to different biological effects [8]. Many factors can influence US treatment outcomes, such as ultrasound exposure duration, heated tissue volume, maximum temperature achieved and rate of temperature increases [11]. This effect is routinely applied in the physiotherapy area to treat osteo-muscular lesions.

2.2 Ultrasound in malignant neoplasm therapy

The first clinical application of ultrasound to malignant neoplasm was performed in 1944 and, since then, several studies have been carried out applying this technique [13]. The consolidation of ultrasound to treat tumors originates in prostate neoplasm treatments that began in the 1990s, by the use of High-intensity focused ultrasound (HIFU), whose intensity applied to tumors may range from 100 to 10,000 W/cm^2 [14].

Almost at the same time, Yumita et al. discovered sonodynamic therapy (SDT), by associating hematoporphyrin derivatives (already applied in PDT) to ultrasound irradiation, observing cell damage up to 50% higher compared to the non-associated treatment [15]. Although it acts in a similar manner as PDT, the exact sonodynamic therapy activation mechanism of a certain molecule (sonosensitizer) is not as well elucidated as in photodynamic therapy. The two main hypotheses concerning SDT mechanisms have been postulated, both directly linked to acoustic cavitation (see above). The thermal effect hypothesis suggests that heat is released, leading to temperatures of up to 10,000 K, with pressures reaching 81 MPa after the collapse of cavitation bubbles, which would be responsible for sonosensitizer activation [16]. The second and currently widely accepted hypothesis is that sonosensitizer activation occurs due to an effect known as sonoluminescence, where light energy is released after the collapse of the cavitation microbubbles [17]. This light energy would be, therefore, responsible for sonosensitizer activation, which leads to the production of free radicals and, consequently, cell death (**Figure 2**) [18]. In addition to the use of low-intensity ultrasound as a treatment using SDT, another interesting feature is the possibility of facilitating the entry of molecules through the plasma membrane, as demonstrated by Harrison and Balcer-Kubiczek in the early 90s when irradiating Chinese hamster ovaries cells with low intensity ultrasound, favoring the entry of adriamycin and amphotericin B, evidenced by increased cell death [19]. Low frequency ultrasound (<100 kHz) is more efficient in increasing skin permeability

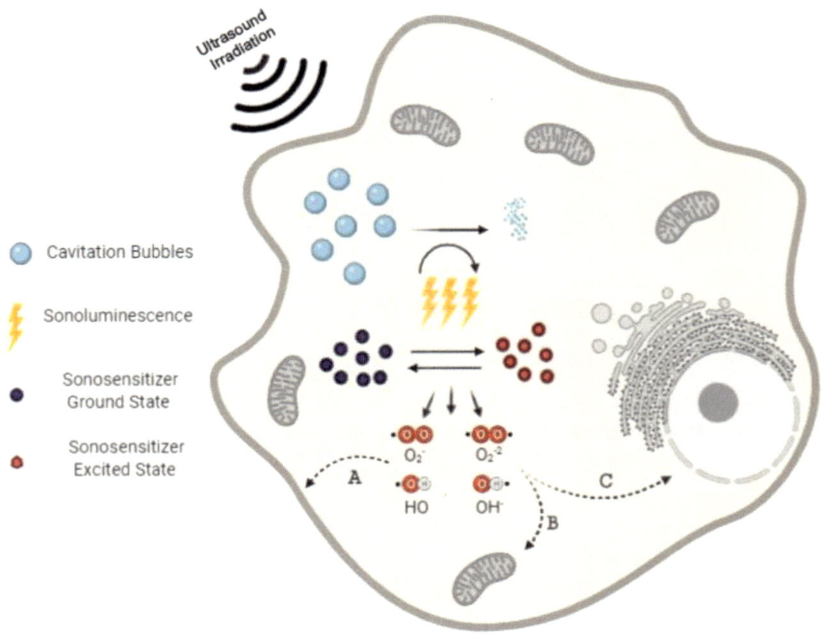

Figure 2.
Scheme representing the potential SDT mechanism. Ultrasound irradiation induces intracellular cavitation bubbles. The collapse of these bubbles, through sonoluminescence, generates an energy that will be responsible for the activation of the sonosensitizer from its fundamental state to an excited state. As the activated sensitizer returns to ground state, the released energy is then transferred to the oxygen present in the cytosol to produce high amounts of ROS, including oxygen peroxide and superoxide ions. These can cause several cell changes that may result in cell death, such as (A) oxidative degradation of lipids, that would damage cell membranes, organelles and vesicles that are made-up of lipids. (B) Damage to the mitochondrial membrane, initiating the apoptotic process mediated by cytochrome C. (C) Direct damage to structures and molecules essential for cellular homeostasis.

than therapeutic ultrasound. This is attributed to the cavitation phenomenon, which is more frequent at low frequencies [20]. Tachibana et al. identified that the blood glucose levels of hairless rats immersed in glasses containing an insulin solution (20 U/mL) and placed in an ultrasound bath (48 kHz) decreased by 50% in 240 minutes [21]. The use of ultrasound as a drug delivery mediator technique represents an important technological advance in many areas. This is no different in PDT treatment, as it may be possible to facilitate tissue molecule entry, reducing the amount of sensitizers to be used in treatments, in addition to allowing a joint sonodynamic and photodynamic therapy effect, since both therapies work in a similar manner.

3. Sono-photodynamic therapy (SPDT) used as a combined therapy

PDT is performed in two main stages. The first comprises patient photosensitizer administration followed by exposing the target region of the therapy to light at an appropriate wavelength to produce reactive oxygen species capable of causing the death of microorganisms or abnormal cells, such as tumors [22]. The wavelength in which the photosensitizer absorbs energy is an important aspect that must be taken into account when choosing the sensitizer. Capella and Capella identified molecules that absorb light between 600 and 800 nm as ideal since, below this range, hemoglobin, the main light-absorbing protein in the blood, would compete for the energy emitted to activate the photosensitizer and, above this range, photons would not have enough energy to participate in photochemical reactions. However, PDT exhibits a major limitation regarding tissue penetration [23]. Bashaktov et al. pointed out that skin light penetration ranges from 1.5 mm to 2.5 mm [24], and Kondo et al. reported that light penetration may reach 7 mm in mucous membranes [25]. In the light of these facts, PDT becomes limited to surface region treatments or treatments for surfaces located close to the irradiating source, demanding invasive techniques in the case of internal tissue and organ treatments. In this scenario, sonodynamic therapy may be an alternative, due to the ability of ultrasound to penetrate deeper into the organism, reaching internal tissues and organs. As a result, the combined use of these therapies may be extremely positive. Sono-photodynamic therapy has been considered more effective than the individual therapies as a possible cancer treatment, as verified in a glioma model [26]. The idea is to use both light and sound to activate a sono-photosensitizer, leading to the destruction of tumor cells. Besides the action of US facilitating the sensitizer cell permeability, as described previously, another advantage of the combined use of these two therapies is the possibility of reducing the sensitizer dosage without reducing treatment effects [27], since most assessed sonosensitizers, i.e. porphyrin derivatives, are also photosensitizers [28]. Some *in vitro* studies have already attempted to prove the effectiveness of this therapy. For example, Li et al. studied the effects of SPDT on C6 glioma cells using hematoporphyrin monomethyl ether (HMME) as a sensitizer, by ultrasound and light irradiation, respectively. The C6 glioma cells treated with SPDT exhibited higher growth inhibition than cells treated by the individual therapies [29]. Furthermore, Zhu et al. used SPTD on HEPG2 cells, applying curcumin-loaded poly (L-lactide-co-glycolide) as a sensitizer [30]. Higher apoptosis percentages and better anti-cancer cell proliferation effects were observed in the group treated with SPDT compared to the groups submitted to either SDT or PDT. An *in vivo* study performed by Jin et al. tested the combined therapy on C3H/HeN mice, using ATX-70 and PH-1126 as sensitizers. The percentages of tumor inhibition observed in mice treated with ATX-70 were 92, 77 and 27% when submitted to SPDT, SDT and PDT respectively, and the group treated with the combined therapy exhibited an increase in 120-day survival rates to 60% in five mice, higher than in the SDT and PDT groups. When using PH-1126 as a sensitizer, tumor inhibition results of 98, 76, or 43% were observed for SPDT, SDT and PDT respectively, and the combination therapy increased 120-day survival rates to 88% in eight mice [27]. In addition, the combined therapy has also been tested in humans as summarized in **Table 1**. Li et al. evaluated seven patients with advanced gastric and esophageal adenocarcinoma who, after treatment with SPDT, showed improvement of the condition [31]. Wang et al. studied twelve patients with advanced breast carcinoma and, after treatment with SPDT, reported a median patient survival exceeding 14.5 months [32].

Number of patients	Treatment	Results	References
7	Sensitizers applied sublingually, followed by SPDT once a week	Three patients achieved a complete response, three, a partial response and one, an MR response	Li et al. [31]
12	Sensitizers applied sublingually, followed by SPDT once a week	Two patients achieved a complete response, seven, a partial response and three, a stable disease state	Wang et al. [32]
115	Sensitizers applied sublingually, followed by SPDT once a week	Of the 115 evaluated patients, 70 exceeded the calculated life expectancy	Kenyon et al. [33]

Table 1.
Summary of clinical research results involving SPDT.

Kenyon et al. in a study carried out with 115 patients followed for 4 years, reported a significant life expectancy increase for patients diagnosed with breast, bladder, colorectal, prostate and ovarian cancers, among others [33]. It is important to standardize Sono-Photodynamic therapy experiments according to the sensitizer, the exposure times and light and ultrasound intensities, so that the results may be compared, repeated and discussed worldwide, aiming at minimally invasive applications to neoplasm treatment with minimal patient discomfort.

4. Conclusions

PDT and SDT have great potential to be used as treatments for several diseases, especially cancer. However, when used together (SPDT), their effects can be even more significant. Nonetheless there are many experimental variables that interfere in the outcome of the treatment. This fact leads to difficulties in comparing the results of assays performed by different groups around the world, either *in vitro* or *in vivo*. In order to appraisal the real potential of SPDT, further studies must be carried out in a more standardized manner, controlling the irradiation times, intensities of irradiation by light and ultrasound, type of sensitizer used and even the type and stage of the tumor. Thus, further research in the pre-clinical and clinical areas are crucial. In the case of clinical studies, double blind randomized controlled trials of sonodynamic therapy alone and combined with photodynamic therapy are required.

Author details

Heber Lopes de Mello[1,2], Luiz Anastacio Alves[2*], Evellyn Araujo Dias[2,3], Sabrina de Sá Pereira Magalhães[2,4], Vinicius Cotta-de-Almeida[1] and Rodrigo da Cunha Bisaggio[2,3]

1 Thymus Research Laboratory, Oswaldo Cruz Institute, Fiocruz, Rio de Janeiro, RJ, Brazil

2 Laboratory of Cellular Communication, Oswaldo Cruz Institute, Fiocruz, Rio de Janeiro, RJ, Brazil

3 Biotechnology Departament, Federal Institute of Education, Science and Technology of Rio de Janeiro, Rio de Janeiro, RJ, Brazil

4 Biomedicine Department, Federal University of the State of Rio de Janeiro, Rio de Janeiro, RJ, Brazil

*Address all correspondence to: alveslaa@gmail.com

References

[1] Globocan, WHO, 2020. Available in: <https://www.who.int/health-topics/cancer#tab=tab_1>. Access in: 04 Aug. 2020.

[2] Future Health of our Nation Infographic, CDC National Health Report 2015. Available in: <https://www.cdc.gov/healthreport/infographics/aging/index.htm>. Access in: 04 aug. 2020.

[3] Hanahan D, Weinberg RA. Hallmarks of cancer: The next generation. Cell. 2011;**144**:646-674 https://doi.org/10.1016/j.cell.2011.02.013

[4] Liggett LA, DeGregori J. Changing mutational and adaptive landscapes and the genesis of cancer. Biochim Biophys Acta - Rev Cancer. 2017;**1867**:84-94 https://doi.org/10.1016/j.bbcan.2017.01.005

[5] Sánchez-Danés A, Blanpain C. Deciphering the cells of origin of squamous cell carcinomas. Nature Reviews. Cancer. 2018;**18**:549-561 https://doi.org/10.1038/s41568-018-0024-5

[6] American Cancer Society, 2019. How Surgery Is Used for Cancer. Available in: <https://www.cancer.org/treatment/treatments-and-side-effects/treatment-types/surgery/how-surgery-is-used-for-cancer.html> Access in: 06 aug. 2020

[7] Trendowski M. The promise of sonodynamic therapy. Cancer Metastasis Reviews. 2014;**33**:143-160 https://doi.org/10.1007/s10555-013-9461-5

[8] Kim Y, Rhim H, Choi MJ, Lim HK, Choi D. High-intensity focused ultrasound therapy: An overview for radiologists. Korean Journal of Radiology. 2008;**9**:291 https://doi.org/10.3348/kjr.2008.9.4.291

[9] Dussik KT. Über die Möglichkeit, hochfrequente mechanische Schwingungen als diagnostisches Hilfsmittel zu verwerten 1941.

[10] Lynn JG, Zwemer RL, Chick AJ, Miller AE. A new method for the generation and use of focused ultrasound in experimental biology. The Journal of General Physiology. 1942;**26**:179-193 https://doi.org/10.1085/jgp.26.2.179

[11] ter Haar G. Therapeutic ultrasound. European Journal of Ultrasound. 1999;**9**:3-9 https://doi.org/10.1016/S0929-8266(99)00013-0

[12] Ashokkumar M, Lee J, Kentish S, Grieser F. Bubbles in an acoustic field: An overview. Ultrasonics Sonochemistry. 2007;**14**:470-475 https://doi.org/10.1016/j.ultsonch.2006.09.016

[13] Kremkau FW. Cancer therapy with ultrasound: A historical review. Journal of Clinical Ultrasound. 1979;**7**:287-300 https://doi.org/10.1002/jcu.1870070410

[14] Copelan A, Hartman J, Chehab M, Venkatesan A. High-intensity focused ultrasound: Current status for image-guided therapy. Semin Intervent Radiol. 2015;**32**:398-415 https://doi.org/10.1055/s-0035-1564793

[15] Yumita N, Nishigaki R, Umemura K, Umemura S. Hematoporphyrin as a sensitizer of cell-damaging effect of ultrasound. Japanese J Cancer Res. 1989;**80**:219-222 https://doi.org/10.1111/j.1349-7006.1989.tb02295.x

[16] Misik V, Riesz P. Free radical intermediates in Sonodynamic therapy. Annals of the New York Academy of Sciences. 2006;**899**:335-348 https://doi.org/10.1111/j.1749-6632.2000.tb06198.x

[17] Sazgarnia A, Shanei A, Eshghi H, Hassanzadeh-Khayyat M,

Esmaily H, Shanei MM. Detection of sonoluminescence signals in a gel phantom in the presence of Protoporphyrin IX conjugated to gold nanoparticles. Ultrasonics. 2013;**53**:29-35 https://doi.org/10.1016/j.ultras.2012.03.009

[18] Niedre M, Patterson MS, Wilson BC. Direct near-infrared luminescence detection of singlet oxygen generated by photodynamic therapy in cells In vitro and tissues In vivo¶. Photochemistry and Photobiology. 2002;**75**:382-391 https://doi.org/10.1562/0031-8655(2002)0750382DNILDO2.0.CO2

[19] Harrison GH, Balcer-Kubiczek EK, Eddy HA. Potentiation of chemotherapy by low-level ultrasound. International Journal of Radiation Biology. 1991;**59**:1453-1466 https://doi.org/10.1080/09553009114551301

[20] Tezel A, Sens A, Tuchscherer J, Mitragotri S. Frequency dependence of sonophoresis. Pharmaceutical Research. 2001;**18**:1694-1700 https://doi.org/10.1023/A:1013366328457

[21] Tachibana K, Tachibana S. Transdermal delivery of insulin by ultrasonic vibration. The Journal of Pharmacy and Pharmacology. 1991;**43**:270-271 https://doi.org/10.1111/j.2042-7158.1991.tb06681.x

[22] Berg K, Madslien K, Bommer JC, Ofterbro R, Winkelman JW, Moan J. Light induced relocalization of sulfonated meso-tetraphenylporphines in NHIK 3025 cells and effects of dose fractionation. Photochemistry and Photobiology. 1991;**53**:203-210 https://doi.org/10.1111/j.1751-1097.1991.tb03924.x

[23] Capella MAM, Capella LS. A light in multidrug resistance: Photodynamic treatment of multidrug-resistant Tumors. Journal of Biomedical Science. 2003;**10**:361-366 https://doi.org/10.1159/000071155

[24] Bashkatov AN, Genina EA, Kochubey VI, Tuchin VV. Optical properties of human skin, subcutaneous and mucous tissues in the wavelength range from 400 to 2000 nm. Journal of Physics D: Applied Physics. 2005;**38**:2543-2555 https://doi.org/10.1088/0022-3727/38/15/004

[25] Kondo K, Miyoshi T, Takizawa H, Kenzaki K, Sakiyama S, Tangoku A. Photodynamic therapy for submucosal tumor of the central bronchus. The Journal of Medical Investigation. 2005;**52**:208-211 https://doi.org/10.2152/jmi.52.208

[26] Tserkovsky DA, Alexandrova EN, Chalau VN, Istomin YP. Effects of combined sonodynamic and photodynamic therapies with photolon on a glioma C6 tumor model. Experimental Oncology. 2012;**34**:332-335

[27] Jin Z, Miyoshi N, Ishiguro K, Umemura S, Kawabata K, Yumita N, et al. Combination effect of photodynamic and Sonodynamic therapy on experimental skin squamous cell carcinoma in C3H/HeN mice. The Journal of Dermatology. 2000;**27**:294-306 https://doi.org/10.1111/j.1346-8138.2000.tb02171.x

[28] Chen H, Zhou X, Gao Y, Zheng B, Tang F, Huang J. Recent progress in development of new sonosensitizers for sonodynamic cancer therapy. Drug Discovery Today. 2014;**19**:502-509 https://doi.org/10.1016/j.drudis.2014.01.010

[29] Li JH, Chen ZQ, Huang Z, Zhan Q, Ren FB, Liu JY, et al. In vitro study of low intensity ultrasound combined with different doses of PDT: Effects on C6 glioma cells. Oncology Letters. 2013;**5**:702-706 https://doi.org/10.3892/ol.2012.1060

[30] Zhu J-X, Zhu W-T, Hu J-H, Yang W, Liu P, Liu Q-H, et al. Curcumin-loaded poly(L-lactide-co-glycolide) microbubble-mediated Sono-photodynamic therapy in liver cancer cells. Ultrasound in Medicine & Biology. 2020;**46**:2030-2043 https://doi.org/10.1016/j.ultrasmedbio.2020.03.030

[31] Li LQ, Wang X, Zhang IW, Mitchell D. Primary clinical use of the sono-photo-dynamic therapy for advanced esophagocadiac and gastric adenocarcinoma. Journal Of Clinical Oncology. 2014;**32** http://dx.doi.org/10.1200/jco.2014.32.15_suppl.e15024

[32] Wang X, Zhang W, Xu Z, Luo Y, Mitchell D, Moss RW. Sonodynamic and photodynamic therapy in advanced refractory breast cancer. Journal of Clinical Oncology. 2012;**8**:283-287 https://doi.org/10.1200/jco.2012.30.27_suppl.118

[33] Kenyon J, Fulle R, Lewis T. Activated cancer therapy using light and ultrasound - a case series of Sonodynamic photodynamic therapy in 115 patients over a 4 year period. Curr Drug Ther. 2009;**4**:179-193 https://doi.org/10.2174/157488509789055036

Chapter 4

Clinical Usage of Photodynamic Therapy

Niral M. Patel and Ali I. Musani

Abstract

This chapter will provide a brief overview of the fundamentals of photodynamic therapy with an emphasis on its use in a clinical setting. Beginning with the history and fundamental science underlying photodynamic therapy and delving into clinical uses. There will be a primary focus on understanding the use of photodynamic therapy under currently approved clinical indications along with their limitations. There are a number of approved therapeutic indications for photodynamic therapy, but there are important limitations and contraindications when applying this therapy. Photodynamic therapy, as applied to the clinical treatment of cancer will be the primary focus with further emphasis on endoluminal and specifically endobronchial cancer as the primary case study.

Keywords: photodynamic therapy, lung cancer, esophageal cancer, Barrett's esophagus, interventional pulmonology, interventional gastroenterology

1. Introduction

Photodynamic therapy is a minimally invasive approach for the treatment of malignancy [1, 2]. It involves selective uptake of a photosensitizing agent, which is then activated by specific wavelengths of light [3, 4]. This results in oxidative damage to the cells by the production of reactive oxygen species [5, 6]. This results in targeted cellular destruction [5, 6]. Along with this direct cellular destruction, there are local inflammatory effects as well as vascular thromboemboli formation, which allow for a further delayed therapeutic effect [5, 6]. The thromboemboli effect blocks blood flow to the target and thereby results in ischemia [5–7]. Photodynamic therapy has been approved across the world for a number of different clinical indications [5, 6]. This chapter will review the mechanisms and clinical utility of photodynamic therapy.

A photosensitizer in this context is an agent, often a porphyrin which reacts to light in the 500–800 nanometer range depending upon the specific agent utilized [7]. The earliest described photodynamic effect was in 1900 by Raab, Von Tappeiner coined the term photodynamic therapy [3, 5]. Over time, hematoporphyrins were noted to result in tumor fluorescence [3]. This was gradually studied further and refined until the nature of the porphyrins was better understood. Light exposure following cellular uptake resulted in cellular damage and destruction [6]. Over time the fundamentals of this damage were better understood. Depending upon the exact photosensitizer, different mechanisms of damage have been proposed. The major mechanisms of damage are singlet oxygen and free radical formation inducing: apoptosis, autophagy, and necrosis [6, 8, 9]. Apoptosis is a form of controlled cellular death which in this case is induced when photosensitizers cause damage to mitochondria or the proteins of bcl-2 [6]. These are major regulators of the cellular death pathway. Autophagy allows for the gradual destruction of cellular components in an ordered manner [8]. However, necrosis is a less orderly effect and can often result in unintended tissue damage due to the disorganized manner of tissue destruction [6, 8].

Over time, many different photosensitizers have been discovered, but of these, only a few have seen broad clinical approval and use [5, 6, 10]. Each photosensitizer is reactive at a specific wavelength of light. Hematoporphyrin (HPD) was the first photosensitizer approved by the FDA in 1995 for the indication of esophageal cancer. HPD was a hematoporphyrin mixture containing monomers and chains of varying lengths [3, 5, 6]. Photofrin (porfimer sodium) is a refined version of HPD with monomers removed, and it is one of the most common clinically used agents, see **Figure 1** [3, 5, 6]. Photosensitizers are primarily porphyrin-based and contain multiple ring structures [3, 5, 6, 11]. These can be applied locally or injected systemically, and over a period of time they will be selectively taken up by cells [3, 5, 6, 11]. Porfimer sodium is part of the first generation of photosensitizers developed in the 1970s and early 1980s [5, 10, 12]. Later generations were developed as the characteristics of the agents were chemically refined [5, 10, 12]. These later generation agents also tended to have decreased duration of systemic photosensitivity [3, 5, 6, 11]. The second generation has been refined to target longer wavelengths of light, thus allowing for deeper tissue penetration of the activating wavelength of light and, therefore greater effect [5, 6, 11]. In conjunction with the increased penetration of longer wavelengths of light, the light source can be embedded into the tissue to allow for an alternative way to increase the effect [6, 11].

Photodynamic therapy has approved indications for superficial or early-stage malignancies as well as late-stage malignancies [5, 6]. These indications intuitively make sense as light penetration is a vital component of this therapy. Given that later stages of malignancy typically spread systemically via blood or lymphatic spread, photodynamic therapy has limited utility in those cases unless it is for a local effect. For example, photodynamic therapy has been well described as an alternative therapy in addressing central airway obstructions in lung cancer [13]. Central airway obstructions are typically manifestations of late-stage cancer, but photodynamic

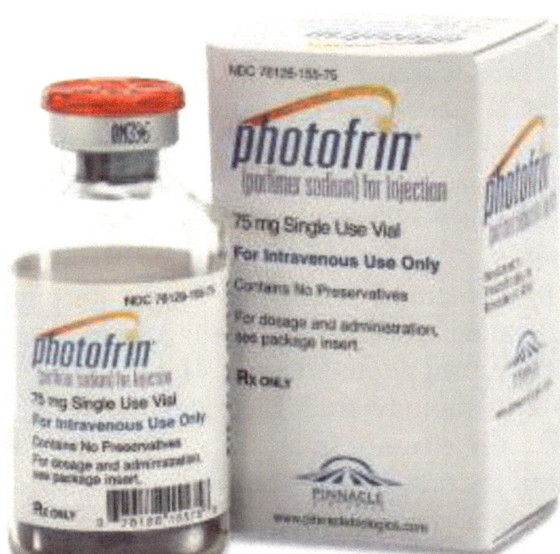

Figure 1.
Comercially available porfimer sodium. Photo used with permission from Pinnacle Biologics.

therapy can be used to clear the tumor obstructing the airway even when it does not have the ability to affect the entirety of the metastatic tumor burden [1, 2, 13]. In many ways, this focused local effect is a significant advantage over alternative treatments which can have greater side effects [1, 2, 13]. These cases of central airway obstruction can be challenging and having an option to provide a delayed and gradual effect that specifically targets tumor cells can be a vital therapeutic intervention. Skin and endoluminal malignancy treatment are approved indications for photodynamic therapy, but this chapter will primarily focus on endoluminal malignancy and especially endobronchial malignancy. Of the photosensitizing agents commercially available, Protomir sodium is the most well studied and widely available, and the best understood.

Photodynamic therapy usage in lung cancer is used as the primary example for a few reasons. The primary being that in many ways. it is the most challenging application. The esophagus consists of a single cylindrical region where the therapy is applied, and blockage of it is not life threatening. Utilization of photodynamic therapy on the skin similarly has limited side effects. However, utilization of photodynamic therapy within the pulmonarysystem is limited to only some surfaces, and damage to this tissue has the potential for life threatening complications. Therefore, understanding the practical applications of photodynamic therapy within the context of lung cancer can be extrapolated to other vital organs.

2. Contraindications of photodynamic therapy

Photodynamic therapy and porfimer sodium, in particular, has a set of contraindications that are worth noting. Porfimer sodium and really any photodynamic therapy cannot be used therapeutically in individuals with porphyria [14, 15]. These individuals have one of a group of diseases that allow for an increased accumulation of porphyrins utilized by the human body in hemoglobin production, and these porphyrins increase photosensitivity [16]. Given the foundation of photodynamic therapy is localized photosensitivity by means of porphyrins, this contraindication is reasonable [3]. Other contraindications are existing tracheoesophageal/bronchoesophageal fistulas [17]. These are abnormal connections between the airway and the esophagus. Tumor eroding into the airway are also contraindicated given the risks that will be described below [17]. Additionally, given the delayed time scale of photodynamic therapy, usage in emergency situations when therapy must be delivered immediately would not be optimal [17].

3. Fundamentals of lung cancer

Throughout the world, lung cancer is one of the most prevalent cancers worldwide; it is the most commonly occurring cancer in men and the third most common in women [18]. The best treatment responses to lung cancer are early detection, diagnosis, and treatment [18, 19]. Photodynamic therapy has a robust role in both early and late-stage lung cancers [20]. Lung cancer has significant morbidity and mortality, and there has been strong interest and research in identifying treatments to improve the morbidity and mortality associated with this disease process [18, 19, 21]. Frequently, management of lung cancer is discussed in local meetings at tumor boards allow physicians of different specialties to determine the optimal next stage of diagnosis or treatment [21]. Knowing the risks and benefits of photodynamic therapy in this context can allow for discussion of the optimal role it can play in treatment.

4. Fundamentals of photodynamic therapy for lung cancer

In the United States, the FDA has approved the usage of photodynamic therapy (porfimer sodium) for endobronchial malignancy [17]. Within the airway, this treatment is applied to non-small cell lung cancer that is not otherwise treatable by surgery or radiation therapy [17]. Beyond this, the limitation to therapy is solely the ability to illuminate the desired areas of disease with the correct wavelength of light [3, 6, 11, 22]. This, therefore limits therapy to lesions that are primarily visible on bronchoscopy. Standard bronchoscopy is able to visualize airways out to the fourth or fifth generation of airways [23]. The airways of the human go out past twenty generations which can limit utility to only the larger central airways [24]. There have been preliminary studies utilizing electromagnetic navigational bronchoscopic approaches to treat more distal malignancies, but these are still early studies [25]. There are also tools now available, including robotic bronchoscopic platforms that allow for navigation, direct visualization, and intervention down to the ninth generation of airways [26]. Although not directly studied with photodynamic therapy, these recent developments could greatly expand the role of photodynamic therapy in lung cancer.

Currently, the major roles for photodynamic therapy in lung cancer are utilizing it early-stage carcinoma in situ or in central airway lesions [1, 2, 13, 20, 27]. There have been multiple off-label uses and case series reporting success in other disease processes, such as in tracheal papillomatosis [28]. This is a relatively benign but recurrent papillomatosis disease of the trachea causing partial obstruction overtime with significant risk for malignant transformation of the underlying papillomas [28]. Although not directly approved for this indication, as will be discussed, endoluminal obstruction in an early or premalignant disease process is not too far from the currently approved indications [28].

Photodynamic therapy can also target the vasculature that feeds areas of malignancy [5]. This can require illumination with the appropriate wavelength of light up to 30 minutes after exposure/injection to the photosensitizer [5, 7]. This ensures the photosensitizers are still circulating and in the vasculature near the target malignant cells [5, 7]. This approach is more often used in ocular conditions such as macular degeneration to target neovascularization as well as cutaneous lesions of the skin [5]. Photodynamic therapy targeting vasculature has demonstrated efficacy in animal models of solid tumors [7]. However, additional studies need to be performed.

There has been increasing interest in the local injection of photosensitizers directly into tumors [5, 12]. Although only early studies have been done, this has demonstrated efficacy in tumors as small as 8 mm in diameter [12]. However, again these are results from early studies. In general, there are many areas of research both clinical and in basic science for photodynamic therapy. However, clinical utilization often has stringent criteria [17]. Therefore, the focus on the currently approved indications will be to better understand where growth in clinical utilization of this technique will need to occur. Given the requirements for safely delivering therapy to patients, understanding these limitations can help guide the future direction of clinical and translational research. Lung cancer will be utilized as a primary model given the unique characteristics of its prevalence and complexity, and esophageal cancer use will be contrasted to it.

5. Approach to photodynamic therapy in lung cancer

Airway lesions must first be identified then confirmed bronchoscopically to ensure the lesions can be reached and light can be applied to the desired areas.

Additionally, it is important to note the anatomy of the area surrounding the lesions. If the lesion location is adjacent to the large blood vessels surrounding the airway, the risk of massive hemoptysis should be considered prior to administering therapy [29]. This is also true for large central airway tumors that may have large vascular beds [29, 30]. As necrosis occurs, these perforating vessels can potentially lead to significant bleeding. The risk of further airway compromise in an already partially compromised airway (i.e. from the central airway tumor) is already significant in these scenarios. This is a greater consideration when there is malignancy both intrinsic and extrinsic to the airway. Additionally, there is a risk of fistula formation into the surrounding structures of the thorax such as: the esophagus, mediastinum, or blood vessels (pulmonary artery, superior vena cava, innominate vein, etc.) [31]. It should also be noted that mediastinal anatomy, especially airways and blood vessels will shift out of their traditional anatomic locations in the presence of large tumor burden. Being aware of these changes can be vital when reviewing a patient for consideration of photodynamic therapy. Depending upon the shape and course of the lesions, consideration should be given to the anticipated inflammatory effects during photodynamic therapy as the process of controlled and uncontrolled cell death occurs. The areas particularly at risk are the trachea, carina, and main stem bronchi [17, 29]. In these cases, long or circumferential tumors would be at a higher risk of obstructing the airway given the expansion associated with edema that would be anticipated with photodynamic therapy [17]. Additionally, individuals with impaired liver and/or renal function can have delayed clearance of porfimer sodium [17]. This delayed clearance can prolong the period of photosensitivity beyond 90 days when it would typically be ~30 days [5, 12, 28].

Skin/systemic photosensitivity is the most significant and common adverse effect associated with photodynamic therapy [17]. Following the injection of the photosensitizer, it is important to ensure that patients are able to protect their skin until the photosensitizer is fully cleared [17]. This can be as short as two weeks and sometimes as long as three months [5, 6, 12]. Ensuring patients remain indoors for this period to prevent serious collateral skin damage from occurring is vital to safely administering this therapy [17]. Porfimer sodium has not been extensively studied in pregnant and lactating women, but there are animal studies that have demonstrated adverse effects [17]. This has led to porfimer sulfate having an FDA pregnancy category of C, ie animal studies demonstrating adverse fetus effects without any well-controlled human studies, but the benefits may warrant consideration in this population. Similarly, there are no studies on lactation either, so it is not known if porfimer sulfate is secreted in breast milk [17].

Porfimer sodium is injected systemically at a dosage of 2 mg/kg intravenously over 3–5 minutes; this is considered time zero [2, 28]. From this point onwards, the patient will be extremely photosensitive and must wear protective clothing. Additionally, there can be ocular sensitivity, so it is important for patients to wear dark glasses that transmit <4% of white light over the next 30 days [17]. Over the next 2–3 days from time zero, the porfimer sodium will preferentially localize to the desired areas of malignancy over this period of time [5, 6]. Next, the patient will be brought in for a bronchoscopy for the second stage of the treatment [17]. This typically will occur 40–50 hours from time zero [1, 2]. Upon reidentification of the lesions of interest, here a laser light diffuser illuminating at a wavelength of 620 nm with 200 J/cm for the length of the diffuser is utilized, **Figure 2** shows available diffusers [17]. The duration of illumination is eight minutes and twenty seconds (five hundred seconds) [17]. If the tissue of the lesion is soft and allows, the fiber can be positioned interstitially, otherwise the fiber remains within the lumen of the airway for the five hundred seconds of illumination [17]. During this period all

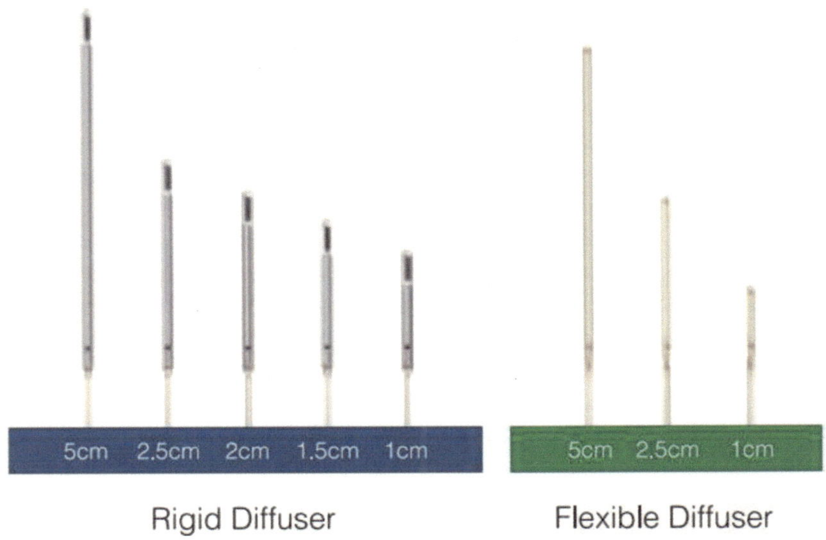

Figure 2.
Comercially available laser diffuser fibers for endobronchial use. Photo used with permission from Pinnacle Biologics.

individuals, including the patient receiving therapy, in the procedure room wear eye protection. Following endoillumination of the desired lesions, it is often advisable to have the patients hospitalized for observation [17]. As the tumor sloughs off, it can often be necessary to debride the necrotic tissue to prevent obstruction of the airway [17]. This is recommended to be done 48–72 hours after the light treatment, or 88–122 hours from time zero [17]. If it is clinically indicated a second light treatment can be performed 96–120 hours from time zero [17]. Given there is an overlap between when tissue debridement is performed and when a second light therapy can be indicated, they are sometimes performed simultaneously. Although the tumor debridement is recommended to be 48–72 hours from light therapy, there can often be a very robust tissue response, and the debridement may need to be done sooner and multiple times before the photodynamic effect is fully realized. Given that airway obstruction can be an emergent and life-threatening condition if not intervened upon quickly, there is a strong reason to keep patients hospitalized for the duration of this therapy.

Following the first injection of Porfimer sodium, subsequent injections and light exposures can be repeated as described above up to three times [17]. However, each treatment must be separated by thirty days. If radiation therapy was performed at any point there should be a period of approximately four weeks from the completion of radiation before photodynamic therapy is attempted [17]. After exposure to porfimer sodium, exposure to sunlight can cause a significant skin reaction, but indoor light can help clear the residual photosensitizer [17]. The duration of the of photosensitivity period can vary from patient to patient, and should be individualized, but a minimum of thirty days should be considered [17]. To determine if there is any residual photosensitivity, patients can be instructed to expose an area of skin to sunlight for approximately ten minutes and then observe for any skin reaction over the subsequent twenty-four hours. As it may be difficult to remember exactly where the exposure was, using a pen or marker to outline the sun-exposed area can help identify this area. Following treatment, chest discomfort secondary to the associated inflammatory effect may require temporary analgesia until the inflammation subsides [17].

6. Esophageal cancer and high-grade Barrett's esophagus

Similar to lung cancer, the dosing for porfimer sodium is 2 mg/kg [17]. The laser light diffuser utilized however, is different. In esophageal cancer a laser light diffuse of 200 J/cm is utilized, and in Barrett's esophagus, a laser light diffuser of 130 J/cm is used, see **Figure 2** for current available laser light diffusers [17]. High-grade Barrett esophagus is the final precancerous stage before progressing to esophageal cancer [32]. Typically, high- grade Barrett esophagus is treated by surgical resection [32]. Treatment of high-grade Barrett's esophagus is an approved indication for photodynamic therapy if surgical resection is not an option [17, 33]. Treatment of esophageal cancer is an approved treatment for photodynamic therapy if there is complete obstruction of the esophagus by tumor or a partial obstruction that cannot adequately be treated by laser therapy/debridement [17, 33]. Given that the esophagus travels just posterior to the trachea and mainstem bronchi, the risks of fistula formation are the same and primarily to the trachea, blood vessels, and mediastinum. Specifically, if a tumor has already spread into these structures, there is a higher risk of fistula formation as the malignant cells are destroyed from photodynamic therapy. Esophageal varices are veins within the esophagus that are enlarged. These veins are at high risk for bleeding and rupture at baseline, and photoactivation of the photosensitizer in these veins could lead to significant bleeding [17]. Specifically, if these varices are >1 cm in diameter, the risk is likely too great [17]. Following treatment of Barrett esophagus, there is a risk of esophageal strictures resulting in food dysphagia (inability to swallow) [34]. In research studies these strictures occurred in 38% of subjects within six months of initiating photodynamic therapy. This is typically treated with dilation of the stricture, but it may require other treatments, depending upon the severity [17].

In esophageal cancer the timeline from injection to photoactivation of the photosensitizer is the same as in lung cancer. The time of injection (time zero) to photoactivation (40–50 hours from time zero) to potential second photoactivation (96–120 hours) is the same [17]. However, the duration of the treatment is different, the exposure to light is 12.5 minutes (750 seconds) [17]. A minimum of 30 days between injections of porfimer sodium is recommended with similar distancing between radiation therapy and photodynamic therapy [17]. Additionally, just as in lung cancer, endoscopic re-evaluation between treatments is recommended to ensure no complications have occurred such as fistula formation [17]. Barrett's esophagus has similar injection to photoactivation of the photosensitizer is the same as in lung cancer and esophageal cancer [17]. The time of injection (time zero) to photoactivation (40–50 hours from time zero) is the same [17]. The duration of treatment with light can however vary depending upon the length of the laser light diffuser utilized to deliver therapy with a maximum length of 7 cm treated at any one time [17]. In high-grade Barrett's esophagus, the time interval between injections of porfimer sodium is a minimum of 90 days [17].

7. Building a photodynamic therapy program

In building a program that utilizes photodynamic therapy, a collaborative and team-based approach is often vital. This is especially true in cases immediately after light exposure when interventions may need to be done at any hour of the day depending upon the reaction to photdynamic therapy. In the world of Oncology, there are frequent meetings amongst local specialists to discuss how best to diagnose and treat suspected cancers. These tumor boards meet regularly to review patient cases and determine next steps [21]. Given that photodynamic therapy uses similar equipment, it is reasonable to share equipment across a single institution to maximize utility. Depending upon the country/locale it is administered cost of the drug, approval by insurance/regulatory agencies, and equipment costs can easily add up significantly. Porfimer sodium is sold commercially as Photofirin and is sold by Concordia Healthcare Corporation. Its retail cost in the United States is > $20,000 per dose. Between the cost of the drug, facility fees, physician fees, and the need for frequent short term follow up the upfront costs may be high. The upfront costs of utilizing this therapy can be difficult to overcome, but a shared resource model can help overcome this given the benefits provided. With a robust clinical program, there is always room to expand the research aspect of photodynamic therapy, whether it is basic research, translational research, or clinical research.

8. Conclusion

In the years since photodynamic therapy was first discovered and developed through today, it has gone through numerous iterations. From the early identification of fluorescence to the discovery of selective uptake and tissue destruction with light exposure, the field of photodynamic therapy has had great potential. The number of publications has increased year over year, and there are no signs of this decreasing in the near future. From a biochemical perspective, its mechanism of action is unique and it shows great promise for the future as a scientific tool as well as a therapeutic one. However, as a therapeutic instrument there are currently limited indications, and even amongst these indications there are both obvious and subtle advantages and disadvantages in its use. Fully understanding the limitations of the current clinical role of photodynamic therapy can allow for future research and development to better address the current shortcomings and allow for even more widespread use of this technology.

Author details

Niral M. Patel[1,2]* and Ali I. Musani[2]

1 Division of Pulmonary Diseases and Critical Care Medicine, University of California Irvine, Orange, CA, USA

2 Division of Pulmonary Sciences and Critical Care Medicine, University of Colorado, Denver, CO, USA

*Address all correspondence to: niral.patel@uci.edu

References

[1] Bilaceroglu, S., *Endobronchial Ablative Therapies.* Clin Chest Med, 2018.**39**(1): p. 139-148.

[2] Seaman, J.C. and A.I. Musani, *Endobronchial ablative therapies.* Clin Chest Med, 2013.**34**(3): p. 417-25.

[3] Kessel, D., *Photodynamic Therapy: A Brief History.* J Clin Med, 2019.**8**(10).

[4] Kessel, D., *Components of hematoporphyrin derivatives and their tumor-localizing capacity.* Cancer Res, 1982.**42**(5): p. 1703-6.

[5] Dolmans, D.E., D. Fukumura, and R.K. Jain, *Photodynamic therapy for cancer.* Nat Rev Cancer, 2003. **3**(5): p. 380-7.

[6] dos Santos, A.F., et al., *Photodynamic therapy in cancer treatment - an update review.* Journal of Cancer Metastasis and Treatment, 2019. **5**: p. 25.

[7] Huang, Z., et al., *Photodynamic therapy for treatment of solid tumors--potential and technical challenges.* Technol Cancer Res Treat, 2008. **7**(4): p. 309-20.

[8] Kessel, D., *Apoptosis, Paraptosis and Autophagy: Death and Survival Pathways Associated with Photodynamic Therapy.* Photochem Photobiol, 2019. **95**(1): p. 119-125.

[9] Agarwal, M.L., et al., *Photodynamic therapy induces rapid cell death by apoptosis in L5178Y mouse lymphoma cells.* Cancer Res, 1991. **51**(21): p. 5993-6.

[10] McFarland, S.A., et al., *Metal-based photosensitizers for photodynamic therapy: the future of multimodal oncology?* Curr Opin Chem Biol, 2020. **56**: p. 23-27.

[11] Dougherty, T.J., et al., *Photodynamic therapy.* J Natl Cancer Inst, 1998. **90**(12): p. 889-905.

[12] Huang, Z., et al., *Photodynamic therapy of cancer — Challenges of multidrug resistance.* Journal of Innovative Optical Health Sciences, 2015. **08**(01): p. 1530002.

[13] Diaz-Jimenez, J.P., et al., *Efficacy and safety of photodynamic therapy versus Nd-YAG laser resection in NSCLC with airway obstruction.* Eur Respir J, 1999. **14**(4): p. 800-5.

[14] Babes, A., et al., *Photosensitization in Porphyrias and Photodynamic Therapy Involves TRPA1 and TRPV1.* J Neurosci, 2016. **36**(19): p. 5264-78.

[15] Sylantiev, C., et al., *Acute neuropathy mimicking porphyria induced by aminolevulinic acid during photodynamic therapy.* Muscle Nerve, 2005. **31**(3): p. 390-3.

[16] Bissell, D.M., K.E. Anderson, and H.L. Bonkovsky, *Porphyria.* N Engl J Med, 2017. **377**(9): p. 862-872.

[17] *Pinnacle Biologics. Photofrin (porfimer sodium) [Injection Label]. U.S. Food and Drug Administration Revised 06/2008.*

[18] Dela Cruz, C.S., L.T. Tanoue, and R.A. Matthay, *Lung cancer: epidemiology, etiology, and prevention.* Clin Chest Med, 2011. **32**(4): p. 605-44.

[19] Colt, H.G., et al., *Follow-up and surveillance of the patient with lung cancer after curative-intent therapy: Diagnosis and management of lung cancer, 3rd ed: American College of Chest Physicians evidence-based clinical practice guidelines.* Chest, 2013. **143**(5 Suppl): p. e437S-e454S.

[20] Simone, C.B., 2nd, et al., *Photodynamic therapy for the treatment of non-small cell lung cancer.* J Thorac Dis, 2012. **4**(1): p. 63-75.

[21] Kay, F.U., et al., *Revisions to the Tumor, Node, Metastasis staging of lung cancer (8(th) edition): Rationale, radiologic findings and clinical implications.* World J Radiol, 2017.**9**(6): p. 269-279.

[22] Minnich, D.J., et al., *Photodynamic laser therapy for lesions in the airway.* Ann Thorac Surg, 2010.**89**(6): p. 1744-8; discussion 1748-9.

[23] Leong, S., et al., *Diagnostic bronchoscopy--current and future perspectives.* J Thorac Dis, 2013. **5 Suppl 5**: p. S498-510.

[24] Patwa, A. and A. Shah, *Anatomy and physiology of respiratory system relevant to anaesthesia.* Indian J Anaesth, 2015. **59**(9): p. 533-41.

[25] Musani, A.I., et al., *Photodynamic therapy via navigational bronchoscopy for peripheral lung cancer in dogs.* Lasers Surg Med, 2018. **50**(5): p. 483-490.

[26] Murgu, S.D., *Robotic assisted-bronchoscopy: technical tips and lessons learned from the initial experience with sampling peripheral lung lesions.* BMC Pulm Med, 2019. **19**(1): p. 89.

[27] Jayadevappa, R., et al., *Outcomes of patients with advanced non-small cell lung cancer and airway obstruction treated with photodynamic therapy and non-photodynamic therapy ablation modalities.* J Thorac Dis, 2019. **11**(10): p. 4389-4399.

[28] Glisinski, K., et al., *Photodynamic therapy for the treatment of tracheobronchial papillomatosis: A multicenter experience.* Photodiagnosis Photodyn Ther, 2020. **30**: p. 101711.

[29] MacRosty, C.R., et al., *Fatal Hemoptysis in a Patient With Left Mainstem Bronchus Squamous Cell Carcinoma Treated With Photodynamic Therapy: A Case Report and Review of the Literature.* J Bronchology Interv Pulmonol, 2019. **26**(4): p. e60-e63.

[30] Johnstone, C. and S.E. Rich, *Bleeding in cancer patients and its treatment: a review.* Ann Palliat Med, 2018. **7**(2): p. 265-273.

[31] Liu, W. and J. Deslauriers, *Mediastinal divisions and compartments.* Thorac Surg Clin, 2011. **21**(2): p. 183-90, viii.

[32] Naini, B.V., R.F. Souza, and R.D. Odze, *Barrett's Esophagus: A Comprehensive and Contemporary Review for Pathologists.* Am J Surg Pathol, 2016. **40**(5): p. e45-66.

[33] Wu, H., T. Minamide, and T. Yano, *Role of photodynamic therapy in the treatment of esophageal cancer.* Dig Endosc, 2019. **31**(5): p. 508-516.

[34] Overholt, B.F., M. Panjehpour, and J.M. Haydek, *Photodynamic therapy for Barrett's esophagus: follow-up in 100 patients.* Gastrointest Endosc, 1999. **49**(1): p. 1-7.

Chapter 5

Anatomically Adjustable Device for Large-Area Photodynamic Therapy

Alessandra Keiko Lima Fujita, Daniel José Chianfrome, Vinicius Sigari Moreira, Anderson Luiz Zanchin, Priscila Fernanda Campos de Menezes and Vanderlei Salvador Bagnato

Abstract

The illumination system composed of LEDs is an anatomically adjustable device of high intensity that can be applied in different areas of the body. It can be applied in health care, as in the dermatological and esthetic treatments. The device improved the treatment of pathological diseases (e.g. actinic keratosis) since disseminated lesions were reached in a single application, thus reducing the time of the procedure and ensuring homogeneous light distribution. It was compared with a smaller and non-adjustable illumination device and evaluated in the treatment of actinic keratosis. The results showed its versatile application and a uniform adjustment to body curvatures.

Keywords: light-emitting diodes, anatomical LED system, photodynamic therapy, actinic keratosis

1. Introduction

Topical photodynamic therapy (PDT) using 5-aminolevulinic acid (ALA) and its variants as the methyl-aminolevulinate (MAL) is a well-established technique that requires a light source appropriate to a specific application, such as cancer types and precancerous lesions [1, 2]. ALA and its variants are the main precursors of protoporphyrin IX (PpIX), which is an endogenous photosensitizer (PS) and it is part of the heme biosynthesis pathway. PpIX selectively sensitizes the diseased cells, and when it is excited by light of a certain wavelength, interact with molecular oxygen producing reactive cytotoxic species, causing cells death by necrosis, apoptosis or autophagy. However, for PDT to work is required, a PS, the wavelength to excite the PS, and the molecular oxygen present in the tissue [3].

Lasers and light-emitting diodes (LEDs) are suitable light sources for PDT applications. But fiber-optic-lasers are more appropriate for light endoscopes device, or even for intraoperative cavities illumination. In general, illumination devices have light emitters of fixed geometry. An exception is the recently developed fabric-like material made with single-mode optical fibers adjustable to a specific application or anatomic site [4–6].

Several authors have reported PDT applications in dermatology for not only non-melanoma skin cancer but esthetic treatments [7–10]. Therefore, laser devices with optical fibers are not convenient, since large areas and anatomic sites must be considered.

On the other hand, Light Emitting Diodes (LEDs) are an alternative illumination system and can deliver the necessary intensities for PDT performance at lower costs. LED devices have already been used in PDT for the treatment of skin cancer and esthetic procedures [11–16], however, its field of illumination is limited and it is not anatomically adjustable to the body, which hampers the treatment of areas not reached by the light. Moreover, it is not effective for the treatment of large lesions located in the head, neck, legs, and arms, due to its non-conformability, which causes the illumination not to be homogenous. An example is the treatment of actinic keratosis (AK), which are lesions more likely to occur on the face and scalp due to high exposure to the sun [6–10].

The treatment of AK with photodynamic therapy requires illumination of the entire region at the same intensity. In this case, the anatomical device enables the use of the PDT procedure and optimizes the application time.

The topical application of the ALA prodrug and its derivatives in PDT can be used by several light sources, so long as the photosensitive agents are activated by the wavelengths. Because the PpIX accumulated by the application of the prodrug has absorption peaks in the Soret band and four minor peaks in the Q band, 510 nm, 545 nm, 580 nm, and 630 nm. Thus, blue light-emitting at 450 nm and red light-emitting at 630 nm from LED devices can be applied for the activation of PpIX. However, blue light penetrates superficial layers of the skin and red-light deeper layers of the skin [17–20].

Our main concern was to produce a flexible LED illumination system of high-power that operates at 450 ± 10 nm and 630 ± 10 nm wavelengths; therefore, the device was tested by engineers and in clinical applications (AKs treatment and esthetic dysfunctions) [20, 21].

2. Illumination systems: small, fixed and adjustable array

Figure 1a shows LINCE® (MMOptics, São Carlos, SP, Brazil) device, it is treatment system and comprised of a circular probe (on the left) with approximately 9.0 cm^2 area that emits at 630 nm ± 10; on the right, it is a diagnostic system, which emits at 405 ± 10 nm and collects the image of the protoporphyrin IX formation induced by a topical application of a precursor on the skin. **Figure 1b** displays a square illumination of LINCE® accessory in a 61 cm^2 area, with LEDs (light-emitting diodes) emitting at 630 ± 10 nm.

The system is recommended for small lesions, such as superficial or nodular Basal Cell Carcinoma (BCC). It was developed in the Brazilian Skin Cancer PDT program, currently, already it is used in the clinics. [1, 4, 13–15].

The device was designed for improving the large area attachment of LINCE® accessory and providing an extra accessory that can multiply the possibilities of the Clinical PDT treatment. It was developed in cooperation with MMOptics industry (São Carlos, SP, Brazil) and Technological Support Laboratory (São Carlos Institute of Physics, University of São Paulo, São Carlos, SP, Brazil) and assembled by rectangular modules (up to 10, in principle).

However, a version with 5 modules composing a 192 cm^2 area of illumination (**Figure 2a**) was employed in this study. It consists of five LEDs (Luxeon Rebel, Lumileds Company) boards, thus totaling 30 LEDs emitting at 630 ± 10 nm, and 25

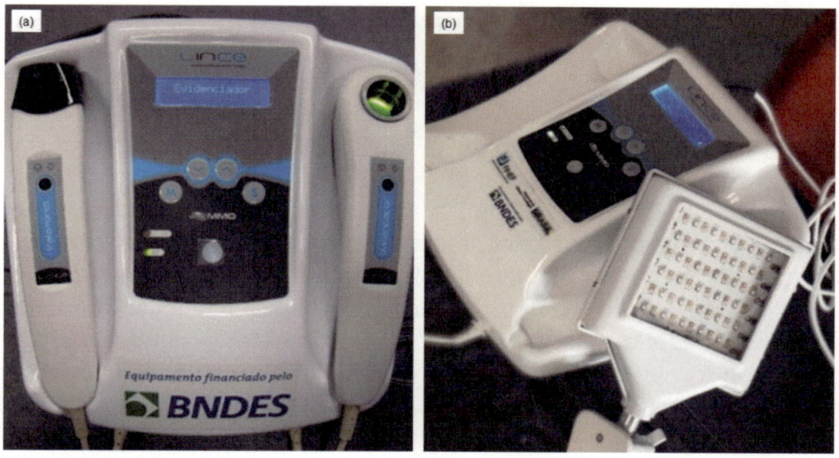

Figure 1.
(a) LINCE® equipment (MMOptics – Brazil): left - treatment system emitting at 630 nm; right - diagnostic system emitting at 405 ± 10 nm. (b) Square illumination of the LINCE® accessory emitting at 630 ± 10 nm.

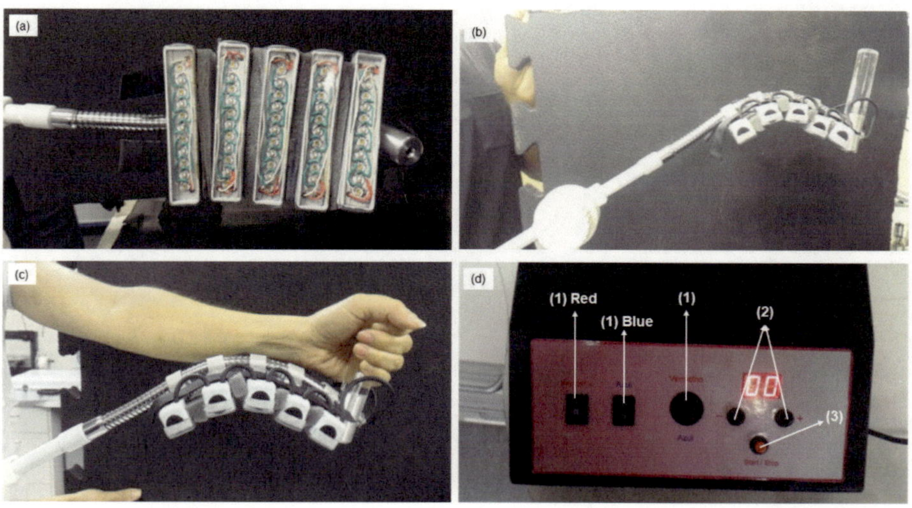

Figure 2.
Anatomically adjustable device. (a) Front of the equipment, where the LEDs are coupled and protected by plastic covers. (b) Side of the device, with an acrylic tube that facilitates its handling. (c) Adaptation of its curvature to the body by the acrylic tube. (d) Electronic box with the sequence of the drive buttons.

LEDs emitting at 450 ± 10 nm. A flexible tube was added for adapting the equipment to regions of the body (**Figure 2b**), and a handle facilitated its use in areas of curvature (**Figure 2c**) and avoided the bending of the plates with LEDs. Power sources of 16 V for emission at 450 ± 10 nm, and 5 V for emission at 630 ± 10 nm, both with 3 A electric current, are connected to the device. Below is the description of the power buttons (**Figure 2d**):

1. On/off button for the selection of the wavelength (450 nm or 630 nm).

2. Timer button for the selection of the illumination time in minutes.

3. Start/Stop button.

4. Button that turns on the equipment according to the wavelength selected (1).

5. Button that disables the equipment if pressed for a few seconds.

Figure 3 shows the way the equipment can be used in different parts of the body, according to an adequate anatomic configuration.

Figure 4 shows LINCE® (MMOptics, São Carlos, SP, Brazil) lighting system and its accessory (the 61 cm^2 fixed array) for the treatment of large areas. LINCE® is not adequate for treatments that require illumination of a larger area, since it does not have good applicability - it must be pushed away, which reduces the intensity and increases the application time. LINCE® accessory (the 61 cm^2 fixed array) has a larger area; however, it is fixed and does not fit the body anatomy. The delivered dose decreases when it moved away from the patient's skin, and a longer time is

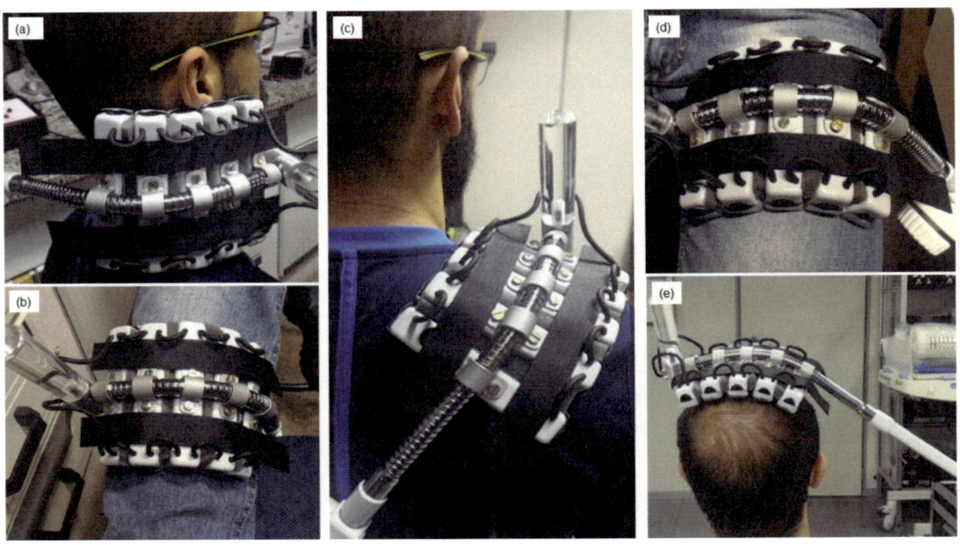

Figure 3.
Possible configurations of the device for different regions of the body. (a) Neck; (b) shin; (c) back; (d) quadriceps and (e) head.

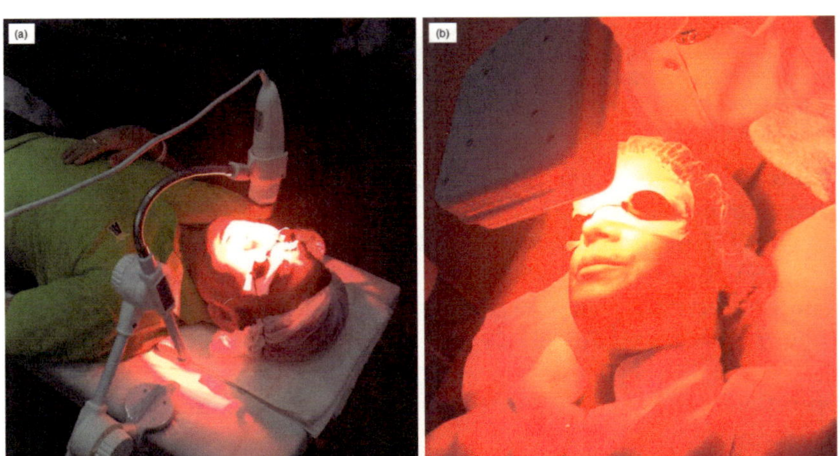

Figure 4.
Images of a treatment performed on the face. Devices emit at 630 nm. (a) LINCE® (MMOptics, São Carlos, SP, Brazil) - illumination system for treatment. (b) LINCE® accessory.

necessary for the achievement of the desired effect. In addition, the irradiance delivered on the target tissue is not homogeneous.

Figure 5 shows the PDT treatment for AK and acne vulgaris by the anatomical device.

AKs lesions often appear scattered in a specific region of the body most exposed to the sun. The device optimizes the PDT treatment so that it covers extensive regions and delivers the necessary intensity. **Figure 5a** shows the device used for the treatment of AKs at the back of the hand. The device enabled the treatment of both hands concomitantly. **Figure 5b** displays the device being used in patients with actinic keratosis on top of the head. The shape of the device adjusted to the anatomy of the region promotes uniform illumination and covers the entire area of lesions, thus reducing the number of exposures needed to treat larger areas effectively.

Figure 5c and **d** show the device being used for the treatment of acne vulgaris in the face. It was leaned against the treated area so that the desired intensity and fluency rate could be delivered. The equipment was moved a little away from the patient to allow a clearer photograph and the area treated. A flat device would not treat the surface so closely and uniformly.

2.1 Optical characteristics - adjustable array

The light distribution was measured using the laser power meter (LabMax-TOP, Coherent Inc., Santa Clara, USA). It has a 0.5 cm^2 circular area sensor and the wavelength was configured for the collection of the intensity measured. The light distribution was measured 5 cm away from the equipment, and the power meter

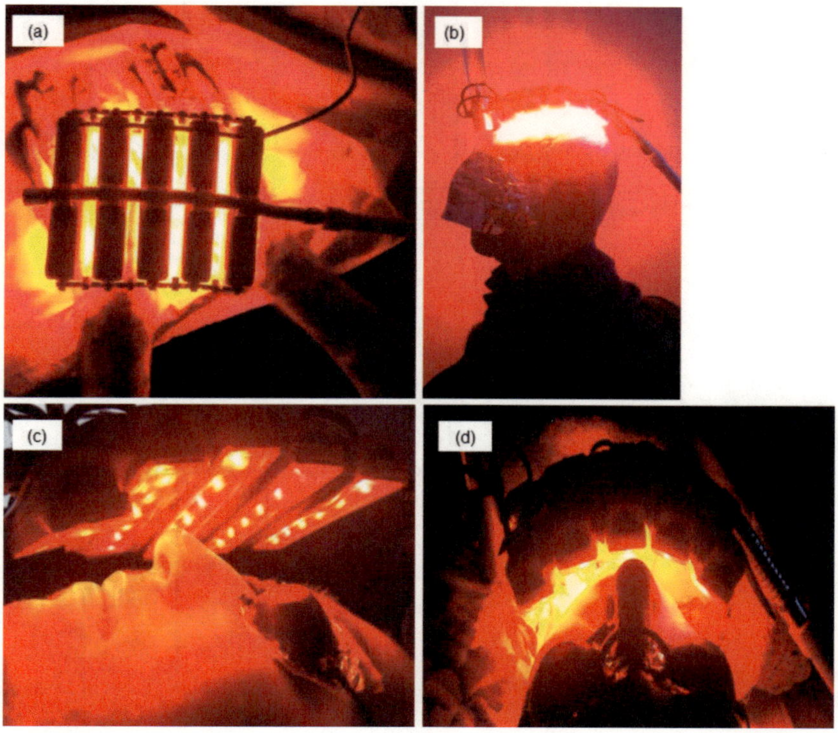

Figure 5.
(a) AK treatment with the anatomical device at the back of the hand. Both hands can be treated concomitantly. (b) AK treatment with the anatomical device in the head region, covering its whole region. (c) and (d) PDT procedure for acne vulgaris on the face.

sensor was scanned throughout the device area. The distance from each point collected was the diameter of the power meter detector.

Figure 6 shows the measurement of intensity (collected point to point) of the light emission of the anatomical device.

The device remained on for 20 minutes to perform the warm-up test, and it did not heat up, which has proven the light-emitting surface causes no thermal damage to the skin.

Planar irradiance distribution was mapped out at a range of distances from the light source. Measurements were collected from the distance zero until 5 cm of the laser power meter, varying each 1 cm (**Figure 7**). The covered area of the measurements corresponds to 192 cm^2 (13 × 15 cm). The intensity fluctuates with a small decay at the boundary for both wavelengths. We calculated the average intensity, considering a continuous emitting surface (**Figure 8**). The intensity at any z-axis from the emitting surface can be evaluated through the integration of all elementary emitters.

To calculate the intensity at a certain position (x, y, z) above the surface, we can proceed with the sum of the contributions of all the emitters distributed on the surface. Imagine that in each position determined by the coordinates (x', y') there is an emitting element. The contribution of all of them to the intensity at the point

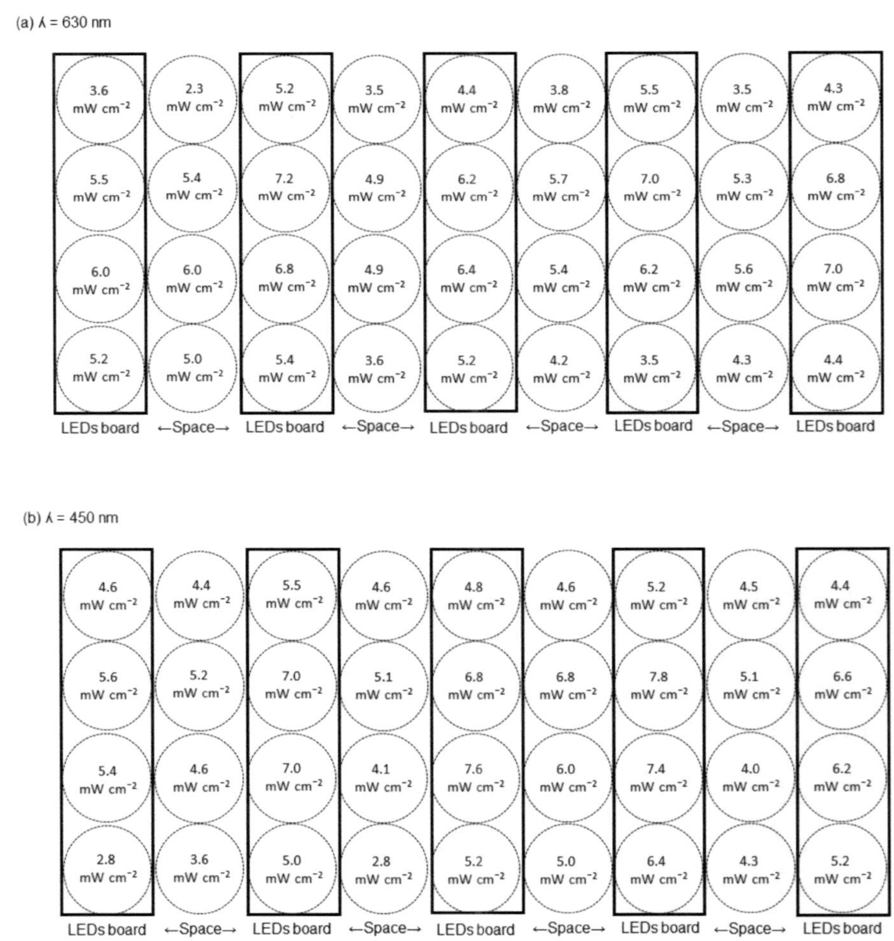

Figure 6.
Intensity measurements were collected from point to point in the anatomical device area. (a) Intensity emitting at 630 ± 10 nm and (b) intensity emitting at 450 ± 10 nm.

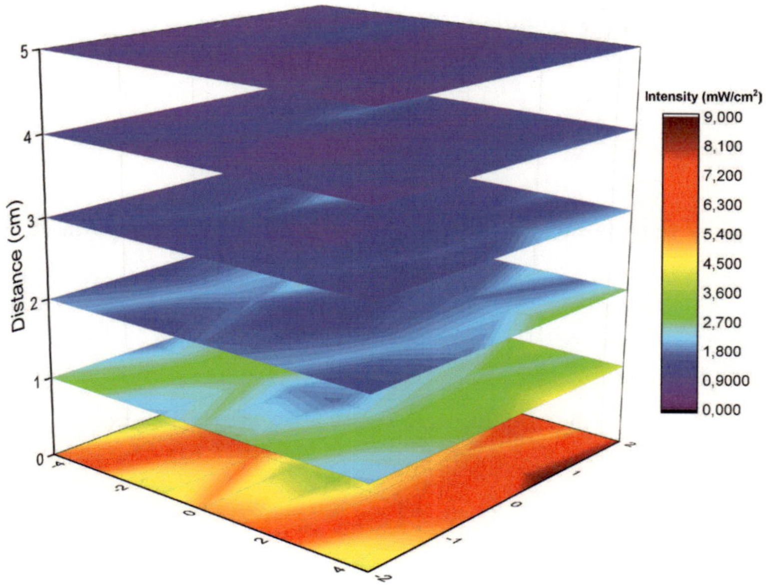

Figure 7.
Intensity versus distance. The intensity was measured by LabMax-TOP laser power meter (Coherent Inc., Santa Clara, USA). Measurements were collected every 1 cm from the device up to 5 cm and scanned throughout the device area.

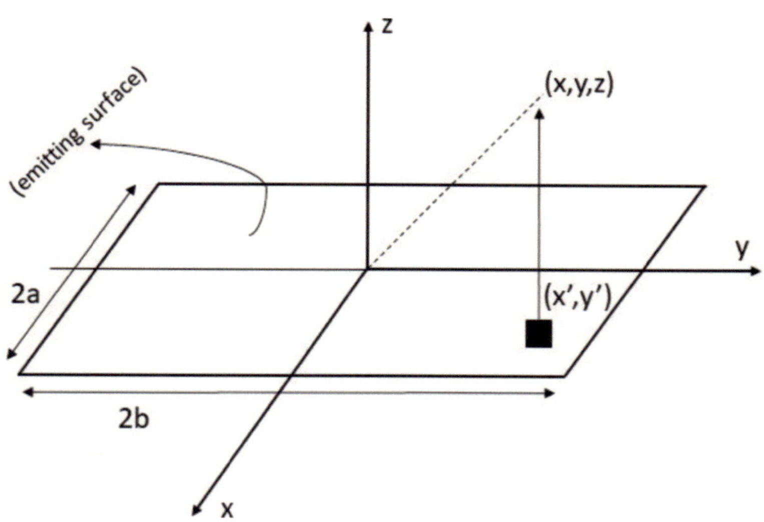

Figure 8.
Average intensity calculated by the integral of the elementary emitters at any point of the intensity (x',y').

outside the surface (x, y, z) is then given by the integral of all elements, covering the entire area that contains emitters. Considering as in **Figure 8**, where we represent in a simplified way the position of the issuer and the point considered, we have the integral:

$$I(x,y,z) = Io \iint_{al\,surface} \frac{dx'dy'}{(x-x')^2 + (y-y')^2 + z^2} \tag{1}$$

If we consider a special point of interest, the central point of the distribution (x = 0 and y = 0), we have that the previous integral is reduced to:

$$I(z) = Io \iint_{al\,surface} \frac{dx'dy'}{x^2 + y^2 + z^2} \tag{2}$$

If I_0 is close to the emitters intensity (z → 0), the intensity at point (x, y, z) is given by (3)

$$I(x, y, z) = I_0 \int_{-a}^{+a}\int_{-b}^{+b} \frac{dx'dy'}{(x - x')^2 + (y - y')^2 + (z - z')^2}.$$

At the center of the illuminating area (x = y = 0), at any distance z

$$I(z) = I_0 \int_{-a}^{+a}\int_{-b}^{+b} \frac{dx'dy'}{x'^2 + y'^2 + z'^2} \tag{4}$$

The integral can be solved by traditional approximation and results in a center average intensity of

$$I(z) = \pi I_0 \ln\left(\frac{\frac{4ab}{\pi} + z^2}{z^2}\right) \tag{5}$$

The calibration of I_0 at certain z provides a center intensity at a distance z from the device shown in **Figure 9**.

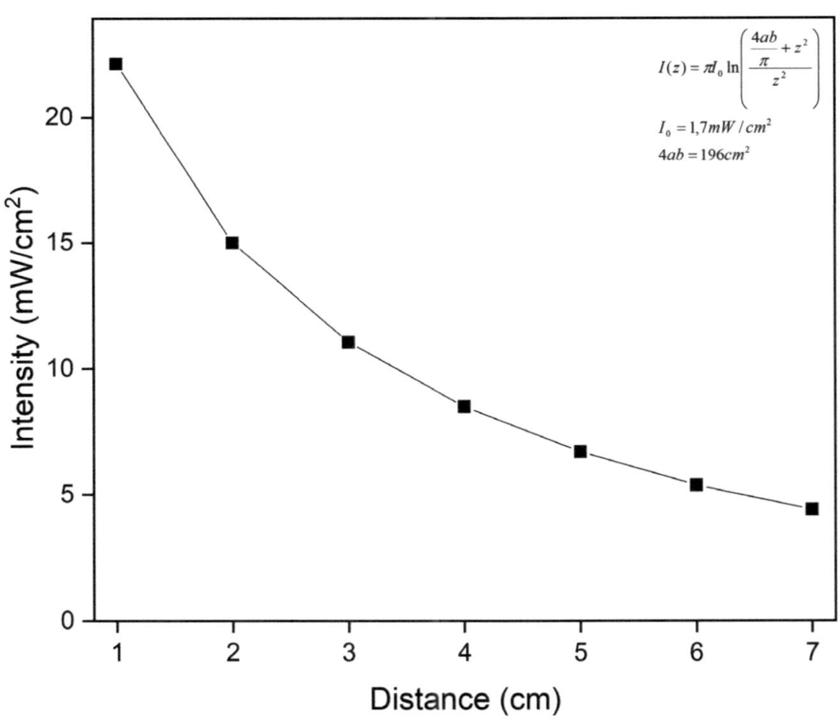

Figure 9.
Intensity decay caused by an increase in the distance from the device to the target tissue.

The ideal distance for the treatment is up to 1 cm because since the presence of the emitter is dominant in this distance, the intensity fluctuates. Therefore, if the expected average is considered the center intensity, the dose can be obtained from **Figure 9**, and for each 1 s illumination, the intensity (mW/cm^2) corresponds to the 10^{-3} J/cm^2 total dose delivered. At a 1 cm distance, the total dose delivery is 1.32 J/cm^2 energy, while at 5 cm distance, it decays to 0.39 J/cm^2.

Generally, the total dose applied in the PDT procedures ranges from 30 to 100 J/cm^2, so that for device equates a 22 to 66-minute application time, respectively. This time increases if the illumination distance increases. Those times are equivalent to 450 ± 10 nm and 630 ± 10 nm emissions.

3. Clinical demonstration: anatomical device (adjustable array)

LINCE® accessory (fixed array) and the anatomical device (adjustable array) were designed towards meeting the clinical needs for the PDT application in the AK treatment. However, esthetics and rehabilitation procedures that use low-power laser have been intensively studied, and more versatile devices with larger illumination areas have attracted more health professionals. The development of a device that enables the choice of wavelength is fundamental for the adoption of the appropriate procedure for a given treatment.

Two patients with a clinical diagnosis of AK were recruited to be treated with PDT using the anatomical device (**Figure 10**). The protocol applied was ALA-20% cream; incubation time 1 h 30 min; total dose 50 J/cm^2, emission at 630 ± 10 nm. After one month, no residual lesion was observed in the nose; the scalp region showed a residual lesion, which indicates an 85% elimination.

The anatomical device (adjustable array) was able to cover all extension of the lesions treated on the nose and scalp. The emission surface was leaning against the treatment region and there was no heating, which enabled the delivery of the adequate intensity.

LINCE® accessory (the 61 cm^2 fixed array) was observed that excessive heating occurred when applied in contact with the treatment area, causing greater

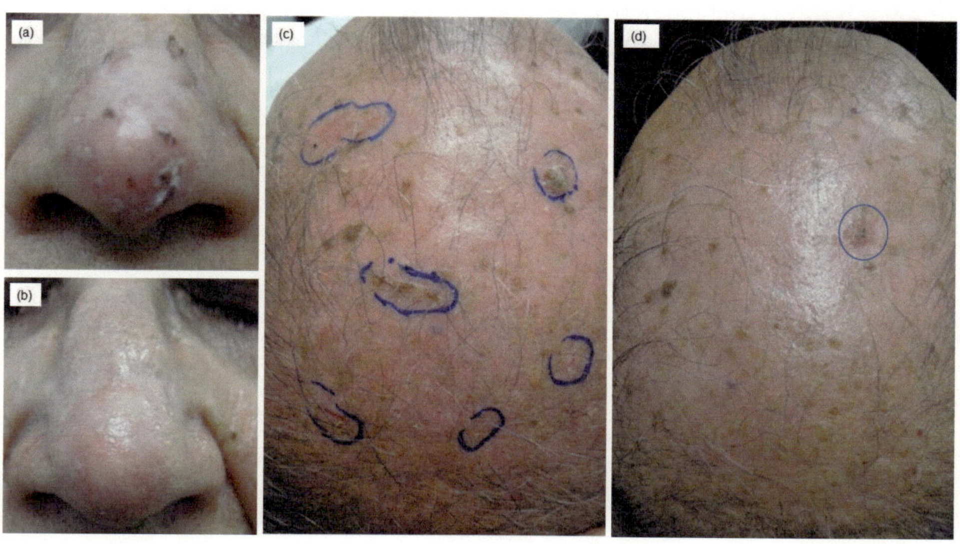

Figure 10.
(a) AK lesion on the nose. (b) 30 days after the PDT procedure - no residual lesion. (c) Approximately six AKs lesions scattered on the scalp region. (d) 30 days after the PDT procedure - a residual lesion.

discomfort to the patient. This is due to its geometry of heat dissipation because it has more LEDs per area than the anatomical device (192 cm^2 adjustable array). In the anatomical device, the LEDs are divided between the boards, thus obtaining a better air circulation mechanism and more heat dissipation. Therefore, the anatomical device is more comfortable for the patient and it is possible to apply it in contact with the treated area and operating at high intensity without causing excessive heating.

4. Conclusion

LINCE® (MMOptics, São Carlos, SP, Brazil) device has become excellent commercial equipment for the PDT treatment for non-melanoma skin cancer in Brazil. Thereby, the development of an anatomical device with a larger illumination area becomes more efficient to treat extensive lesions.

The anatomical device was designed to optimize the PDT procedure in AK lesions scattered in a specific region of the body and in body sites, where a machine is required for the obtaining of the curvature according to the anatomy of the treated region. The device treated extensive lesions and reached their entire extension. It suffered no heating during treatments, therefore the thermal energy dissipation in this shape was more effective, and caused no sensation of thermal discomfort to the patient.

The anatomical device can be used for several dermatological clinical applications, including esthetic procedures for facial, body, and capillary treatments.

Further clinical tests will be conducted and, if necessary, the device will undergo modifications towards improvements in clinical procedures.

Acknowledgements

The authors acknowledge the financial support provided by BNDES (09.2.1458.1), FINEP (01.14.0242.00), MMOptics industry (São Carlos, SP, Brazil), São Paulo Research Foundation - FAPESP (2013/07276-1), CEPOF (2009/54035-4 – EMU) and INCT (2014/50857-8).

They are also indebted to the Technological Support Laboratory (São Carlos Institute of Physics, University of São Paulo, São Carlos, SP, Brazil) for technological support.

Conflict of interest

The author Anderson Luiz Zanchin is employee at MMOptics Ltda.

Author details

Alessandra Keiko Lima Fujita[1*], Daniel José Chianfrome[1], Vinicius Sigari Moreira[1], Anderson Luiz Zanchin[2], Priscila Fernanda Campos de Menezes[1] and Vanderlei Salvador Bagnato[1,3]

1 São Carlos Institute of Physics, University of São Paulo, São Carlos, SP, Brazil

2 MMOptics industry, São Carlos, SP, Brazil

3 Hagler Fellow, Texas A&M University, College Station, Texas, USA

*Address all correspondence to: alessandra.keiko@gmail.com

References

[1] Grecco C, Buzzá HH, Stringasci MD, et al. Single LED-based device to perform widefield fluorescence imaging and photodynamic therapy. Proc. SPIE 9531, Biophotonics South America. 2015; 4:953121.

[2] Buzzá HH, da Silva AP, Vollet Filho JD, et al. Photodynamic therapy: progress toward a scientific and clinical network in Latin America. Photodiagnosis Photodyn Ther. 2016; 13:261-266.

[3] Kennedy JC and Pottier RH. Endogenous protoporphyrin-IX, a clinically useful photosensitizer for photodynamic therapy. J Photochem Photobiol B: Biol. 1992; 14:275-292.

[4] Moseley H. Light distribution and calibration of commercial PDT LED arrays. Photochem Photobiol Sci. 2005; 4(11):911-914.

[5] Mordon S, Cochrane C, Tylcz, JB, et al. Light emitting fabric technologies for photodynamic therapy. Photodiagnosis Photodyn Ther. 2015; 12(1):1-8.

[6] Oniszczuk A, Wojtunik-Kulesza KA, Oniszczuk T, et al. The potential of photodynamic therapy (PDT)—Experimental investigations and clinical use. Biomed Pharmacother. 2016; 83:912-929.

[7] Kim M, Jung HY, Park HJ. Topical PDT in the treatment of benign skin diseases: principles and new applications. International journal of molecular sciences. 2015; 16(10): 23259-23278.

[8] Vollet Filho JD, Andrade CT, Buzza HH, et al. PDT and emerging therapies for Actinic Keratosis—A resource letter. Photodiagnosis Photodyn Ther. 2017; 17:205-207.

[9] Lehmann P. Methyl aminolaevulinate–photodynamic therapy: a review of clinical trials in the treatment of actinic keratoses and nonmelanoma skin cancer. Br J Dermatol. 2007; 156(5):793-801.

[10] Wen X, Li Y, Hamblim MR. Photodynamic therapy in dermatology beyond non-melanoma cancer: An update. Photodiagnosis Photdyn Ther. 2017; 19:140-152.

[11] da Costa MM, Andrade CT, Inada NM, et al. Development and application of a homemade device for fluorescence diagnosis. Sociedade Brasileira de Laser em Medicina e Cirurgia. 2010; 2(14):8-12.

[12] Inada NM, da Costa MM, Guimarães OC, et al. Photodiagnosis and treatment of condyloma acuminatum using 5-aminolevulinic acid and homemade devices. Photodiagnosis Photodyn Ther. 2012; 9(1):60-68.

[13] da Silva AP, Chiandrone DJ, Tinta, JW, et al. Development and comparison of two devices for treatment of onychomycosis by photodynamic therapy. J Biomed Opti. 2015; 20(6):061109.

[14] Ramirez DP, Kurachi C, Inada NM, et al. Experience and BCC subtypes as determinants of MAL-PDT response: preliminary results of a national Brazilian project. Photodiagnosis Photodyn Ther. 2014; 11(1), 22-26.

[15] Blanco KC, Moriyama LT, Inada NM, et al. Fluorescence guided PDT for optimization of the outcome of skin cancer treatment. Front Phys. 2015; 3:30.

[16] Blanco KC, Inada NM, Silva AP, et al. A Multicenter Clinical Study of Expected and Unexpected Side Reactions During and After Skin Cancer Treatment by Photodynamic Therapy. Skinmed. 2017; 15(2):113-118.

[17] Zelickson B, Counters J, Coles C, et al. Light patch: preliminary report of a novel form of blue light delivery

for the treatment of actinic keratosis. Dermatologic surgery. 2005; 31(3):375-378.

[18] Antoniou C, Dessinioti, C, Sotiriadis D, et al. A multicenter, randomized, split-face clinical trial evaluating the efficacy and safety of chromophore gel-assisted blue light phototherapy for the treatment of acne. Int J Dermatol. 2016; 55(12): 1321-1328.

[19] Gholam P, Bosselmann I, Enk A, et al. Impact of red versus blue light on tolerability and efficacy of PDT: a randomized controlled trial. J Dtsch Dermatol Ges 2018; 16(6):711-717.

[20] Menezes PF, Requena MB, Lizarelli RFZ, et al. Blue LED irradiation to hydration of skin. In Biophotonics South America. 2015; 9531:95311W. International Society for Optics and Photonics.

[21] Pinto Mdo C, Fujita AKL, de Menezes PF, et al. Photodynamic therapy with 5-aminolevulinic acid (ALA) in the treatment of acne: A case study. Clin Dermatol Res Ther. 2017; 1(1):114.

Chapter 6

Application of Photodynamic Therapy in the Treatment of Osteonecrosis of the Jaw

Marko Vuletić, Božana Lončar Brzak, Igor Smojver, Luka Marković, Mato Sušić and Dragana Gabrić

Abstract

Osteonecrosis as term represents the death of bone tissue in the body and causes of necrosis can be different. Medication-related osteonecrosis of the jaws (MRONJ) is nowadays known as an inability of the alveolar bone to respond to a local trauma and it can result in severe local and systemic complications. In the etiology of medication-related osteonecrosis there are antiangiogenic and antiresorptive agents which have great effect on alveolar bone, producing an imbalance between resorption (osteoclastic activity) and deposition (osteoblastic activity). The exact mechanisms of development are not todays completely resolved. It is thought that it is a result from combination of medication interactions, microbiological contamination of the area and local tissue trauma. Typical signs and symptoms are painful mucosal lesions, swelling, exposed necrotic bone in the jaws, discomfort and dysesthesias. There is currently no gold standard or clearly defined treatment protocol for the disease itself. Process of treatment is demanding and main goal is to eliminate pain, control infection of soft and hard tissue and minimize progression of osteonecrosis. Besides the conventional surgical treatment, photodynamic therapy can be a viable supportive tool of initial and advanced stages of osteonecrosis and may contribute to improvements of patient's quality of life.

Keywords: osteonecrosis, osteoclasts, bone, surgical procedure, photodynamic therapy

1. Introduction

Osteonecrosis as term represents the death of bone tissue in the body and causes of necrosis can be different. If it is associated with a reduced or complete absence of blood supply, this process is called avascular necrosis of the bone and is most commonly associated in the literature with the femur bone [1].

Radiotherapy (radiation) can also adversely affect bone tissue due to compromised angiogenesis resulting in avascular necrosis with hypoxic, hypocellular, and hypovascular lesions, termed osteoradionecrosis [1]. In 2003, when 36 cancer patients receiving treatment with pamidronate or zoledronate developed a painful bone exposure of the mandible, of the maxilla or both, which was unresponsive to medical and surgical treatment, a new type of osteonecrosis of the jawbone associated with bisphosphonate was called osteonecrosis of the jaw (BRONJ) [2].

Over time, precisely in 2010, new drugs have been identified, such as denosumab for causing osteonecrosis, that do not belong to the group of bisphosphonates so the name has changed to medication-related osteonecrosis of the jaw (MRONJ) [3]. MRONJ is an uncommon condition that can occur after exposure to medication to prevent bone complications, such as bisphosphonates or denosumab or other agents as angiogenesis inhibitors [4]. In most cases it manifests as exposed bone in the maxillofacial region, although non-exposed MRONJ has also been recognized [5–8].

The purpose of this chapter was to describe medication-related osteonecrosis of the jaw, the theory of its development, clinical picture, classification, epidemiology and modalities of treatment, including biostimulative and antimicrobial photodynamic therapy, of medication-related osteonecrosis of the jaw.

2. The process of bone remodeling

Bone remodeling is a physiological process that lasts lifetime and is characterized by the interaction of bone-forming cells - osteoblasts and bone-resorbing cells - osteoclasts. The remodeling process begins with the activation of osteoclasts (multinuclear cells of the monocyte–macrophage system) which are located on the bone surface and with the formation of acidic medium, they dissolve mineralized bone with the breakdown of proteins of the remaining bone matrix. This resorption process takes between two and four weeks. After the resorption process, osteoblasts replace osteoclasts (cells of mesenchymal origin) which synthesize osteoid and organic matrix over a period of two to four months, as a prerequisite for bone mineralization or calcium hydroxyapatite mineral investment [2]. Finally, when osteoblasts are implanted in the bone matrix, they become osteocytes [3]. The presence of osteocytes is extremely important for bone vitality because they can recognize and respond to a variety of mechanical stimuli by regulating the differentiation of osteoblasts and osteoclasts. The remodeling process is regulated by various mechanisms, of which the most important is the RANK/RANKL/Osteoprotergin system. Osteoblasts secrete osteoprotergin, which prevents osteoclast differentiation from precursor cells and thus inhibits resorption. On the other hand, RANKL (Receptor Activator of NF-kb Ligand) along with M-CSF (Macrophage Colony-Stimulating Factor) stimulates osteoclast differentiation and maturation from precursor cells [4]. If this physiological process is disturbed, and this is especially important with increased expression of RANKL, resorption occurs. RANKL is produced by osteoblasts and activated T lymphocytes.

During remodeling and healing of bone fractures, osteoblasts activate various bone morphogenetic proteins that stimulate the production of VEGF (Vascular Endothelial Growth Factor) factor, which is necessary for the formation of new blood vessels, or angiogenesis [5].

The process of physiological remodeling can be disrupted in a variety of diseases and conditions associated with hyperactivated osteoclasts that have a high potential for bone destruction, which can result in hypercalcemia, decreased bone density, and consequent spontaneous fractures. The most common metabolic disease of the skeletal system is osteoporosis which is characterized by osteoclast hyperactivity with loss of bone quality. Malignant diseases of the breast, prostate, lungs, kidneys and thyroid often metastasize to bone. Complications of bone metastases include bone pain, fractures, hypercalcemia, and cachexia. Once formed in the bones, malignant cells stimulate bone resorption where various growth factors, released during bone destruction from the bone matrix, serve them for further growth and proliferation. In addition to growth factors, VEGF factor is also important for later tumor growth. Multiple myeloma, a malignant hematological disease, which is manifested by the presence of lytic lesions in the bone, has a similar mechanism of bone destruction. In the treatment of these diseases, antiresorptive drugs that directly or indirectly inhibit osteoclasts and antiangiogenic drugs that inhibit VEGF are used.

3. Medications-related osteonecrosis of the jaw (MRONJ)

There are two groups of drugs that may cause medication-related osteonecrosis of the jaw. The first group includes antiresorptive drugs, specifically bisphosphonates and denosumabs, and the second group consists of antiangiogenic drugs that include bevacizumab (Avastin) which is humanized monoclonal antibody and also sunitinib (Sutent) which acts as a thyroxine kinase inhibitor [9–13].

3.1 Antiresorptive drugs

The first type of drugs is antiresorptive drugs, which include bisphosphonates and denosumabs. They have a similar mechanism of action and a similar potency of causing osteonecrosis.

3.1.1 Bisphosphonates

Bisphosphonates are medications that act as analogs of pyrophosphate, which is a natural inhibitor of bone metabolism. The mechanism of their action has not yet been fully elucidated, but they are inhibitors of osteoclast activity and inductors of their apoptosis, reducing the process of bone remodeling. Bisphosphonates are incorporated into the hydroxyapatite bone matrix, at the site of the OH group of bisphosphonates, using the P-C-P compound, which alters bone microstructure by slowing bone growth and reducing the amount of mineral dissolution in bone. Unlike osteoclasts, osteoblastic activity does not decrease, but remains preserved, which results in an increase in bone mass. There are currently three generations of bisphosphonates on the market. The first generation of nitrogen-free bisphosphonates has the least potential for jaw osteonecrosis. The main side effect of bisphosphonate therapy is osteonecrosis of the jaw [2]. Other side effects that may occur in bisphosphonate therapy are: gastrointestinal disorders (nausea and vomiting), atypical femoral fractures, esophageal inflammation with consequent mucosal erosions, secondary hyperparathyroidism, atrial fibrillation, eye outbursts, muscle pain and others [14–17]. Bisphosphonates are excreted by the kidneys, after accumulation at sites of active remodeling (both jaws). Their characteristic is also rapid deposition in the bones and their long retention in the same (the half-life of zoledronic acid is 11.2 years in the bones) [18]. There are two types of bisphosphonate administration, oral and intravenously.

Oral bisphosphonates are medications that are most commonly prescribed in the treatment of osteoporosis and osteopenia, also they are the medications of choice for bone diseases that occur less frequently, such as Paget's disease, osteogenesis imperfecta, chronic recurrent multifocal osteomyelitis and for prevention heterotopic ossifications mostly of the spinal cord [19, 20]. They are also indicated in treatment of chronic kidney disease, kidney transplantation, in rheumatoid diseases related with systemic bone loss such as rheumatoid arthritis, spondylarthritis or SAPHO (synovitis, acne, pustulosis, hyperostosis, osteitis) syndrome and in non-inflammatory rheumatoid diseases, as aseptic osteonecrosis, neuropathic osteoarthropenia, and fibrous dysplasia [21]. Unlike intravenous bisphosphonates, have a lower potential for osteonecrosis.

Intravenous bisphosphonates are the most potent in causing osteonecrosis [22]. They are used in the treatment of various conditions associated with malignant diseases such as hypercalcemia caused by cancer and for treatment of bone metastases (secondaryism) [23]. Secondaryism in bones are releasing cytokines and growth factors, which enhance the effectiveness of osteoclasts and consequently bone resorption, which favors tumor growth. Intravenous bisphosphonates stimulate antitumor immune mechanisms, which inhibit growth, migration, and secondary formation, most commonly in breast and prostate cancer. This type of bisphosphonates is very common used in treatment of lytic lesion and for prevention of massive bone resorption in multiple myeloma. Patients with this diagnosis are often treated with aggressive chemotherapy which one of many side-effects is osteonecrosis. Despite the mentioned facts, these medications have positive effect on patient's quality of life [24].

3.1.2 Denosumab

Denosumab are humanized monoclonal antibodies directed to a RANK ligand (modeling regulator) that inhibit osteoclasts and reduce bone resorption [25]. It is used for treatment of osteoporosis in which there is an increased risk of bone fractures, in osteoporosis where there is bone loss due to the use of various drugs and in the treatment of malignant bone lesions diseases. Denosumab therapy is a better option than bisphosphonate therapy, especially with renal dysfunction. The potency of denosumabs to induce osteonecrosis alone has been shown to be approximately similar to the potency of zoledronic acid which is the most potent bisphosphonate [26, 27].

Denosumabs are administered subcutaneously and, unlike bisphosphonates, do not accumulate in bone, so that their effect on bone remodeling is reversible and lasts approximately six months [28].

3.2 Antiangiogenic drugs

Antiangiogenic medications prevent the formation of new blood vessels binding to various signaling molecules that inhibit angiogenesis.

3.2.1 Bevacizumab

Bevacizumab is humanized monoclonal antibody that binds selectively to a protein called vascular endothelial growth factor (VEGF) in the blood and lymph vessels. It is used in the treatment of malignant diseases of the kidneys, gastrointestinal tract, lungs and glioblastoma [9, 10].

3.2.2 Sunitinib

Sunitinib is used in the treatment of gastrointestinal tumors, metastatic renal cell carcinomas cells and neuroendocrine tumors of the pancreas. It works by inhibiting thyroxine kinase function. In combination with chemotherapy or bisphosphonates, they have high risk of inducing osteonecrosis [29].

4. Mechanism of development MRONJ

The exact mechanisms of development MRONJ are not todays completely resolved. It is thought that its development is a result from combination of medication interactions, microbiological contamination of the area and local tissue trauma [30]. In the literature there are few hypotheses of the development of this specific disease.

4.1 Inhibition of bone resorption and remodeling

Antiresorptive medications inhibit osteoclast function and differentiation, leading to their apoptosis, and this results in reduced bone remodeling [31]. In addition to acting on osteoclasts, antiresorptive medications also reduce the activity of osteoblasts, keratinocytes and fibroblasts [32, 33]. Of all the bones, the jaws are the most susceptible to remodeling, so osteonecrosis specifically occurs on them.

4.2 Inflammation or infection

In the pathogenesis of medication-related osteonecrosis, inflammation plays a significant role development. Advanced periodontal disease and tooth extraction are one of the main triggers for occurrence of necrosis. Pathohistological analysis of bone parts, which are affected with osteonecrosis, decontamination with various bacteria is present, especially *Actinomyces* species in 70–100% of cases [34]. The main role in development of MRONJ has bacterial decontamination [35, 36]. Bisphosphonates have synergistic effect with bacteria because they increase the possibility of bacterial adhesion to hydroxyapatite found in the bone, resulting in the invasion of microorganisms into the bone itself afterwards the bone loses blood supply, becomes avascular and necrotic.

4.3 Inhibition of angiogenesis

Inhibition of angiogenesis means inhibition of growth, migration and differentiation of new endothelial cells in forming blood vessels. Medications that inhibit angiogenesis, due to ischemia or lack of blood supply to the bone secondary create osteonecrosis [37].

4.4 Soft tissue toxicity

One of theory of medication-related osteonecrosis is that drugs directly negatively affect fibroblasts producing toxicity of the oral mucosa. In vitro studies, increased apoptosis has been reported, especially in oral epithelial cells, after application bisphosphonates. Bone exposure and impaired healing caused by tissue toxicity play an important role in the development of osteonecrosis [38].

4.5 Immune dysfunction

Antiresorptive drugs together with other immunosuppressants such as corticosteroids, chemotherapy or methotrexate increases the possibility of osteonecrosis [3]. Ruggiero et al. [3] stated that in the beginning of investigating the influence of bisphosphonates on wound healing in animal models, to induce osteonecrosis, steroids were combined with bisphosphonates. Inflammation, delayed healing, mucosal ulceration, exposed bone, fistula and histologic necrosis are well documented symptoms in different animal species and in humans exposed to surgical procedures after application chemotherapy with antiresorptive drugs. Methotrexat is standard or first line drug for therapy of rheumatoid arthritis. It can be an iatrogenic cause of lymphoproliferative disorders in immunodeficient or immunosuppressed patients, resulting with osteonecrosis of the jaw in some cases [35].

4.6 Low pH values

Depending on the pH value, bisphosphonates can bind to hydroxyapatite in the bone or leave it and activate. At neutral pH the bisphosphonates are bound to hydroxyapatite and at reduced pH values bisphosphonates are released and activated from it [37, 38]. Bone resorption mechanism takes place in the Howship's lacunae. In situations when the pH remains low, potentially leads to toxic levels of bisphosphonates which have a negative effect on osteoclasts and other cells as well. By acting on different types of cells, there is suppression of remodeling, suppression of angiogenesis, increasing the toxicity of the oral mucosa, which contributes creating an infection with developing the osteonecrosis [38].

5. Epidemiology of development MRONJ

The incidence of drug osteonecrosis depends on a variety of factors.

5.1 Method of application

The way of medication administration is an important factor in assessing the risk of developing osteonecrosis. Bisphosphonates taken orally have been shown to be more benign than bisphosphonates administered intravenously [3, 39]. The prevalence of medication related osteonecrosis in oral bisphosphonates is much lower (ranging from 0.1% to 0.05%) than the prevalence of intravenous bisphosphonates and denosumab (ranging from 2% to 10). Prevalence increases after invasive surgical procedure and also increases with the duration of therapy. The largest prevalence of medication-related osteonecrosis has been described in patients with multiple myeloma [22, 40].

5.2 Duration of therapy

An important factor in the development of medication related osteonecrosis is the duration of the antiresorptive therapy. The literature states that after each year of therapy, the risk of medication osteonecrosis doubles [41].

5.3 Dosage

Medications that cause MRONJ can be prescribed every day, once weekly, once a month, once every three months or once every six months. Incidence of osteonecrosis increases with a higher dose [42–45].

5.4 Potency

Almost every antiresorptive medication shows its potency in causing osteonecrosis [42].

5.5 Accumulation in the body

Zoledronic acid and denosumab have similar potency of inducing osteonecrosis. They are different in the time of accumulation in the body. Bisphosphonates accumulate in bones, where they persist for a long time, their half-life last up to 11.2 years, while unlike bisphosphonates, denosumabs do not accumulate in the bones and are eliminated from the body after only 6 months [28, 46].

5.6 Local factors

Dental procedures that are invasive, such as dentoalveolar surgery, increase the risk of MRONJ up to seven times [3]. From local factors dentoalveolar surgery is considered the most risky factor for the development of medication-related osteonecrosis with an incidence of 60 to 65% [31, 47]. In other dental procedures such as endodontic or periodontal, the incidence of medication-related osteonecrosis is less. Dental diseases that the patient has already overcome, such as periodontitis, peri-implantitis, various inflammatory conditions of the jaw and poor oral hygiene are among the additional risk factors conducive to the development of MRONJ [47, 48].

5.7 Anatomical factors

It is known that medication related osteonecrosis occurs more often in the lower jaw in 73% of cases relative to the upper jaw, where it occurs in 22.5% of cases, while the incidence of osteonecrosis in both jaws simultaneously only in 4.5% of cases [3]. It also turned out that MRONJ more often develops in places with the thinnest layer of mucosa, and these are the lingual side of the lower jaw and the various exostoses and toruses found in the oral cavity [3, 47]. Wearing a prosthesis is also doubling the risk of developing MRONJ.

5.8 Systemic factors

A significant risk factor for the development of MRONJ is the patient's basic disease [49]. An increased risk of medication-related osteonecrosis has been shown in women, mostly due to osteoporosis or breast cancer. A risk of MRONJ significantly increases if, in addition to antiresorptive therapy are added additional drugs that act immunosuppressively, such as chemotherapeutics or corticosteroids. Studies show that MRONJ occurs in 40% of cases in patients who have been or are still on chemotherapy, in 25% cases of patients on corticosteroid therapy and in 10% of patients with diabetes [50, 51]. Anemia, systemic lupus, hypothyroidism, renal failure, rheumatoid arthritis, hypertension and smoking are also conditions that contribute to an increased risk of osteonecrosis [52, 53].

5.9 Genetics

The risk of developing osteonecrosis is also associated with gene predisposition. Some studies have shown an association between the FDPS (farnesyl diphosphate synthase gene) which encodes a key enzyme of the mevalonate pathway and the development of osteonecrosis of the jaw. That is why are tested rs2297480, a SNP region on the FDPS gene. Studies have been conducted in patients who have suffered from multiple myeloma or metastatic carcinomas and have been treated with zoledronate acid [54].

5.10 Biomarkers for risk assessment

Bone markers have been shown to be useful for assessing the risk of developing osteonecrosis [47]. C-terminal telopeptide (CTX) and N-terminal telopeptide (NTX) are demonstrated as the two main bone markers that measure osteoclast activity, i.e., degradation of osteoclasts and osteoblasts [47].

6. Prevention of MRONJ

6.1 Before starting antiresorptive therapy

Before starting antiresorptive therapy, it is important to make an initial dental examination with a detailed history and radiologically and clinically evaluate the patient's condition. An orthopantomogram is recommended of the radiological techniques. The goal of preventive screening is to remove any potential conditions that could lead to the formation of osteonecrosis during therapy. It is necessary to remove all incurable teeth or teeth with a poor prognosis, cure acute or chronic infections, cysts, tumors and other pathological conditions of the jaw. If the patient has a prosthesis, it is necessary to examine the sharp edges or possible painful areas ("blistering") that may adversely affect the mucosa. If teeth need to be extracted, it is advisable to wait a minimum of three weeks to achieve acceptable soft tissue healing, or preferably four to six weeks to achieve sufficient bone healing before initiating antiresorptive therapy [3].

Patients need to be educated about the risk of developing osteonecrosis, motivate them to strengthen oral hygiene and more frequent control (at least four times a year).

6.2 After therapy/during therapy

Depending on the duration and manner of taking antiresorptive drugs, it is necessary to make a detailed treatment plan that includes a consultation with a competent doctor for possible withdrawal of therapy.

Invasive surgical procedures (extraction, endodontic surgery) are reported as an increased risk of creating necrosis itself. In high-risk patients (high-potency drugs, adjunctive therapy), for the development of osteonecrosis, tooth extraction is not recommended and instead of extraction, endodontic treatment is recommended with root smoothing and cement coating. However, if invasive surgery is required as indicated for severe periodontitis, movable teeth, root fractures, then it is advisable to use the recommended guidelines [3].

A. Oral bisphosphonates.

1. If the patient is on therapy for less than four years and is not on adjunctive therapy (corticosteroids or angiogenic drugs), antiresorptive therapy does not need to be removed.

2. If the patient is on therapy for less than four years and prescribes adjunctive therapy (corticosteroids or angiogenic drugs) or is on therapy for more than four years or without adjunctive therapy, then consultation with a physician is required to discontinue bisphosphonate therapy at least two months before surgical treatment and continuation of bisphosphonate therapy when adequate bone healing is achieved (usually three months after the surgical treatment) [3].

B. Denosumabs.

Denosumabs are most commonly taken subcutaneously every six months. If invasive surgery is required, it is recommended to do it three weeks before the next application of the drug itself. It should be in mind that denosumabs are extremely potent drugs for the formation of osteonecrosis, but they, unlike bisphosphonates, are eliminated from the tissues after six months [3].

C. Parenteral bisphosphonates.

The previous recommendation was to discontinue therapy six months before the procedure and three months after, but this is especially difficult in malignant patients (due to the severity of the underlying disease) and discontinuation of therapy has not been scientifically proven to reduce the risk of osteonecrosis. It is recommended that the patient be referred to a specialist institution for the most at-risk group. Poor soft tissue healing should be in mind in patients receiving chemotherapy, especially three to four weeks after chemotherapy when mucositis of the oral mucosa is most common [3].

7. Clinical aspect of MRONJ

To diagnose medication related osteonecrosis of the jaws the following criteria must be filled:

1. Current or previous therapy with antiresorptive or antiangiogenic medications;

2. Exposed bone or appearance of a fistula in the jaw (intraoral or extraoral) that persists longer from eight weeks;

3. The patient is not irradiated and has no proven metastasis in the jaw bones [3, 55].

Medication-related osteonecrosis significantly impairs the quality of life of the patient and represents problems with speech, chewing, swallowing, feeding, often there is pain in the swollen mucosa, as well as chronic sinusitis [3]. In almost 94% of cases of medication-related osteonecrosis, exposed bone is present [56]. It is also the main feature of osteonecrosis (**Figure 1**). Variations can be different, from the small exposed edges around the empty alveoli all the way to complete involvement of one or both jaws [57]. We often find next to the exposed bone and signs of inflammation of the surrounding soft tissues that present as swelling that may or may not be purulent. The most lesions are asymptomatic, and when the patient develops pain,

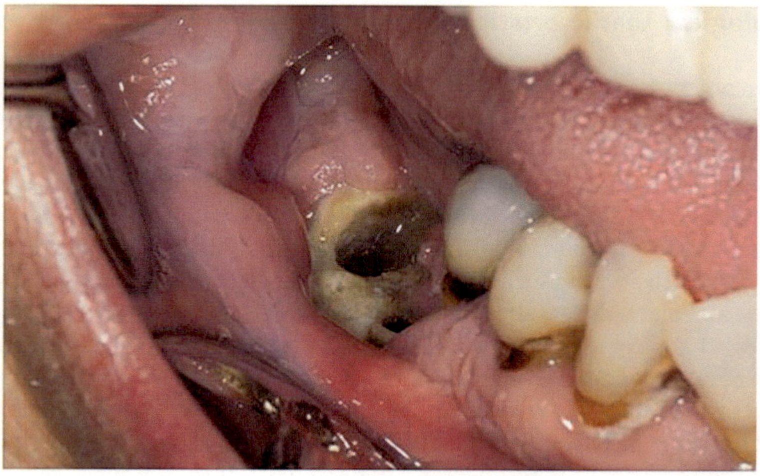

Figure 1.
Clinical appearance of MRONJ-exposed bone (Zometa).

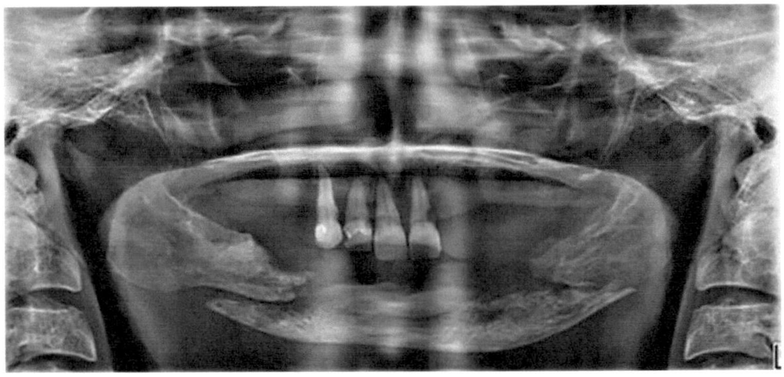

Figure 2.
Spontaneous bilateral mandibular fracture (Aredia).

we often find signs of acute inflammation in the surrounding tissue. In two-thirds of cases, medication-related osteonecrosis is found in the lower jaw [58]. The reason for this is a thinner mucosa than in the upper jaw and poorer blood supply to the lower jaw. Patients suffering from malignant diseases are most predisposed to MRONJ so it is very important to estimate whether the symptoms of progression are consequences osteonecrosis itself or are symptoms of secondaryism. After removal of the necrotic part of the bone, it is recommended to send materials for pathohistological analysis to determine the persistence of necrosis or some other lesions.

7.1 The course of the disease

The course of the disease itself can vary. Lesions can be limited and at dormancy stage or can spread to surrounding structures. MRONJ can spread all the way to the mandibular canal or maxillary sinus. In such cases, there are symptoms such as numbness, sinus infection and even the formation of oroantral communication. By spreading necrotic lesions it can also lead to pathological fractures of the jaw, which are serious, therapeutic and functional problems. Pathological fractures (**Figure 2**) are not common, they occur in 3% of patients who are treated from MRONJ [3].

8. Radiological characteristics of MRONJ

The involvement of the region by medication-related osteonecrosis can be assessed by radiographic analysis. This type of imaging is also useful in monitoring the disease and in diagnosing complications that occur in osteonecrosis such as fractures and sinusitis. By radiological analysis we can detect different stages of the disease and even the zero stage. Two-dimensional panoramic images (**Figure 3**) are recommended as an initial radiographic technique that give an excellent overview of the bones, teeth and the surrounding structure. Sclerosis found in the lamina dura of the alveolar ridge, after radiological examination, is the most common radiological change at risk patients. We can also find others radiological changes that are not so common, namely: sclerosis of the marginal parts of the jaw (most commonly in the mandible), narrowing of the mandibular canal, difficult or complete absence of healing of postextraction alveoli, radiolucent regions around the bone corresponding to osteolysis and necrotic bone sequesters that occur in the later stages of medication-related osteonecrosis [59–61]. More precisely, the lesion can be represented by one of the three-dimensional display techniques such as computed

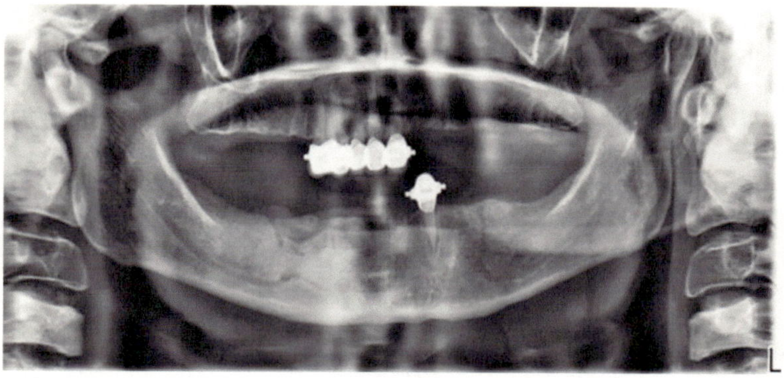

Figure 3.
MRONJ in a patient with multiple myeloma and treated with zoledronic acid (Zometa).

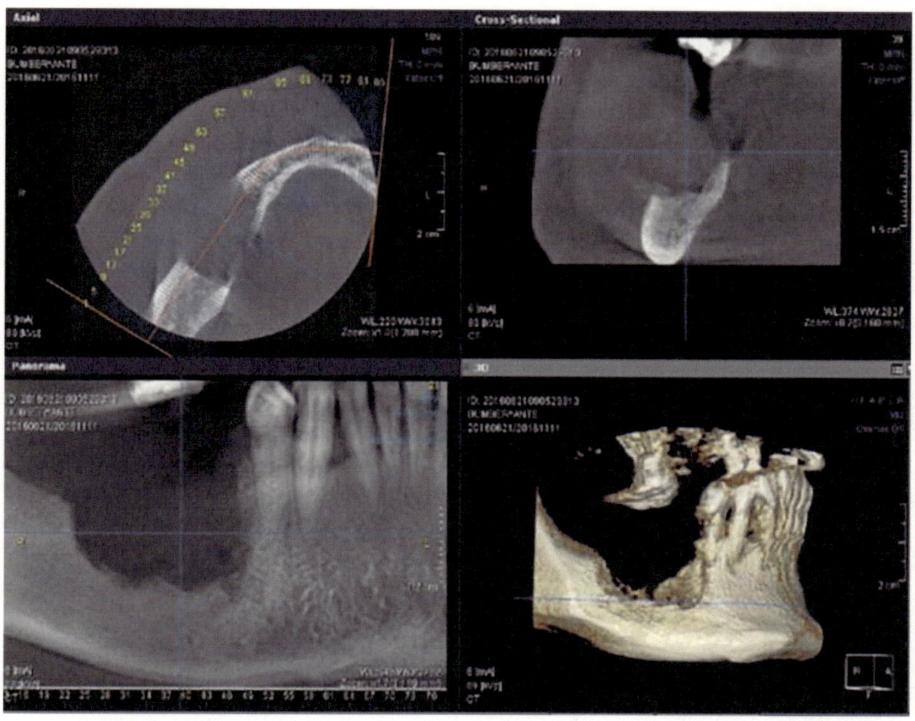

Figure 4.
CBCT scan (of same patient as in ***Figure 1****) after surgical treatment.*

tomography or cone-beam computed tomography. In the CBCT scan (**Figure 4**) we can get more precise data on the localization and on the progression of the disease and useful data on the surrounding bone structures. At early diagnosis of MRONJ, magnetic resonance (MRI), single-photon emission computed tomography (SPECT) and positron emission tomography with computed tomography (PET/CT) were also proved as an excellent diagnostic tool [59, 62–67].

9. Classification of MRONJ

The disease, according to the clinical picture and the appearance of symptoms of osteonecrosis, is classified into four stages [3].

9.1 Stage 0

This stage of disease includes patients who have not clinically developed osteonecrosis but have nonspecific symptoms or radiological signs that may be associated with therapy. Symptoms associated with stage zero are: unexplained odontalgia, dull pain of lower jaw extending toward the temporomandibular joint, sinus pain that may be associated with inflammation and narrowing of the bone wall toward the sinus [3]. Clinical findings that may indicate stage zero are: unexplained tooth loss unrelated to chronic periodontal disease, periapical/periodontal fistula unrelated to pulp necrosis or caries, unexplained gingival swelling. Radiological signs are: loss of alveolar bone or resorption not related to chronic periodontitis, changes in the composition of the trabeculae, difficult (delayed) wound healing after tooth extraction, sclerosing regions of the alveolar part (thickening of the lamina dura, or reduction of the space belonging to the periodontal ligament) or surrounding part of the bone [66–68].

Zero-stage therapy is symptomatic and conservative, aimed at remediation of predisposing conditions that can cause osteonecrosis (remediation of caries, periodontal diseases, other pathological conditions, inadequate dentures). It is also necessary to exclude other diseases such as fibroseal lesions, chronic sclerosing osteomyelitis and others.

Patients need to be educated about the disease, about adequate oral hygiene and encouraged to have more frequent check-ups (at least every two months).

9.2 Stage 1

Stage one of the disease describes clinically exposed necrotic bone or the appearance of a fistula that forms from the bone, however patients have no symptoms and no signs of acute infection. The time required for proper diagnosis of the first stage of disease is eight weeks from appearance of exposed bone or fistula [3].

First-stage therapy is primarily aimed at monitoring the lesion. If necrotic bone sequesters or sharp bone margins occur, they should be removed. Monitoring the condition of the surrounding mucosa is extremely important for further prognosis of the disease.

It is also necessary to educate and motivate patients for frequent checkups.

9.3 Stage 2

Stage two describes clinically exposed necrotic bone or the appearance of a fistula that forms from bone with signs of acute infection accompanied by pain [3].

Stage two therapy is initially aimed at repairing the inflammation and antibiotic therapy is often attributed to it in combination with antimicrobial washes (most commonly chlorhexidine). Necrotic bone is often contaminated with bacteria to form biofilms that may be resistant to antibiotic therapy. After repairing the inflammation, it is necessary to remove the necrotic part of the bone and the inflamed mucosa.

9.4 Stage 3

Stage three describes clinically exposed necrotic bone or the appearance of a fistula that forms from bone with signs of acute infection accompanied by pain and at least one of these signs: spreading necrosis outside the dental alveolus (lower edge and ascending part of mandible, maxillary sinus, toward the cheekbone), the appearance of extraoral fistula, osteolysis of the lower border of the lower jaw and the bottom of the maxillary sinus with the appearance of oroantral communication and the appearance of pathological fractures [3].

Third-stage therapy focuses on palliative therapy that includes debridement or resection of the lesion in combination with antibiotic therapy to eliminate acute infection and pain. Therapy directly depends on the health condition of the patient. If larger resections are performed, reconstruction is performed by different reconstructive methods (fibula graft) with or without obturator.

10. MRONJ treatment protocol

There is currently no gold standard or clearly defined treatment protocol for the disease itself.

If osteonecrosis of the jaw occurs, it is recommended that the patient be referred to an oral or maxillofacial surgery specialist for further treatment.

The goals of therapy are aimed at eliminating inflammation and pain by preventing or slowing the progression of the disease. Before treatment, it is necessary to take a detailed medical and dental history and consult a doctor about the possible removal of the drug. Treatment depends on the degree of the disease and is initially focused on antibiotic therapy in combination with antimicrobial therapy and analgesics. Surgical techniques for removing the necrotic part of the bone include sequestration, ridge modeling, resection of the jaw with various reconstructive methods [3].

American Association of Oral and Maxillofacial Surgeons (AAOMS) recommends starting conservative therapy before surgery [3]. Conservative therapy serves to control the disease itself and is achieved by antibiotic therapy and chlorhexidine rinsing. They believe that elective surgery can lead to further disease progression. If the disease progresses then surgery needs to remove the necrotic lesion. On the other hand, European guidelines recommend the initial surgical removal of the necrotic part of the bone regardless of the degree of the disease for several reasons: the necrotic part of the bone cannot be revitalized and it is the entrance door for colonization of bacteria and fungi [69–71]. Histological processing is recommended to demonstrate necrosis and differential diagnosis in the form of bone metastases, osteomyelitis (inflammatory bone condition) or osteoradionecrosis (radiation-related ischemic bone necrosis) [72].

Surgical procedures have been scientifically proven to perform better compared to a conservative approach [73–76]. Conservative treatment consists of more frequent follow-up examinations (once or twice a week) for months, which is a burden for patients. It should be in mind that frequent check-ups are difficult for oncology patients.

The success of the therapy is achieved when the necrotic part of the bone is removed and when the mucosal integrity of the tissue is established. Treatment of MRONJ should be divided into bone and soft tissue repair. After removal of the necrotic part of the bone or tooth extraction, it is necessary to keep in mind the smoothing or modeling of sharp sclerotic bone edges of the wound because they remodel very slowly and can potentiate the development of necrosis (**Figure 5**). After removal of the necrotic part, it is necessary to process the soft tissue. The aim is to achieve optimal marginal closure of the wound in the form of preventing the penetration of microorganisms, i.e., contamination of the surrounding bone. Mucosal integrity is achieved by primary suturing of the wound without tension. Some surgeons recommend double covering the exposed portion of the bone with a muscle flap (*m. mylohyoideus*) or buccal fat pad flap [77–79]. For larger defects, reconstruction with a microvascular skin or bone graft is recommended, however, it should be considered that the transplanted bone is also rich in antiresorptive drugs. Major reconstructions depend on the health status of the patients.

The necrotic portion of the bone relative to the surrounding healthy bone tissue may be clearly limited (sequestration formation) or may be diffusely incorporated into healthy bone tissue. Clearly demarcated sequesters are easily removed during surgery, while diffuse parts are difficult to remove due to the unclear boundary of necrotic from vital bone tissue [80, 81]. Bone bleeding was previously thought to be a sign of vitality (which makes it easier for surgeons to work) however, this has proven to be wrong. For the treatment of diffuse lesions, the use of fluorescence in combination with tetracycline is recommended [82, 83].

11. Photodynamic therapy and MRONJ

There are various additional methods of treatment, in addition to surgical treatment, that promote healing of the lesion. For this purpose oxygen therapy (ozone, hyperbaric chamber), hormone therapy (parathyroid hormone), growth factor (**Figure 6**) therapy (PRP, PRF, PRGF, BMP), mesenchymal stem cell therapy and a combination of pantophilin and tocopherol [84–88] are used.

Vescovi et al. [89] in 2006 described the application of low-level-laser therapy (LLLT) as possible treatment of osteonecrosis of the jaw. The effect of lasers is classified in two categories, regarding its mW range: biostimulation (LLLT) and photodynamic therapy (PDT). Main difference between this two types is that in biostimulation therapy (LLLT) the laser acts directly on the tissue and aims to

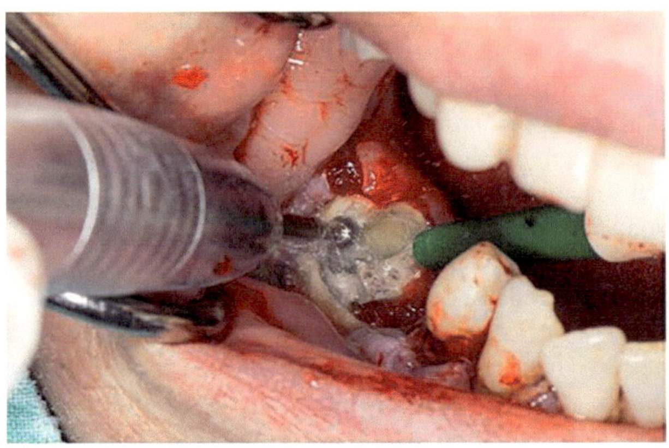

Figure 5.
Surgical treatment- modeling of sharp sclerotic bone edges.

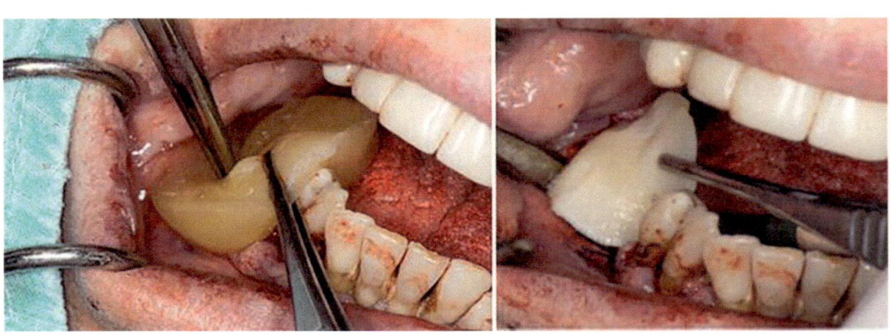

Figure 6.
Augmentation using autologous growth factors; PRGF technique, F2 and F1 phase.

support tissue healing, while in photodynamic therapy (PDT) it acts on chemical medium (photosensitizer) (**Figure 7**) which induces cell (e.g. bacteria) and tissue damage as a chemical effect [90].

LLLT has from clinical point of view become adjuvant medical tool for enhancing wound-healing process, so some clinical studies reported laser-induced stimulation especially of soft tissue healing such as ulcers and postoperative wound dehiscences [91, 92]. Stein et al. [93]. in their *in vitro* study confirmed that low energy laser irradiation promotes proliferation and maturation of human osteoblasts, while stimulating effect of LLLT is explained by an increase of ATP in affected cells [94].

Photodynamic therapy (PDT) is being increasingly used in the management of MRONJ in combination with other therapeutic choices [90].

In the beginning photodynamic therapy (PDT) was used particularly to treat cancer and several studies have shown its antimicrobial potency [95–98]. Analyzing the effects of PDT on osteoblasts growth, study by Zancanela et al. [99] showed that PDT results in biostimulation of osteoblastic cell cultures or a cytotoxic effect depends of the applied dose. PDT has well documented clinical impact as adjuvant local treatment of ulcers and infected wounds, and potential indications for therapy of periodontitis and peri-implantitis, but treatment of MRONJ still in phase of collecting clinical results [100–105]. Treatment concept of MRONJ with PDT describes its use for symptomatic treatment in stage 0, preoperatively to reduce bacterial load and in cases with healing deficiencies, while in stages 1, 2 and 3 it is used after surgical treatment. Also it may be used as adjuvant conservative intervention for palliative therapy of compromised patients or in cases to avoid progression of disease when patients refuse surgery.

While application of LLLT for therapy of MRONJ has been described in numerous studies, there are few studies mainly focused on impact of photodynamic therapy of preventing occurrence of MRONJ. Vescovi et al. [89] used Nd:YAG laser biostimulation in addition to medical and surgical therapy and demonstrate a better healing tendency due to bony ablation, bactericidal and detoxification effect [106, 107]. Da Guarda et al. [108] reported a case of successful MRONJ treatment with the GaAIAs diode laser in combination with bone curettage. Summarizing the literature, use of LLLT is beneficial for treatment of MRONJ, although till today there are no large studies that proves significant improvement.

One of promoting factor in mechanism of MRONJ is presence of microflora. Species such as *Fusobacterium, Eikenella, Bacillus, Actinomyces, Staphylococcus,* and *Streptococcus* are predisposed to survive in oxygen depleted areas of necrotic bone that lack blood supply [109, 110]. Although the identification of microbial biofilms

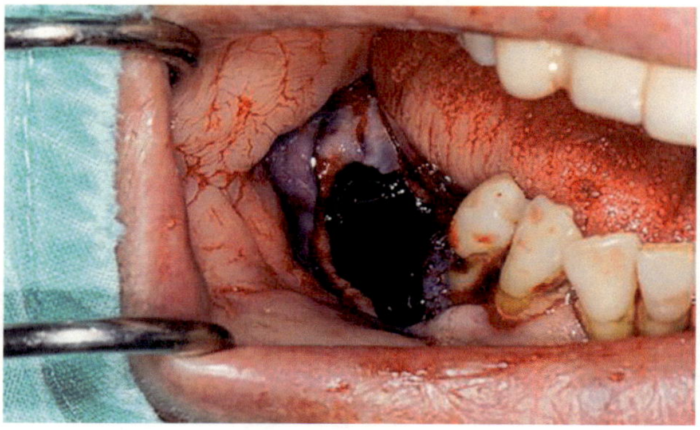

Figure 7.
Application of chemical medium (photosensitizer)- toluidine blue.

and *Actinomyces* species as the leading bacterial pathogen isolated from patients with MRONJ, there is unclear definitive treatment and no data reffering to bactericidal activity of laser therapy against *Actinomyces* species in MRONJ lesions.

The most used PDT system is one with mobile diode laser and dye (HELBO) with methylene blue (MB) (**Figure 8**). It has shown very promising results during surgical procedures or as adjuvant therapy in cases of postoperative wound dehiscences in patients with MRONJ. Photosensitizers's antimicrobial activity is mediated by singlet oxygen, which has high chemical reactivity and results with a direct effect on extracellular molecules. The polysaccharides present in extracellular matrix of a bacterial biofilm are sensitive to photodamage, so breaking biofilms can interrupt colonization and prevent antibiotic resistance [111].

Although is surgical treatment first option to deal with MRONJ, appliance of photodynamic therapy has several advantages. Before surgery usually we treat symptoms of MRONJ infection, such as swelling, purulent discharge and pain. They can be managed by bio-stimulative effect of the laser, especially those with advanced primary disease or those suffering from other sickness resulting in a general poor health [90]. PDT might be very sufficient in early stages of osteonecrosis promoting secondary granulation and formation of mucosal coverage, so surgery can be avoid. Unfortunately there are no controlled studies opposing PDT and LLLT to evaluate use of photosensitizer. Appliance of photodynamic therapy immediately after surgery could decrease complications of impaired healing of the wound (**Figure 9**).

In conclusion, although MRONJ is considered difficult to treat and may even be recalcitrant to therapy, photodynamic therapy can be a viable supportive tool

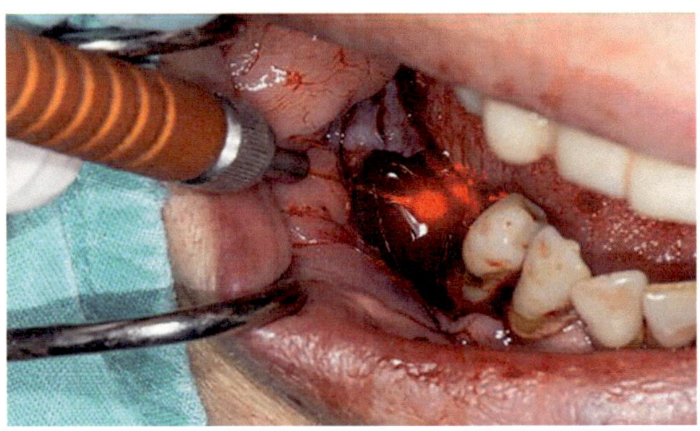

Figure 8.
Antimicrobial photodynamic therapy using low-power diode laser (aPDT mode, LaserHF, Hagernnnnn Werken).

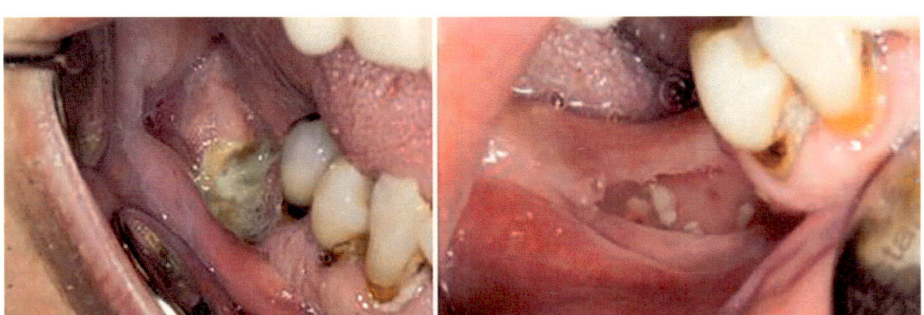

Figure 9.
MRONJ before and 2 months after treatment with combined therapy (surgery/aPDT/PRGF).

of initial and advanced stages of MRONJ, as an adjuvant treatment before or after surgery or primary treatment in cases without surgery indicated.

Conflict of interest

The authors declare no conflict of interest.

Author details

Marko Vuletić[1], Božana Lončar Brzak[2], Igor Smojver[3], Luka Marković[4], Mato Sušić[1] and Dragana Gabrić[1]*

1 Department of Oral Surgery, School of Dental Medicine, University of Zagreb, Clinical Hospital Center Zagreb, Croatia

2 Department of Oral Medicine, School of Dental Medicine, University of Zagreb, Clinical Hospital Center Zagreb, Croatia

3 Special Hospital St. Catherine, Zagreb, Croatia

4 Department of Periodontology, School of Dental Medicine, University of Zagreb, Private Dental Clinic, Pula, Croatia

*Address all correspondence to: dgabric@sfzg.hr

References

[1] Marx RE. Pamidronate (Aredia) and zoledronate (Zometa) induced avascular necrosis of the jaws: a growing epidemic [Letter]. J Oral Maxillofac Surg. 2003;61:1115.

[2] Bartl R, Frisch B, von Tresckow E, Bartl C. Bisphosphonates in medical practice actions, side effects, indication, strategies. Berlin/New York; Springer: 2007.

[3] Ruggiero SL, Dodson TB, Fantasia J, et al. American Association of Oral Maxillofacial Surgeons position paper on medication-related osteonecrosis of the jaw-2014 update. J Oral Maxillofac Surg. 2014; 72:1938-1956.

[4] Khan AA, Morrison A, Hanley DA, et al. Diagnosis and management of osteonecrosis of the jaw: a systematic review and international consensus. J Bone Miner Res. 2015;30:3-23.

[5] Fassio A, Bertoldo F, Idolazzi L, Viapiana O, Rossini M, Gatti D. Drug-induced osteonecrosis of the jaw: the state of the art. Reumatismo. 2017;69:9-15.

[6] Fedele S, Bedogni G, Scoletta M, et al. Up to a quarter of patients with osteonecrosis of the jaw associated with antiresorptive agents remain undiagnosed. Br J Oral Maxillofac Surg. 2015;53:13-17.

[7] Schiodt M, Reibel J, Oturai P, Kofod T. Comparison of nonexposed and exposed bisphosphonate-induced osteonecrosis of the jaws: a retrospective analysis from the Copenhagen cohort and a proposal for an updated classification system. Oral Surg Oral Med Oral Pathol Oral Radiol. 2014;117:204-213.

[8] Patel S, Choyee S, Uyanne J, et al. Non-exposed bisphosphonate-related osteonecrosis of the jaw: a critical assessment of current definition, staging, and treatment guidelines. Oral Dis. 2012;18:625-632.

[9] Troeltzsch M, Woodlock T, Kriegelstein S, Steiner T, Messlinger K. Physiology and pharmacology of nonbisphosphonate drugs implicated in osteonecrosis of the jaw. J Can Dent Asoc. 2012;78:c85.

[10] Ortega J, Vigil CE, Chodkiewicz C, Current progress sin targeted therapy for colorectal cancer. Cancer control. 2010;17:7-15.

[11] Hopp RN, Pucci J, Santos-Silva AR, Jorge J. Osteonecrosis after administration of intravitreous bevacizumab. J Oral Maxillofac Surg. 2011;70:632-635.

[12] Estilo CL, Fornier M, Farooki A, Carlson D, Bohle 3rd G, Huryn JM. Osteonecrosis of the jaw related to bevacizumab. J Clin Oncol. 2008;26:4037-4038.

[13] Mena AC, Pulido EG, Guillen-Ponce C. Understanding the molecular-based mechanism of action of the tyrosine kinase inhibitor: sunitinib. Anticancer Drugs. 2010;21:S3-11.

[14] Diel IJ, Bergner R, Grötz KA. Adverse effects of bisphosphonates: current issues. J Support Oncol. 2007;5:475-482.

[15] Honig S, Chang G. Osteoporosis: an update. Bull NYU Hosp Jt Dis. 2012;70:140-144.

[16] Shkolnikova J, Flynn J, Choong P. Burden of bisphosphonate-associated femoral fractures. ANZ J Surg. 2013;83:175-181. doi:10.1111/ans.12018

[17] Orozco C, Maalouf NM. Safety of bisphosphonates. Rheum Dis Clin North

Am. 2012;38:681-705. doi:10.1016/j.rdc.2012.09.001

[18] Lasseter KC, Porras AG, Denker A, Santhanagopal A, Daifotis A. Pharmacokinetic considerations in determining the terminal elimination half-lives of bisphosphonates. Clin Drug Investig. 2005;25:107-114. doi:10.2165/00044011-200525020-00003

[19] Hampson G, Fogelman I. Clinical role of bisphosphonate therapy. Int J Womens Health. 2012;4:455-469. doi:10.2147/IJWH.S24783

[20] Abdelmoula LC, Ben M'barek R, Ben Hadj Yahia C, et al. Indications des bisphosphonates dans les affections osseuses autres que l'ostéoporose [Bisphosphonates: indications in bone diseases other than osteoporosis]. Tunis Med. 2011;89:511-516.

[21] Otto S, Pautke C, Van den Wyngaert T, Niepel D, Schiødt M. Medication-related osteonecrosis of the jaw: Prevention, diagnosis and management in patients with cancer and bone metastases. Cancer Treat Rev. 2018;69:177-187. doi:10.1016/j.ctrv.2018.06.007

[22] Then C, et al. Incidence and risk factors of bisphosphonate related osteonecrosis of the jaw in multiple myeloma patients having undergone autologous stem cell transplantation. Onkologie. 2012;35:658-664.

[23] Zavras AI. The impact of bisphosphonates on oral health: lessons from the past and opportunities for the future. Ann NY Acad Sci. 2011;1218:55-61.

[24] Berenson JR, Hillner BE, Kyle RA, et al. American Society of Clinical Oncology clinical practice guidelines: the role of bisphosphonates in multiple myeloma. J Clin Oncol. 2002;20:3719-3736. doi:10.1200/JCO.2002.06.037

[25] Cummings SR, San Martin J, McClung MR, Siris ES, Eastell R, Reid IR, et al. Denosumab for prevention of fractures in postmenopausal women with osteoporosis. N Engl J Med. 2009;361:756-765.

[26] Van den Wyngaert T, Claeys T, Huizing MT, Vermorken JB, Fossion E. Initial experience with conservative treatment in cancer patients with osteonecrosis of the jaw [ONJ] and predictors of outcome. Ann Oncol. 2009;20:331-336.

[27] Henry DH, Costa L, Goldwasser F, Hirsh V, Hungria V, Prausova J, et al. Randomized, double-blind study of denosumab versus zoledronic acid in the treatment of bone metastases in patients with advanced cancer [excluding breast and prostate cancer] or multiple myeloma. J Clin Oncol. 2011;29:1125-1132.

[28] Rx List Inc. Denosumab.[Internet] Available at: www.rxlist.com/prolia-drug/clinicalpharmacology.htm. Accessed 2020. August 10 th.

[29] Estilo CL, Fornier M, Farooki A, Carlson D, Bohle G 3rd, Huryn JM. Osteonecrosis of the jaw related to bevacizumab. J Clin Oncol. 2008;26:4037-4038. doi:10.1200/JCO.2007.15.5424

[30] Wimalawansa SJ. Insight into bisphosphonate-associated osteomyelitis of the jaw: pathophysiology, mechanisms and clinical management. Expert Opin Drug Saf. 2008;7:491-512.

[31] Marx RE, Sawstari Y, Fortin M, et al. Bisphosphonate-induced exposed bone [osteonecrosis/osteoporosis] of the jaws: risk factors, recognition, prevention, and treatment. J Oral Maxillofac Surg. 2005 Nov; 63:1567-1575.

[32] Walter C, Klein MO, Pabst A, Al-Nawas B, Duschner H,

Ziebart T. Influence of bisphosphonates on endothelial cells, fibroblasts, and osteogenic cells. Clin Oral Investig. 2010;14:35-41.

[33] Walter C, Pabst A, Ziebart T, Klein M, Al-Nawas B. Bisphosphonates affect migration ability and cell viability of HUVEC, fibroblasts and osteoblasts in vitro. Oral Dis. 2011;17:194-199.

[34] Hansen T, Kunkel M, Springer E, Walter C, Weber A, Siegel E, Kirkpatrick CJ. Actinomycosis of the jaws-histopathological study of 45 patients shows significant involvement in bisphosphonate-associated osteonecrosis and infected osteoradionecrosis. Virchows Arch. 2007;451:1009-1017.

[35] Landesberg R, Woo V, Cermers S, et al. Potential pathophysiological mechanisms in osteonecrosis of the jaw. Ann NY Acad Sci. 2011;1218:62-79.

[36] Yoneda T. Bisphosphonate-related osteonecrosis of jaw: position paeper form the Allied Task Force Committee of Japanese Society for Bone and Mineral Research, Japan Osteoporosis Society, Japanese Society of Periodontology, Japanese Society of Oral and Maxillofacial Radiology, and Japanese Society of Oral and Maxillofacial Surgeons. J Bone Miner Metab. 2010:28:365-383.

[37] Thumbigere-Math V, Sabino MC, Gopalakrishnan R, et al. Bisphosphonate-related osteonecrosis of the jaw: clinical features, risk factors, management, and treatment outcomes of 26 patients. J Oral Maxillofac Surg. 2009;67:1904-1913. doi:10.1016/j.joms.2009.04.051

[38] Otto S, Hafner S, Grötz KA. The role of inferior alveolar nerve involvement in bisphosphonate-related osteonecrosis of the jaw. J Oral Maxillofac Surg. 2009;67:589-592. doi:10.1016/j.joms.2008.09.028

[39] Khosla S, Burr D, Cauley J, et al. Bisphosphonate-associated osteonecrosis of the jaw: report of a task force American Society for Bone and Mineral Research. J Bone Miner Res. 2007 Oct; 22:1479-1491.

[40] Lo JC, O'Ryan FS, Gordon NP, Yang J, Hui RL, Martin D, et al. Prevalence of osteonecrosis of the jaw in patients with oral bisphosphonate exposure. J Oral Maxillofac Surg. 2010;68:243-253.

[41] Jadu F, Lee L, Pharoah M, Reece D, Wang L. A retrospective study assessing the incidence, risk factors and comorbidities of pamidronate-related necrosis of the jaws in multiple myeloma patients. Ann Oncol. 2007;18:2015-2019.

[42] Thumbigere-Math V, Tu L, Huckabay S, Dudek AZ, Lunos S, Basi DL, et al. A retrospective study evaluating frequency and risk factors of osteonecrosis of the jaw in 576 cancer patients receving intravenous bisphosphonates. Am J Clin Oncol. 2012;35:386-392.

[43] Hoff AO, Toth BB, Altudag K, Johnson MM, Warneke CL, Hu M, et al. Frequency and risk factors associated with osteonecrosis of the jaw in cancer patients related with intravenous bisphosphonates, J Bone Miner Res. 2008;23:826-836.

[44] Fehm T, Beck V, Banys M, Lipp HP, Hairass M, Reinert S, et al. Bisphosphonate-induced osteonecrosis of the jaw [ONJ]: incidence and risk factors in patients with breast cancer and gynecological malignancies. Gynecol Oncol. 2009;112:605-609.

[45] Then C, Horauf N, Otto S, Pautke C, von Tresckow E, Rohnisch T, et al. Incidence and risk

factors of bisphosphonate-related osteonecrosis of the jaw in multiple myeloma patients having undergone autologous stem cell transplatation. Onkologie. 2012;35:658-664.

[46] Lasseter KC, Porras AG, Denker A, et al. Pharmacokinetic considerations in determining the terminal elimination half-lives of bisphosphonates. Clin Drug Investig. 2005;25:107-114.

[47] Marx RE, Cillo JE, Jr., Ulloa JJ. Oral bisphosphonate-induced osteonecrosis: risk factors, prediction of risk using serum CTX testing, prevention, and treatment. J Oral Maxillofac Surg. 2007;65:2397-2410.

[48] Aghaloo TL, Kang B, Sung EC, et al. Periodontal disease and bisphosphonates induced osteonecrosis of the jaws in the rat. J Bone Miner Res. 2011;26:1871-1882.

[49] Neviaser AS, Lane JM, Lenart BA, et al. Low-energy femoral shaft fractures associated with alendronate use. J Orthop Trauma. 2008; 22:346-350.

[50] O'Ryan FS, Lo JC. Bisphosphonate-related osteonecrosis of the jaw in patients with oral bisphosphonate exposure: clinical course and outcomes. J Oral Maxillofac Surg. 2012;70:1844-1853.

[51] Di Fede O, Fusco V, Matranga D, Solazzo L, Gabriele M, Gaeta GM, et al. Osteonecrosis of the jaws in patients assuming oral bisphosphonates for osteoporosis: a retrospective multihospital-based study of 87 Italian cases. Eur J Intern Med. 2013;11.

[52] Malden N, Lopes V. An epidemiological study of alendronate-related osteonecrosis of the jaws. A case series from the south-east of Scotland with attention given to case definition and prevalence. J Bone Miner Metab. 2012;30:171-182.

[53] Diniz-Freitas M, Lopez-Cendrun JL, Fernandez-Sanroman J, Garcia-Garcia A, FernandezFeijoo J, Diz-Dios P. Oral bisphosphonate- related osteonecrosis of the jaws: clinical charasteristics of a series of 20 cases in Spain. Med Oral Patol Oral Cir Bucal. 2012;17:751-758.

[54] Zhong DN, Wu JZ, Li GJ. Association between CYP2C8 [rs1934951] polymorphism and bisphosphonate-related osteonecrosis of the jaws in patients on bisphosphonate therapy: a meta-analysis. Acta Haematol. 2013;129:90-95. doi:10.1159/000342120

[55] American Association of Oral and Maxillofacial Surgeons. Position paper on bisphosphonate-related osteonecrosis of the jaws. J Oral Maxillofac Surg. 2007;65:369-376.

[56] Otto S, Schreyer C, Hafner S, Mast G, Ehrenfeld M, Stürzenbaum S, et al. Bisphosphonaterelated osteonecrosis of the jaws- characteristics, risk factors, clinical features, localization and impact on oncological treatment. J Craniomaxillofac Surg. 2012;40:303-309

[57] Otto S. Medication Related Osteonecrosis of the Jaw: Bisphosphonates, Denosumab, and New Agents. Berlin, Heidelberg. Springer 2015; 220 p.

[58] Assaf AT, Zrnc TA, Riecke B, Winker J, Zustin J, Friedrich RE, et al. Intraoperative efficiency of fluorescence imaging by Visually Enhanced Lesion Scope [VELscope®] in patients with bisphosphonate related osteonecrosis of the jaw [MRONJ]. J Craniomaxillofac Surg. 2013;42:157-164.

[59] Arce K, Assael LA, Weissman JL, et al. Imaging findings in bisphosphonate-related osteonecrosis of jaws. J Oral Maxillofac Surg. 2009;67:S75-84.

[60] Bedogni A, Blandamura S, Lokmic Z, et al. Bisphosphonate-associated jaw bone osteonecrosis: a correlation between imaging techniques and histopathology. Oral Surg Oral Med Oral Pathol Oral Radiol Endod. 2008;105:358-364

[61] Bianchi SD, Scoletta M, Cassione FB, et al. Computerized tomographic findings in bisphosphonate-associated osteonecrosis of the jaw in patients with cancer. Oral Surg Oral Med Oral Pathol Oral Radiol Oral Endod. 2007;104:249-258.

[62] Chiandussi S, Biasotto M, Dore F, Cavalli F, Cova MA, Di Lenarda R. Clinical and diagnostic imaging of bisphosphonate-associated osteonecrosis of the jaws. Dentomaxillofac Radiol. 2006;35:236-243.

[63] O'Ryan FS, Khoury S, Liao W, Han MM, Hui RL, Baer D, et al. Intravenous bisphosphonate-related osteonecrosis of the jaw: bone scintigraphy as an early indicator. J Oral Maxillofac Surg. 2009;67:1363-1372.

[64] Tsao C, Darby I, Ebeling PR, Walsh K, O'Brien-Simpson N, Reynolds E, et al. Oral health risk factors for bisphosphonate-associated jaw osteonecrosis. J Oral Maxillofac Surg. 2013;71:1360-1366.

[65] Saad F, Brown JE, Van Poznak C, Ibrahim T, Stemmer SM, Stopeck AT, et al. Incidence, risk factors, and outcomes of osteonecrosis of the jaw: integrated analysis from three blinded active-controlled phase III trials in cancer patients with bone metastases. Ann Oncol. 2012; 23:1341-1347.

[66] Hutchinson M, O'Ryan F, Chavez V, Lathon PV, Sanchez G, Hatcher DC, et al. Radiographicfindingsinbisphosphonate-treated patients with stage 0 disease in the absence of bone exposure. J Oral Maxillofac Surg. 2010;68:2232-2240.

[67] Aghaloo TL, Dry SM, Mallya S, Tetradis S. Stage 0 osteonecrosis of the jaw in a patient on denosumab. J Oral Maxillofac Surg. 2014;72:702-716.

[68] Farias DS, Zen Filho EV, de Oliveira TF, Tinôco-Araújo JE, Sampieri MB, Antunes HS, et al. Clinical and image findings in bisphosphonate-related osteonecrosis of the jaws. J Craniofac Surg. 2013;24:1248-1250.

[69] Groetz KA, Piesold JU, Al-Nawas B. Bisphosphonatassoziierte Kiefernekrose [BP-ONJ] und andere Medikamenten-assoziierte Kiefernekrosen. AWMF online www.awmf.org. 2012.

[70] Schipmann S, Metzler P, Rossle M, Zemann W, von Jackowski J, Obwegeser JA, et al. Osteopathology associated with bone resorption inhibitors – which role does Actinomyces play? A presentation of 51 cases with systematic review of the literature. J Oral Pathol Med. 2013;42:587-593.

[71] Sedghizadeh PP, Kumar SK, Gorur A, Schaudinn C, Shuler CF, Costerton JW. Identification of microbial biofilms in osteonecrosis of the jaws secondary to bisphosphonate therapy. J Oral Maxillofac Surg. 2008;66:767-775.

[72] Otto S, Schuler K, Ihrler S, Ehrenfeld M, Mast G. Osteonecrosis or metastases of the jaw or both? Case report and review of the literature. J Oral Maxillofac Surg. 2010;68:1185-1188.

[73] Lesclous P, Grabar S, Abi Najm S, Carrel JP, Lombardi T, Saffar JL, et al. Relevance of surgical management of patients affected by bisphosphonate-associated osteonecrosis of the jaws. A prospective clinical and

radiological study. Clin Oral Investig. 2014;18:391-399.

[74] Stockmann P, Vairaktaris E, Wehrhan F, Seiss M, Schwarz S, Spriewald B, et al. Osteotomy and primary wound closure in bisphosphonate-associated osteonecrosis of the jaw: a prospective clinical study with 12 months follow-up. Support Care Cancer. 2010;18:449-460.

[75] Voss PJ, Joshi Oshero J, Kovalova-Muller A, Veigel Merino EA, Sauerbier S, Al-Jamali J, et al. Surgical treatment of bisphosphonate-associated osteonecrosis of the jaw: technical report and follow up of 21 patients. J Craniomaxillofac Surg. 2012;40:719-725.

[76] Carlson ER, Basile JD. The role of surgical resection in the management of bisphosphonate-related osteonecrosis of the jaws. J Oral Maxillofac Surg. 2009;67:85-95.

[77] Lemound J, Eckardt A, Kokemuller H, von See C, Voss PJ, Tavassol F, et al. Bisphosphonate-associated osteonecrosis of the mandible: reliable soft tissue reconstruction using a local myofascial fl ap. Clin Oral Investig. 2012;16:1143-1152.

[78] Mast G, Otto S, Mucke T, Schreyer C, Bissinger O, Kolk A, et al. Incidence of maxillary sinusitis and oroantral fistulae in bisphosphonate-related osteonecrosis of the jaw. J Craniomaxillofac Surg. 2012;40:568-571.

[79] Gallego L, Junquera L, Pelaz A, Hernando J, Megias J. The use of pedicled buccal fat pad combined with sequestrectomy in bisphosphonate-related osteonecrosis of the maxilla. Med Oral Patol Oral Cir Bucal. 2012;17:236-241.

[80] Advisory Task Force on Bisphosphonate-Related Ostenonecrosis of the Jaws, American Association of Oral and Maxillofacial Surgeons. J Oral Maxillofac Surg. 2007;65:369-376.

[81] Khosla S, Burr D, Cauley J, Dempster DW, Ebeling PR, Felsenberg D, et al. Bisphosphonate-associated osteonecrosis of the jaw: report of a task force of the American Society for Bone and Mineral Research. J Bone Miner Res. 2007;22:1479-1491.

[82] Wang J, Goodger NM, Pogrel MA. Osteonecrosis of the jaws associated with cancer chemotherapy. J Oral Maxillofac Surg. 2003;61:1104-1107.

[83] Harris WH. A microscopic method of determining rates of bone growth. Nature. 1960;188:1039-1049.

[84] Cella L, Oppici A, Arbasi M, Moretto M, Piepoli M, Vallisa D, et al. Autologous bone marrow stem cell intralesional transplantation repairing bisphosphonate related osteonecrosis of the jaw. Head Face Med. 2011;7:16.

[85] Curi MM, Cossolin GS, Koga DH, Zardetto C, Christianini S, Feher O, et al. Bisphosphonate-related osteonecrosis of the jaws–an initial case series report of treatment combining partial bone resection and autologous platelet-rich plasma. J Oral Maxillofac Surg. 2011;69:2465-2472.

[86] Dayisoylu EH, Ungor C, Tosun E, Ersoz S, Duman MK, Taskesen F, et al. Does an alkaline environment prevent the development of bisphosphonate-related osteonecrosis of the jaw? An experimental study in rats. Oral Surg Oral Med Oral Pathol Oral Radiol. 2014;117:329-334.

[87] Cheung A, Seeman E. Teriparatide therapy for alendronate- associated osteonecrosis of the jaw. N Engl J Med. 2010;363:2473-2474.

[88] Dayisoylu EH, Senel FC, Ungor C, Tosun E, Cankaya M, Ersoz S, et al. The effects of adjunctive parathyroid hormone injection on bisphosphonate-related osteonecrosis of the jaws: an animal study. Int J Oral Maxillofac Surg. 2013;42:1475-1480.

[89] Vescovi P, Merigo E, Meleti M, Manfredi M. Bisphosphonate-associated osteonecrosis [BON] of the jaws: a possible treatment? J Oral Maxillofac Surg 2006;64:1460-1462.

[90] Rugani P, Truschnegg A, Acham S, Kirnbauer B, Jakse N. Use of Photodynamic Therapy in Treatment of Bisphosphonate-related Osteonecrosis of the Jaws: Literature Review and Case Series. J Anal Bioanal Tech. 2013;S1:006. doi:10.4172/2155-9872.S1-006

[91] Mester E, Mester AF, Mester A. The biomedical effects of laser application. Lasers Surg Med. 1985;5:31-39.

[92] Liao HF, Chen QJ, Yi JL, Feng Z, Zhang XR, et al. Semiconductor low level laser irradiation for exposure of hydroxyapatite orbital implants. Zhonghua Zheng Xing Wai Ke Za Zhi. 2004;20:177-179.

[93] Stein A, Benayahu D, Maltz L, Oron U. Low-level laser irradiation promotes proliferation and differentiation of human osteoblasts in vitro. Photomed Laser Surg. 2005;23:161-166.

[94] Karu T, Pyatibrat L, Kalendo G. Irradiation with He-Ne laser increases ATP level in cells cultivated in vitro. J Photochem Photobiol B. 1995;27:219-223.

[95] Hamblin MR, Hasan T. Photodynamic therapy: a new antimicrobial approach to infectious disease? Photochem Photobiol Sci. 2004;3:436-450.

[96] Meisel P, Kocher T. Photodynamic therapy for periodontal diseases: state of the art. J Photochem Photobiol B. 2005;79:159-170.

[97] Komerik N, MacRobert AJ. Photodynamic therapy as an alternative antimicrobial modality for oral infections. J Environ Pathol Toxicol Oncol. 2006;25:487-504.

[98] Donnelly RF, McCarron PA, Tunney MM, David Woolfson A. Potential of photodynamic therapy in treatment of fungal infections of the mouth. Design and characterisation of a mucoadhesive patch containing toluidine blue O. J Photochem Photobiol B. 2007;86:59-69.

[99] Zancanela DC, Primo FL, Rosa AL, Ciancaglini P, Tedesco AC. The effect of photosensitizer drugs and light stimulation on osteoblast growth. Photomed Laser Surg. 2011;29:699-705.

[100] Morley S, Griffiths J, Philips G, Moseley H, O'Grady C, et al. Phase IIa randomized, placebo-controlled study of antimicrobial photodynamic therapy in bacterially colonized, chronic leg ulcers and diabetic foot ulcers: a new approach to antimicrobial therapy. Br J Dermatol.2013;168:617-624.

[101] Peplow PV, Chung TY, Baxter GD. Photodynamic modulation of wound healing: a review of human and animal studies. Photomed Laser Surg. 2012;30:118-148.

[102] Simonetti O, Cirioni O, Orlando F, Alongi C, Lucarini G, et al. Effectiveness of antimicrobial photodynamic therapy with a single treatment of RLP068/Cl in an experimental model of *Staphylococcus aureus* wound infection. Br J Dermatol. 2011;164:987-995.

[103] Haas R, Dörtbudak O, Mensdorff-Pouilly N, Mailath G. Elimination of bacteria on different implant surfaces through photosensitization and soft laser. An in vitro study. Clin Oral Implants Res. 1997;8:249-254.

[104] Takasaki AA, Aoki A, Mizutani K, Schwarz F, Sculean A, et al. Application of antimicrobial photodynamic therapy in periodontal and peri-implant diseases. Periodontol 2000. 2009;51:109-140.

[105] Raghavendra M, Koregol A, Bhola S. Photodynamic therapy: a targeted therapy in periodontics. Aust Dent J. 2009;54 Suppl 1:102-109.

[106] Sasaki KM, Aoki A, Ichinose S, Ishikawa I. Ultrastructural analysis of bone tissue irradiated by Er:YAG Laser. Lasers Surg Med. 2002;31:322-332.

[107] Pourzarandian A, Watanabe H, Aoki A, Ichinose S, Sasaki KM, et al. Histological and TEM examination of early stages of bone healing after Er:YAG laser irradiation. Photomed Laser Surg. 2004; 22:342-350.

[108] da Guarda MG, Paraguassú GM, Cerqueira NS, Cury PR, Farias JG, et al. Laser GaAlAs [Î»860 nm] photobiomodulation for the treatment of bisphosphonate-induced osteonecrosis of the jaw. Photomed Laser Surg. 2012;30:293-297.

[109] Hansen T, Kunkel M, Springer E, Walter C, Weber A, et al. Actinomycosis of the jaws--histopathological study of 45 patients shows significant involvement in bisphosphonate-associated osteonecrosis and infected osteoradionecrosis. Virchows Arch. 2007;451:1009-1017.

[110] Sedghizadeh PP, Yooseph S, Fadrosh DW, Zeigler-Allen L, Thiagarajan M, et al. Metagenomic investigation of microbes and viruses in patients with jaw osteonecrosis associated with bisphosphonate therapy. Oral Surg Oral Med Oral Pathol Oral Radiol. 2012;114:764-770.

[111] Konopka K, Goslinski T. Photodynamic therapy in dentistry. J Dent Res. 2007;86:694-707.

Chapter 7

Strategies to Improve Drug Delivery in Topical PDT

Michelle Barreto Requena, Mirian Denise Stringasci, José Dirceu Vollet-Filho and Vanderlei Salvador Bagnato

Abstract

Topical photodynamic therapy (PDT) has been applied to treat premalignant and malignant lesions such as actinic keratosis and non-melanoma skin cancer. A limiting factor of the technique is cream permeation and studies using chemical and physical approaches to overcome it have increased over the years. This chapter is going to explore the main techniques described in the literature used to improve the cream permeation or the photosensitizer (PS) distribution concerning homogeneity. Outcomes-based on animal studies and clinical trials comparing different delivery techniques are going to be presented, highlighting the aspects of invasiveness, costs, harmfulness, and effectiveness of those methods.

Keywords: topical photodynamic therapy, drug delivery, skin cancer, protoporphyrin IX, precursors

1. Introduction

Yet topical photodynamic therapy (PDT) principle is simple and the technique is full of potential to provide an effective treatment for very common malignant and pre-malignant diseases, achieving satisfactory outcomes for a varied number of lesion types with a single approach is not feasible.

Light delivery is successful depending essentially on the ability to provide the best combination of the most suitable wavelength for the drug of choice and the optical properties of the tissue, which determine if light reaches the extension of tissue necessary and if undesired side effects will show up.

Conversely, characteristics on the photosensitizer (PS) accumulation in target tissues are less dependent on direct control of the therapist than light delivery. Further, PS accumulation also defines the light dose (fluency). Therefore, PS accumulation must be properly dealt with in order to provide enhancement of the efficacy of PDT, and presenting the most relevant aspects reported in the literature concerning the strategies to do so is the scope of this chapter.

Topical PDT has been widely applied as a treatment option for pre-malignant lesions such as actinic keratosis (AK) and also for non-melanoma skin cancer (NMSC) lesions [1] such as basal cell carcinoma (BCC) and Bowen disease (BD). The treatment involves the topical application of a PS precursor, followed by the waiting for the drug light interval (DLI) to promote the PS accumulation into the lesion, after which the localized irradiation takes place. Depending on the protocol, this sequence can be repeated with intervals of one week [2–5] or on the same day [6].

The molecules more commonly used worldwide are the aminolevulinic acid (ALA) and its derivative, methyl aminolevulinate (MAL). Both of them can promote protoporphyrin IX (PpIX) endogenous accumulation in cells. The DLI for these drugs can vary from 1 to 4 hours [7], depending on the protocol treatment chosen for the lesion type.

Being clinical PDT still a very empirical field, and since the protocols choices are decisive in determining the therapy outcome, several strategies, both physical and chemical, have been developed aiming to increase the availability of PS *in loco* to increase topical PDT outcome.

2. Drug delivery strategies

Considering the light attenuation by tissue due to the presence of chromophores and to scattering, the wavelength range preferable for PDT is about 650–850 nm, which is known as the 'optical window' for PDT [8]. Once the light penetration can be handled to reach the whole lesion, the remaining concern is to optimize the drug permeation to improve treatment rate success, especially obtaining the improvement of the response of thicker lesions, which shall increase the possibility to make PDT the treatment of choice for those lesions.

Human skin is a complex organ structured to protect the body. The skin layers organization and constitution, as represented in **Figure 1** (*stratum corneum* (SC), epidermis, dermis, and hypodermis) confer its properties of tensile strength and mechanical resistance [9]. For this reason, skin becomes a barrier for the permeation of precursors, which implies an important limitation of topical PDT, with a direct influence on the incubation time and treatment success. The SC is the skin's outermost layer, and it is considered the main barrier to percutaneous absorption.

Although PpIX precursors have a low molecular weight, the PpIX accumulation after as much as three hours of incubation using exclusively topical application of the cream achieves depths up to 1–2 mm. However, the tissue heterogeneities imply in a non-uniform distribution of the produced PpIX, and portions of the lesion do not produce sufficient PS, impairing the treatment effectiveness [10, 11].

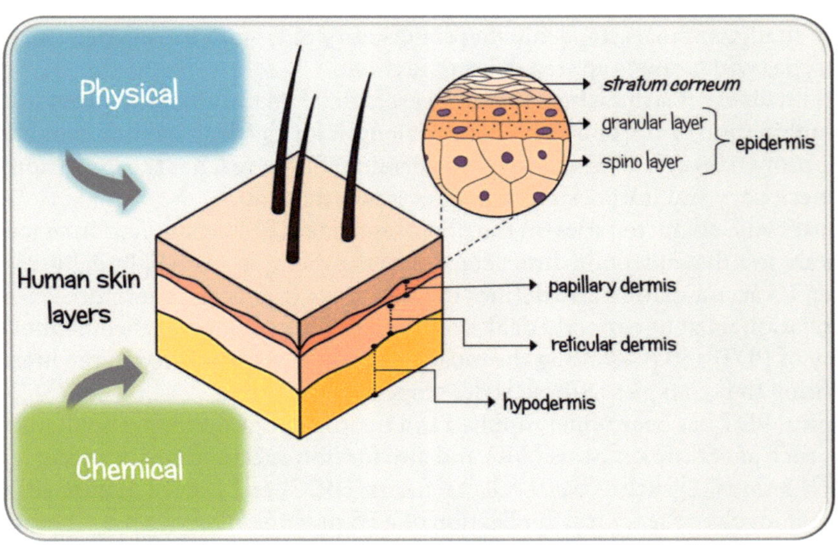

Figure 1.
Representation of human skin layers. Both physical and chemical methods can be explored to overcome the skin barriers and improve topical drug delivery.

Several techniques have been developed to overcome skin barriers and provide penetration enhancement. There are physical and chemical pretreatment strategies to improve drug delivery that can facilitate precursor permeation through skin and into the lesions, allowing PpIX to be produced in deeper layers and also to be distributed more homogeneously.

3. Physical methods

This section presents physical methods based either on creating holes into the skin or on removing the SC to improve drug delivery in topical PDT.

3.1 Tape stripping

This technique consists in applying a tape onto the skin lesions and then to pull it off. By repeating this procedure a number times, which can be repeated using the same piece of tape, part of the SC is removed, reducing it uniformly by about 30%. This procedure is safe, since it is minimally invasive, and involves a low cost to be implemented; as a further advantage, it does not interfere with the intercellular lipids [12–14].

Tape stripping is one of the methods indicated to be applied before PDT; it can be used on patient's lips and also for the preparation of large areas. The recommendation is to choose tapes with strong adhesive properties. According to Christensen *et al.*, each area can be stripped 2–4 times [15]. Some studies reported that removing SC by tape stripping significantly increases the PpIX fluorescence in the tissue but does not change the incubation time required for an effective photosensitizer production [16–18].

3.2 Curettage

The curettage can be performed using a sharp ring curette or a scalpel blade. The purpose is to remove keratotic tissue by surface scraping the lesion. The scrape might be performed in a checkered pattern, performing parallel horizontal followed by perpendicular movements. Due to the possibility of subclinical lesion extensions, it is recommended that the curettage is performed using at least 5-mm margins surrounding the lesion to minimize the possibility of the recurrence. The curettage is also indicated to be applied before PDT [13, 15].

This technique is effective, quite inexpensive, and although it can offer light discomfort during the procedure, it is commonly acceptable both by health professionals and patients [19]. However, it is important to mention that there is a risk of bleeding, and when bleeding takes place, it may displace the cream and lead to a decreased PpIX formation, and thus lower treatment efficacy [20]. Despite this, studies reported that curettage associated with PDT increases the cure rate of treatment compared with no-curettage topical PDT. The combination may be repeated successfully for non-cure or recurrence cases without compromising the cosmetic effect or deteriorating skin structures. The treatment has shown a clearance rate of 91% for superficial BCC (131 lesions treated), 93% for thin nodular BCC (82 lesions), and 86% for thick nodular BCC (86 lesions) [21, 22].

3.3 Debulking

Debulking (or deep curettage) is considered a surgical procedure and it is often used in thicker lesions, reducing as much as possible the total volume. This procedure is usually performed either immediately or a few weeks before PDT [15, 23].

Even though it is considered a more invasive procedure compared with the simple curettage, it can be applied without anesthesia. The cosmetic outcome is considered favorable [23] and allows a significant reduction of the BCC thickness, which makes nodular lesions more responsive to the treatment [24, 25].

Whereas the topical PDT efficiency is about 72% when a previous debulking lesion is not applied, for debulked lesions this efficiency can increase up to 92% [23, 26]. Therefore, the debulking associated with PDT is a relevant option for multiple, pigmented, and nodular lesions, improving clinical response [27].

3.4 Ablative fractional laser

This technique consists of using a laser source to create ablated channels on the lesion surface, vaporizing a small portion of the tissue [28]. Usually, lasers with excitation wavelengths in far-infrared spectrum are used, due to the high absorption by the water in the tissue [29, 30]. The main types used are CO2-laser (10,600 nm), Er:YAG-laser (Erbium yttrium aluminum garnet, 2940 nm), and Er:YSSG-laser (Yttrium scandium gallium garnet, 2790 nm) [13].

The depth of the microchannels created varies according to the laser energy. The energies between 32 mJ and 380 mJ generate microchannels with a depth between 300 μm and 2100 μm [31]. Due to the increased skin penetration, this procedure makes PpIX fluorescence both more intense and homogeneous in deeper skin regions, and this can be controlled by adequately adjusting laser energy density [32, 33].

Studies using CO2 laser associated with PDT for lesions treatments showed an increase of about 20% in the clearance of different protocols comparing the treatment without and with the use of laser, respectively [34–36]. Although it is a reliable and effective method, it is also a more invasive procedure with a high potential for skin damage with scarring, discoloration, and even infection. Besides that, the costs of the devices are considered high compared with the abovementioned techniques [37].

3.5 Microneedles

Needles and especially microneedles (MNs) have been used as a method to enhance drug permeation through SC [38]. MNs have the advantages of being minimally invasive, its application is simple, well accepted by the patients, and it is cost-effective [39]. MNs have been developed with lengths up to 900 μm to avoid penetrating in vascular and nervous regions. Therefore, MNs can penetrate the SC without stimulating pain receptors, which is another advantage [40].

The MNs size cannot be seen by patients, thus reducing possible needle phobia. MNs have strong mechanical properties to enable disruption and penetration through the SC, reaching successfully the deeper skin layers without causing any bleeding due to the small length of needles [13].

There are MNs with different shapes (tetrahedron, pyramidal, conical, beveled tip, or tapered cone) that promote different insertion pathways and permeation into the skin. They also can be divided according to the material, such as solid (metallic) or polymeric (hydrogel or dissolving) types, and can be assembled either as a roller or as low-cost patches. The MNs can also be produced with a drug coating on their surface, to facilitate delivery, or hollow, to promote the delivery through channels [13]. The use of MNs rollers for enhancing penetration of topical cosmeceuticals has been well described and transdermal patches can be used easily by anyone [13, 39].

Some studies described a higher formation of PpIX in deeper skin regions when MNs are used and compared with topical application in animal models [41, 42]. A recent paper by Requena *et al.* explored dissolving MNs containing ALA. The PpIX fluorescence intensity showed to be 5-times higher at 0.5 mm on average compared with cream in *in vivo* tumor mice model [43].

Solid MNs have been commonly used for skin pretreatment before conventional PDT, promoting a good PDT response for actinic keratosis [39]. However, their use for the treatment of BCC or squamous cell carcinoma SCC has not been investigated yet [13].

3.6 Dermograph

The use of dermographs has also been investigated to improve drug delivery. A dermograph is a device currently used in esthetic procedures, which works similarly to a tattoo machine, with simpler handling [44]. The device is composed of a handpiece that couples to different types of needles which oscillate vertically. Usually, both frequency and depth can be adjusted in those devices, according to the application. The holes performed into the skin allow for greater skin penetration of liquids by capillarity [45, 46].

A more homogeneous PpIX distribution and a greater penetration in the tissue were observed for animal model using dermographs compared to the topical application of the cream only [46]. A pilot clinical trial was also performed in nodular BCC lesions using a dermograph for intradermal delivery in PDT, and no recurrence was observed after 28 months of follow-up [46].

3.7 Temperature

Temperature is a parameter with a strong influence on PpIX formation. The increase of the skin temperature (especially in areas that naturally present lower temperatures such as the extremities of the body) during the DLI can improve PDT effectiveness. There are four hypotheses regarding the PpIX formation with the increase of local temperature: increase of ALA penetration in the skin; increase of the conversion rate of ALA to PpIX; increased ALA uptake in the cells due to disruption of the cell membrane, and increase of the amount of skin oxygen due to vasodilation [13, 47].

However, the temperature must be well controlled in order to obtain the desired effect and prevent damage to surrounding tissues [48]. Stringasci *et al.* demonstrated that the most efficient way to increase the production of PpIX and its penetration in the tissue by temperature is to increase the local temperature before applying the cream. This same study reported that the prolonged increase of temperature (during 3 hours) promoted a smaller amount of PpIX accumulation in the skin, unlike other abovementioned hypotheses. That happens because, after increasing the temperature for longer times, cellular metabolism is accelerated which promotes faster elimination of PpIX within the cells [47]. In a clinical study, Willey *et al.* reported the results after PDT treatment of AK on the extremities (head, fingers, and toes) in 18 patients. Skin warming was performed during DLI and was well tolerated, did not promote side effects, and improved PDT efficacy with a clearance rate of 90% after a 1-year follow-up [49].

3.8 Iontophoresis

Iontophoresis is a method based on the use of a voltage gradient applied to an electrolytic formulation, using both a positive (anode) and negative (cathode) electrodes on skin to improve transdermal drug delivery [50]. The advantages of iontophoresis are that it is a non-invasive technique that preserves the skin intact, providing controlled and targeted delivery of the drug. However, regarding PDT, special attention should be taken to ensure that the photosensitizing drug does not enter the systemic circulation, which can cause unexpected side effects [51].

This technique has a potential to decrease the DLI since *ex vivo* experiments demonstrated PpIX accumulation in human SC were achieved faster compared with topical application only [51]. In addition, studies with patients proved that the use of iontophoresis in clinical protocols is an effective method and reduces the incubation time by 1 h [52].

4. Chemical methods

Currently, only three commercial pro-drugs are licensed for topical PDT use: 5-aminolevulinic acid (ALA, Levulan®), methyl aminolevulinate (MAL, Metvix®), and the nanoemulsion containing ALA (nc-ALA, Ameluz®) [53]. Besides the physical methods to improve the delivery of these drugs, there are chemical approaches that have been explored for drug formulation modifications, and the use of agents that modify the heme cycle or enhance PpIX formation. Thus, the chemical methods to improve PpIX availability mostly treat on the effects over these substances.

4.1 Prodrugs

To enhance ALA penetration through the SC, other prodrugs with longer, more lipophilic carbon chains have been explored [54]. In this context, MAL – which has a methyl group associated with the ALA molecule – already presented more lipophilicity properties and increased selectivity.

The use of even more carbon chains has been tested, such as ethyl-ALA, propyl-ALA, butyl-ALA. The main concern about their use is related to the numerous chemical steps necessary to perform the esterification processes for those molecules [55]. The pro-drug hexyl-ALA has been tested in pre-clinical studies [18, 56]. A pilot clinical trial reported that these molecules presented a greater penetration with lower concentrations compared with ALA or MAL which could reduce adverse reactions and decreases the PDT costs [57]. Despite that, ALA and its ester MAL are still the most commonly chosen and investigated molecules to be used as PpIX pro-drugs for PDT.

One aspect explored in literature for the enhancement of the PpIX prodrugs in cells is the addition of iron chelators. Iron has a crucial role in cells within the heme synthetic route, bound to PpIX molecules to form hemoglobin, thus hindering this process preserves the number of available PpIX molecules within cells. Different chelators have been investigated so far as and, such as desferrioxamine, thiosemicarbazones, pyridoxalisonicotinoyl hydrazone, and di-2-pyridyl-derived iron chelators, among others [58–60]. However, yet thiosemicarbazones have been approved for phase II tests [61], the use of these chelators is still under discussion, due to toxicity versus efficacy issues.

4.2 Differentiation-promoting agents

In addition to the drug choice, different vehicles such as creams, gels, patch systems, lotions, liposomes, nanoparticles, powders, and microemulsions have been developed to overcome the penetration issue [13].

The commercial creams Levulan® and Metvix® are prepared with 20% w/w and 16% w/w concentration of prodrug, respectively. Both of them have been widely used with acceptable clearance rates and cosmetic outcomes. Aiming to increase the stability of the cream, the molecule of ALA at 7.8% concentration in a nanoemulsion-based gel has been used to produce the Ameluz® formulation. A multicentric study compared this gel formulation with the Metvix® cream in the treatment of AK, demonstrating similar response and tolerance [62].

A patch is an adhesive system used for topical or systemic drug delivery. For PDT, there is a commercial patch (Alacare®) containing 2 mg of ALA per cm^2. A clinical trial using Alacare® for the PDT treatment of actinic cheilitis (AC) demonstrated high clinical efficacy, good tolerability, and favorable cosmetic effects [63]. However, in the case of thick skin lesions without physical pretreatment, this protocol might be less efficient.

4.3 Nanoformulations

Nanotechnology has an important role in the pharmaceutical industry for the development of new formulations. Studies are concentrated on obtaining drugs with more solubility, biodistribution, bioavailability, uptake, and excretion, decreasing drugs' toxicity, [64] and there are different vehicles to promote drug delivery by nanostructures.

Nanoparticles (NP) used to be defined as a particle with a size up to 100 nm in any direction [65]. Lucky *et al.* described the nanoparticles used in PDT based on their performed functions or tasks as PSs, PS carriers, and PS energy transducers [66].

Among the several NP possibilities, liposomes are one of the most used for topical PDT applications. Liposomes are vesicles made up of one or more phospholipid bilayers oriented concentrically around an aqueous compartment to act as drug carriers. This nanostructure has been explored for topical PDT to enhance the PS penetration into the skin while decreasing its absorption into systemic circulation. Examples of PSs currently encapsulated in liposomes for topical PDT are ALA, temoporfin (mTHPC, commercially available as Foscan®), and methylene blue. In most studies, liposomal ALA induced a higher PpIX synthesis than free ALA non-encapsulated delivery [67].

Other structures are more commonly used for systemic applications of PDT, such as nanofibers and nanomicelles [68, 69] but they are off the scope of this chapter, yet their results are also promising for PDT application.

4.4 Thermogenic and vasodilating substances

Thermogenic and vasodilating substances have been reported as promising to favor the permeation of drugs on the skin [70, 71]. In PDT, vasodilation also increases the oxygen supply in the tissue, which can further optimize the effectiveness of the treatment.

A study was carried out investigating the association of the substances: menthol, methyl nicotinate, and ginger associated with ALA and MAL. The association of methyl nicotinate with MAL demonstrated 50% higher PpIX production after three hours of incubation compared with the cream containing only MAL. These preclinical results are promising as a possible strategy for decreasing the DLI and increase the PpIX production in skin lesions [72].

5. Conclusion

This chapter presented several approaches reported in the literature for the improvement of topical PDT outcome. Some of the techniques here presented to address the task of increasing the availability of PS are increasingly being incorporated to PDT protocols, whereas others are very incipient. Yet, the challenge of making PS available is still an open field, plenty of room for further investigation.

Acknowledgments

We acknowledge support from São Paulo Research Foundation (FAPESP) [grant numbers 2013/07276-1 (CEPOF), 2009/54035-4 (EMU), 2014/50857-8 (INCT)].

Author details

Michelle Barreto Requena[1*], Mirian Denise Stringasci[1], José Dirceu Vollet-Filho[1] and Vanderlei Salvador Bagnato[1,2]

1 Sao Carlos Institute of Physics, University of Sao Paulo (USP), São Carlos, SP, Brazil

2 Hagler Institute for Advance Studies, Texas A&M University, College Station, USA

*Address all correspondence to: requenamichelle@gmail.com

References

[1] Nguyen K, Khachemoune A. An update on topical photodynamic therapy for clinical dermatologists. J. Dermatolog. Treat. 2019

[2] Cabete J, Rafael M, Cravo M, Moura C, Sachse F, Pecegueiro M. Long-term recurrence of nonmelanoma skin cancer after topical methylaminolevulinate photodynamic therapy in a dermato-oncology department. An. Bras. Dermatol. 2015;90(6):846-50.

[3] Buzzá HH, Moriyama LT, Vollet-Filho JD, Inada NM, da Silva AP, Stringasci MD, et al. Overall Results for a National Program of Photodynamic Therapy for Basal Cell Carcinoma: A Multicenter Clinical Study to Bring New Techniques to Social Health Care. Cancer Control [Internet]. 2019 Jan 26;26(1):107327481985688. Available from: http://journals.sagepub.com/doi/10.1177/1073274819856885

[4] Ramirez DP, Kurachi C, Inada NM, Moriyama LT, Salvio AG, Vollet Filho JD, et al. Experience and BCC subtypes as determinants of MAL-PDT response: Preliminary results of a national Brazilian project. Photodiagnosis Photodyn. Ther. 2014;11(1):22-6.

[5] Peris K, Fargnoli MC, Garbe C, Kaufmann R, Bastholt L, Seguin NB, et al. Diagnosis and treatment of basal cell carcinoma: European consensus–based interdisciplinary guidelines. Eur. J. Cancer. 2019;118:10-34.

[6] Ramirez DP, Moriyama LT, de Oliveira ER, Inada NM, Bagnato VS, Kurachi C, et al. Single visit PDT for basal cell carcinoma – a new therapeutic protocol. Photodiagnosis Photodyn. Ther. [Internet]. 2019 Jun;26:375-82. Available from: https://linkinghub.elsevier.com/retrieve/pii/S1572100019301206

[7] Wan MT, Lin JY. Current evidence and applications of photodynamic therapy in dermatology. Clin. Cosmet. Investig. Dermatol. 2014.

[8] Plaetzer K, Krammer B, Berlanda J, Berr F, Kiesslich T. Photophysics and photochemistry of photodynamic therapy: Fundamental aspects. Lasers Med. Sci. 2009;24(2):259-68.

[9] Khavkin J, Ellis DAF. Aging Skin: Histology, Physiology, and Pathology. Facial Plast. Surg. Clin. North Am. 2011. p. 229-34.

[10] LaRochelle EPM, Marra K, LeBlanc RE, Chapman MS, Maytin E V., Pogue BW. Modeling PpIX effective light fluence at depths into the skin for PDT dose comparison. Photodiagnosis Photodyn. Ther. Elsevier; 2019 Mar;25 (January):425-35.

[11] Peng Q, Soler AM, Warloe T, Nesland JM, Giercksky K-E. Selective distribution of porphyrins in skin thick basal cell carcinoma after topical application of methyl 5-aminolevulinate. J. Photochem. Photobiol. B Biol. 2001 Sep;62(3):140-5.

[12] Pellett MA, Roberts MS, Hadgraft J. Supersaturated solutions evaluated with an in vitro stratum corneum tape stripping technique. Int. J. Pharm. 1997;

[13] Champeau M, Vignoud S, Mortier L, Mordon S. Photodynamic therapy for skin cancer: How to enhance drug penetration? J. Photochem. Photobiol. B Biol. [Internet]. 2019 Aug;197:111544. Available from: https://linkinghub.elsevier.com/retrieve/pii/S1011134418312715

[14] SURBER, Christian; SCHWARB FP., SMITH EW. Tape-stripping technique. Drugs Pharm. Sci. 1999. p. 395-410.

[15] Christensen E, Warloe T, Kroon S, Funk J, Helsing P, Soler AM, et al. Guidelines for practical use of MAL-PDT in non-melanoma skin cancer. J. Eur. Acad. Dermatol. Venereol. 2010;24(5):505-12.

[16] Lesar A, Ferguson J, Moseley H. An investigation of the fluorescence induced by topical application of 5-aminolaevulinic acid and methyl aminolaevulinate at different body sites on normal human skin. Photodiagnosis Photodyn. Ther. 2011 Jun;8(2):97-103.

[17] Goff BA, Bachor R, Kollias N, Hasan T. Effects of photodynamic therapy with topical application of 5-aminolevulinic acid on normal skin of hairless guinea pigs. J. Photochem. Photobiol. B Biol. 1992 Aug;15(3):239-51.

[18] van den Akker JTHM, Iani V, Star WM, Sterenborg HJCM, Moan J. Topical Application of 5-Aminolevulinic Acid Hexyl Ester and 5-Aminolevulinic Acid to Normal Nude Mouse Skin: Differences in Protoporphyrin IX Fluorescence Kinetics and the Role of the Stratum Corneum¶. Photochem. Photobiol. 2000;

[19] See J-A, Shumack S, Murrell DF, Rubel DM, Fernández-Peñas P, Salmon R, et al. Consensus recommendations on the use of daylight photodynamic therapy with methyl aminolevulinate cream for actinic keratoses in Australia. Australas. J. Dermatol. 2016 Aug;57(3):167-74.

[20] Nissen C V., Wiegell SR, Philipsen PA, Wulf HC. Short-term chemical pretreatment cannot replace curettage in photodynamic therapy. Photodermatol. Photoimmunol. Photomed. 2016;

[21] Soler AM, Warloe T, Berner A, Giercksky KE. A follow-up study of recurrence and cosmesis in completely responding superficial and nodular basal cell carcinomas treated with methyl 5-aminolaevulinate-based photodynamic therapy alone and with prior curettage. Br. J. Dermatol. [Internet]. 2008 Jul 18;145(3):467-71. Available from: http://doi.wiley.com/10.1111/j.1365-2133.2001.04407.x

[22] Soler AM, Warloe T, TausjØ J, Berner A. Photodynamic therapy by topical aminolevulinic acid, dimethylsulphoxide and curettage in nodular basal cell carcinoma: A one-year follow-up study. Acta Derm. Venereol. 1999;

[23] Thissen MRTM, Schroeter CA, Neumann HAM. SHORT COMMUNICATIONPhotodynamic therapy with delta-aminolaevulinic acid for nodular basal cell carcinomas using a prior debulking technique. Br. J. Dermatol. 2000 Feb;142(2):338-9.

[24] Christensen E, Mørk C, Foss OA. Pre-Treatment Deep Curettage Can Significantly Reduce Tumour Thickness in Thick Basal Cell Carcinoma While Maintaining a Favourable Cosmetic Outcome When Used in Combination with Topical Photodynamic Therapy. J. Skin Cancer. 2011;

[25] Thissen MRTM, Schroeter CA, Neumann HAM. Photodynamic therapy with delta-aminolaevulinic acid for nodular basal cell carcinomas using a prior debulking technique. Br. J. Dermatol. 2000;142(2):338-9.

[26] Arits AHMM, Mosterd K, Essers BAB, Spoorenberg E, Sommer A, De Rooij MJM, et al. Photodynamic therapy versus topical imiquimod versus topical fluorouracil for treatment of superficial basal-cell carcinoma: a single blind, non-inferiority, randomised controlled trial. Lancet Oncol. 2013 Jun;14(7):647-54.

[27] Souza CS, Neves ABS, Felício LAB, Ferreira J, Kurachi C, Bagnato VS. Optimized photodynamic therapy with

systemic photosensitizer following debulking technique for nonmelanoma skin cancers. Dermatologic Surg. 2007;33(2):194-8.

[28] Prakash S, Kumar S. Fabrication of microchannels: A review. Proc. Inst. Mech. Eng. Part B J. Eng. Manuf. 2015 Aug;229(8):1273-88.

[29] Haedersdal M, Sakamoto FH, Farinelli WA, Doukas AG, Tam J, Anderson RR. Pretreatment with ablative fractional laser changes kinetics and biodistribution of topical 5-aminolevulinic acid (ALA) and methyl aminolevulinate (MAL). Lasers Surg. Med. 2014 Aug;46(6):462-9.

[30] Taudorf EH, Haak CS, Erlendsson AM, Philipsen PA, Anderson RR, Paasch U, et al. Fractional ablative erbium YAG laser: Histological characterization of relationships between laser settings and micropore dimensions. Lasers Surg. Med. 2014 Apr;46(4):281-9.

[31] Haak CS, Farinelli WA, Tam J, Doukas AG, Anderson RR, Haedersdal M. Fractional laser-assisted delivery of methyl aminolevulinate: Impact of laser channel depth and incubation time. Lasers Surg. Med. 2012 Dec;44(10):787-95.

[32] Song HS, Jung S-E, Jang YH, Kang HY, Lee E-S, Kim YC. Fractional carbon dioxide laser-assisted photodynamic therapy for patients with actinic keratosis. Photodermatol. Photoimmunol. Photomed. 2015 Nov;31(6):296-301.

[33] Haak CS, Christiansen K, Erlendsson AM, Taudorf EH, Thaysen-Petersen D, Wulf HC, et al. Ablative fractional laser enhances MAL-induced PpIX accumulation: Impact of laser channel density, incubation time and drug concentration. J. Photochem. Photobiol. B Biol. 2016 Jun;159:42-8.

[34] Alexiades M. Randomized, Controlled Trial of Fractional Carbon Dioxide Laser Resurfacing Followed by Ultrashort Incubation Aminolevulinic Acid Blue Light Photodynamic Therapy for Actinic Keratosis. Dermatologic Surg. 2017 Aug;43(8):1053-64.

[35] Haak CS, Togsverd-Bo K, Thaysen-Petersen D, Wulf HC, Paasch U, Anderson RR, et al. Fractional laser-mediated photodynamic therapy of high-risk basal cell carcinomas - a randomized clinical trial. Br. J. Dermatol. 2015 Jan;172(1):215-22.

[36] Choi SH, Kim KH, Song KH. Er:YAG ablative fractional laser-primed photodynamic therapy with methyl aminolevulinate as an alternative treatment option for patients with thin nodular basal cell carcinoma: 12-month follow-up results of a randomized, prospective, comparative trial. J. Eur. Acad. Dermatology Venereol. 2016 May;30(5):783-8.

[37] Preissig J, Hamilton K, Markus R. Current Laser Resurfacing Technologies: A Review that Delves Beneath the Surface. Semin. Plast. Surg. 2012 Nov;26(03):109-16.

[38] McAllister D V., Wang PM, Davis SP, Park J-H, Canatella PJ, Allen MG, et al. Microfabricated needles for transdermal delivery of macromolecules and nanoparticles: Fabrication methods and transport studies. Proc. Natl. Acad. Sci. 2003 Nov;100(24):13755-60.

[39] Clementoni MT, B-Roscher M, Munavalli GS. Photodynamic photorejuvenation of the face with a combination of microneedling, red light, and broadband pulsed light. Lasers Surg. Med. 2010 Feb;42(2):150-9.

[40] Mikolajewska P, Donnelly RF, Garland MJ, Morrow DIJ, Singh TRR, Iani V, et al. Microneedle pre-treatment of human skin improves

5-aminolevulininc acid (ALA)- and 5-aminolevulinic acid methyl ester (MAL)-induced PpIX production for topical photodynamic therapy without increase in pain or erythema. Pharm. Res. 2010;

[41] Jain AK, Lee CH, Gill HS. 5-Aminolevulinic acid coated microneedles for photodynamic therapy of skin tumors. J. Control. Release. 2016 Oct;239:72-81.

[42] Gracielli Sousa RP, de Menezes PFC, Fujita AKL, Requena MB, Govone AB, Escobar A, et al. Microneedles rollers as a potential device to increase ALA diffusion and PpIX production: evaluations by wide-field fluorescence imaging and fluorescence spectroscopy. In: Choi B, Kollias N, Zeng H, Kang HW, Wong BJF, Ilgner JF, et al., editors. 2014. p. 892614. Available from: http://proceedings.spiedigitallibrary.org/proceeding.aspx?doi=10.1117/12.2040618

[43] Requena MB, Permana AD, Vollet-Filho JD, González-Vázquez P, Garcia MR, Faria CMG, et al. Dissolving microneedles containing aminolevulinic acid improves protoporphyrin <scp>IX</scp> distribution. J. Biophotonics [Internet]. 2020 Sep 27;jbio.202000128. Available from: https://onlinelibrary.wiley.com/doi/10.1002/jbio.202000128

[44] Arbache S, de Godoy CE. Microinfusion of drugs into the skin with tattoo equipment. Surg. Cosmet. Dermatology. 2013;

[45] van der Velden EM, Ijsselmuiden OE, Drost BH, Baruchin a M. Dermatography with bleomycin as a new treatment for verrucae vulgaris. Int. J. Dermatol. 1997;36(2):145-50.

[46] Requena MB, Russignoli PE, Vollet-Filho JD, Salvio AG, Fortunato TC, Pratavieira S, et al. Use of dermograph for improvement of PpIX precursor's delivery in Photodynamic Therapy: experimental and clinical pilot studies. Photodiagnosis Photodyn. Ther. [Internet]. 2019 Nov;101599. Available from: https://linkinghub.elsevier.com/retrieve/pii/S1572100019305344

[47] Stringasci MD, Moriyama LT, Vollet-Filho JD, Bagnato VS. Temperature effect on the PpIX production during the use of topical precursors. Photodiagnosis Photodyn. Ther. 2020 Jun;30:101786.

[48] Yang J, Chen AC-H, Wu Q, Jiang S, Liu X, Xiong L, et al. The influence of temperature on 5-aminolevulinic acid-based photodynamic reaction in keratinocytes in vitro. Photodermatol. Photoimmunol. Photomed. 2010 Mar;26(2):83-8.

[49] Willey A, Anderson RR, Sakamoto FH. Temperature-Modulated Photodynamic Therapy for the Treatment of Actinic Keratosis on the Extremities. Dermatologic Surg. 2014 Oct;40(10):1094-102.

[50] Lemos CN, De Souza JG, Simão PS, Lopez RFV. Iontophoresis improved growth reduction of invasive squamous cell carcinoma in topical photodynamic therapy. PLoS One. 2016;

[51] Gratieri T, Kalia YN. Topical Iontophoresis for Targeted Local Drug Delivery to the Eye and Skin. 2014. p. 263-84.

[52] Choi S-H, Kim T-H, Song K-H. Efficacy of iontophoresis-assisted ablative fractional laser photodynamic therapy with short incubation time for the treatment of actinic keratosis: 12-month follow-up results of a prospective, randomised, comparative trial. Photodiagnosis Photodyn. Ther. 2017 Jun;18:105-10.

[53] Wong TH, Morton CA, Collier N, Haylett A, Ibbotson S, McKenna KE, et al. British Association of Dermatologists

and British Photodermatology Group guidelines for topical photodynamic therapy 2018. Br. J. Dermatol. [Internet]. 2019 Apr 2;180(4):730-9. Available from: https://onlinelibrary.wiley.com/doi/abs/10.1111/bjd.17309

[54] Kiesslich T, Helander L, Illig R, Oberdanner C, Wagner A, Lettner H, et al. Real-time analysis of endogenous protoporphyrin IX fluorescence from δ-aminolevulinic acid and its derivatives reveals distinct time- and dose-dependent characteristics in vitro . J. Biomed. Opt. 2014;

[55] Zhu W, Gao Y-H, Song C-H, Lu Z-B, Namulinda T, Han Y-P, et al. Synthesis and evaluation of new 5-aminolevulinic acid derivatives as prodrugs of protoporphyrin for photodynamic therapy. Photochem. Photobiol. Sci. [Internet]. 2017;16(11):1623-30. Available from: http://xlink.rsc.org/?DOI=C7PP00203C

[56] Morrow DIJ, McCarron PA, Woolfson AD, Juzenas P, Juzeniene A, Iani V, et al. Hexyl aminolaevulinate is a more effective topical photosensitiser precursor than methyl aminolaevulinate and 5-aminolaevulinic acids when applied in equimolar doses. J. Pharm. Sci. 2010;99(8):3486-98.

[57] Neittaanmäki-Perttu N, Grönroos M, Karppinen TT, Tani TT, Snellman E. Hexyl-5-aminolaevulinate 0·2% vs. methyl-5-aminolaevulinate 16% daylight photodynamic therapy for treatment of actinic keratoses: results of a randomized double-blinded pilot trial. Br. J. Dermatol. [Internet]. 2016 Feb;174(2):427-9. Available from: http://doi.wiley.com/10.1111/bjd.13924

[58] Lui GYL, Obeidy P, Ford SJ, Tselepis C, Sharp DM, Jansson PJ, et al. The iron chelator, deferasirox, as a novel strategy for cancer treatment: Oral activity against human lung tumor xenografts and molecular mechanism of actions. Mol. Pharmacol. 2013;

[59] Yuan J, Lovejoy DB, Richardson DR. Novel di-2-pyridyl-derived iron chelators with marked and selective antitumor activity: In vitro and in vivo assessment. Blood. 2004;

[60] Richardson DR, Milnes K. The potential of iron chelators of the pyridoxal isonicotinoyl hydrazone class as effective antiproliferative agents II: The mechanism of action of ligands derived from salicylaldehyde benzoyl hydrazone and 2-hydroxy-1-naphthylaldehyde benzoyl hydrazone. Blood. 1997;

[61] Mrozek-Wilczkiewicz A, Serda M, Musiol R, Malecki G, Szurko A, Muchowicz A, et al. Iron Chelators in Photodynamic Therapy Revisited: Synergistic Effect by Novel Highly Active Thiosemicarbazones. ACS Med. Chem. Lett. [Internet]. 2014 Apr 10;5(4):336-9. Available from: https://pubs.acs.org/doi/10.1021/ml400422a

[62] Dirschka T, Ekanayake-Bohlig S, DominicusR,AschoffR,Herrera-CeballosE, Botella-Estrada R, et al. A randomized, intraindividual, non-inferiority, Phase III study comparing daylight photodynamic therapy with BF-200 ALA gel and MAL cream for the treatment of actinic keratosis. J. Eur. Acad. Dermatology Venereol. [Internet]. 2019 Feb;33(2):288-97. Available from: http://doi.wiley.com/10.1111/jdv.15185

[63] Radakovic S, Dangl M, Tanew A. 5-Aminolevulinic acid patch (Alacare) photodynamic therapy for actinic cheilitis: data from a prospective 12-month follow-up study on 21 patients. J. Eur. Acad. Dermatology Venereol. [Internet]. 2020 Sep 10;34(9):2011-5. Available from: https://onlinelibrary.wiley.com/doi/abs/10.1111/jdv.16247

[64] Aditya NP, Vathsala PG, Vieira V, Murthy RSR, Souto EB. Advances in nanomedicines for malaria treatment. Adv. Colloid Interface Sci. [Internet].

2013 Dec;201-202:1-17. Available from: https://linkinghub.elsevier.com/retrieve/pii/S0001868613001292

[65] Strambeanu N, Demetrovici L, Dragos D, Lungu M. Nanoparticles: Definition, Classification and General Physical Properties. Nanoparticles' Promises and Risks [Internet]. Cham: Springer International Publishing; 2015. p. 3-8. Available from: http://link.springer.com/10.1007/978-3-319-11728-7_1

[66] Lucky SS, Soo KC, Zhang Y. Nanoparticles in Photodynamic Therapy. Chem. Rev. [Internet]. 2015 Feb 25;115(4):1990-2042. Available from: https://pubs.acs.org/doi/10.1021/cr5004198

[67] Dragicevic-Curic N, Fahr A. Liposomes in topical photodynamic therapy. Expert Opin. Drug Deliv. [Internet]. 2012 Aug 25;9(8):1015-32. Available from: http://www.tandfonline.com/doi/full/10.1517/17425247.2012.697894

[68] Wu H, Chen N, Wu Z-M, Chen Z-L, Yan Y-J. Preparation of photosensitizer-loaded PLLA nanofibers and its anti-tumor effect for photodynamic therapy in vitro. J. Biomater. Appl. [Internet]. 2013 Feb 15;27(6):773-9. Available from: http://journals.sagepub.com/doi/10.1177/0885328211425706

[69] Jang W-D, Nakagishi Y, Nishiyama N, Kawauchi S, Morimoto Y, Kikuchi M, et al. Polyion complex micelles for photodynamic therapy: Incorporation of dendritic photosensitizer excitable at long wavelength relevant to improved tissue-penetrating property. J. Control. Release [Internet]. 2006 Jun;113(1):73-9. Available from: https://linkinghub.elsevier.com/retrieve/pii/S0168365906001131

[70] Boelsma E, Anderson C, Karlsson AMJ, Ponec M. Microdialysis technique as a method to study the percutaneous penetration of methyl nicotinate through excised human skin, reconstructed epidermis, and human skin in vivo. Pharm. Res. 2000;17(2):141-7.

[71] Sivamani RK, Stoeber B, Wu GC, Zhai H, Liepmann D, Maibach H. Clinical microneedle injection of methyl nicotinate: stratum corneum penetration. Ski. Res. Technol. 2005 May;11(2):152-6.

[72] Stringasci MD, Vollet-Filho JD, Moriyama LT, Kurachi C, Bagnato VS. Investigation of protoporphyrin IX production induced by aminolevulinic acid combined with thermogenic and/or vasodilator substances. In: Hasan T, editor. 17th Int. Photodyn. Assoc. World Congr. [Internet]. SPIE; 2019. p. 216. Available from: https://www.spiedigitallibrary.org/conference-proceedings-of-spie/11070/2525696/Investigation-of-protoporphyrin-IX-production-induced-by-aminolevulinic-acid-combined/10.1117/12.2525696.full

Chapter 8

Photodynamic Treatment of *Staphylococcus aureus* Infections

Christian Erick Palavecino, Camila Pérez and Tania Zuñiga

Abstract

Introduction: *Staphylococcus aureus* is a Gram-positive coconut that causes various life-threatening infections and, in turn, represents a major producer of healthcare-associated infections. This pathogen is highly resistant to antibiotics, which has made it difficult to eradicate in recent decades. Photodynamic therapy is a promising approach to address the notable shortage of antibiotic options against multidrug-resistant *Staphylococcus aureus*. This therapy combines the use of a photosensitizing agent, light, and oxygen to eradicate pathogenic microorganisms. The purpose of this study is to provide relevant bibliographic information about the application of photodynamic therapy as an alternative antimicrobial therapy for *Staphylococcus aureus* infections. Methods: This review was achieved through a bibliographic search in various databases and the analysis of relevant publications on the subject. Results: A large body of evidence demonstrates the efficacy of photodynamic therapy in eliminating biofilm- or biofilm-producing strains of *Staphylococcus aureus*, as well as antibiotic-resistant strains. Conclusion: We conclude that photodynamic therapy against *Staphylococcus aureus* is a recommended antibacterial therapy that may complement antibiotic treatment.

Keywords: photodynamic therapy, *Staphylococcus aureus*, antibiotic resistance

1. Introduction

Staphylococci are a large group of gram-positive cocci, whose diameter varies from 0.5 to 1.5 µm whose grouping resembles grape Clusters. To date, 35 known species and 17 subspecies of the genus *Staphylococcus* have been reported [1]. *Staphylococcus aureus* (*S. aureus*) is a bacterium with wide dissemination; Although it is part of the human body's commensal microbiota, it can cause severe skin infections, localized abscesses, and also may cause osteomyelitis, endocarditis, and other life-threatening diseases. Also, *S. aureus* has become a significant cause of healthcare-associated infections (HAIs) [2]. Besides, *S. aureus* acts as an early colonizer, creating a favorable environment for the adhesion and colonization of bacteria producing biofilms (BF). BFs consist of an array of proteins and polysaccharides that form an extracellular matrix (**Figure 1**). This matrix is considered an essential virulence factor of *S. aureus* strains, as it functions as a barrier against antimicrobial agents and the host's immune system, helping to maintain bacterial colonization [3, 4].

Since the discovery of antibiotics and their application, many bacterial infections have been successfully treated. However, in recent years the resistance of bacteria to antibiotics is emerging and increasing rapidly. *S. aureus* has progressively

IntechOpen

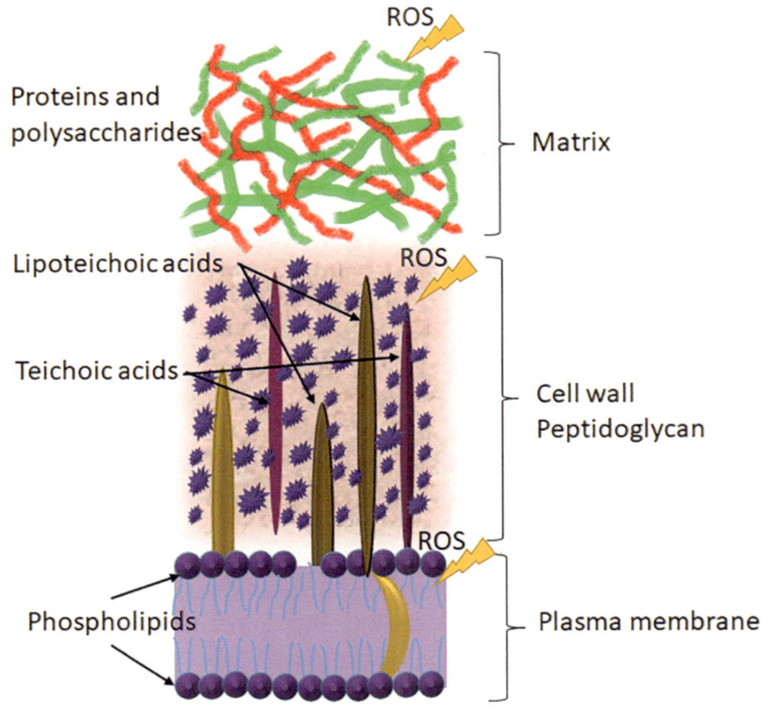

Figure 1.
Target structures from the Gram+ envelope for Photodynamic inactivation. Photodynamic therapy generates ROS that acts unspecifically on macromolecules present in the envelope of Gram + bacteria, such as lipids and proteins of the plasma membrane, peptidoglycan of the cell wall, and the array of proteins and polysaccharides macromolecules of the matrix that forms the biofilm.

gained multiple resistance to antibiotics, such as penicillin, methicillin, and other multiple drugs, leading to infections with frustrated or ineffective antibiotic therapies [5, 6]. The scarce development of new antibiotic added to the progressive increasing in multidrug-resistance of this and other clinically relevant bacteria has been considered by the World Health Organization (WHO) as one of the most pressing global threats to human health in the 21st century and described the situation as a global crisis and impending catastrophe of a return to the pre-antibiotic era. In this regard, the WHO published a list of microorganisms that should be investigated with priority to generate new antimicrobial drugs [7]. According to this list, *S. aureus,* with resistance to methicillin or vancomycin, is ranked second with high priority [7].

S. aureus displays various resistance mechanisms; for example, resistance to penicillin is mediated by hydrolytic enzymes called beta-lactamases. Beta-lactamases confer resistance to all penicillins except isoxazolyl penicillins (oxacillin, methicillin, cloxacillin, and nafcillin), as well as sensitivity to combinations of beta-lactams with beta-lactamase inhibitors (clavulanic acid, tazobactam, and sulbactam), or cephalosporins and carbapenems [8]. Resistance to methicillin, nafcillin, and oxacillin is independent of beta-lactamase production. This resistance is mediated by the *mec*A gene acquisition, which is translated into a new penicillin-binding protein (PBP2a). PBP2a decreases *S. aureus*'s affinity for methicillin and, therefore, allows it to survive treatments with this antibiotic [9]. Strains of *S. aureus* that express the *mec*A gene are called methicillin-resistant *S. aureus* (MRSA). MRSA strains are resistant to all beta-lactams (except 5th generation cephalosporins) and usually to aminoglycosides, erythromycin, clindamycin, tetracyclines, sulfonamides, quinolones, and rifampicin. While colonization of MRSA in a healthy individual is generally not serious, it can be life-threatening for patients with deep wounds, intravenous catheters, or other invasive instruments, as well as secondary infections in patients with a weakened immune system. Following the guidelines of the Clinical and Laboratory Standards Institute (CLSI), there are strains of *S. aureus* that present low-level or borderline resistance, for example, to oxacillin (BORSA) or vancomycin (VISA). The BORSA is characterized by a minimum inhibitory concentration (MIC) of oxacillin at the resistance cut-off point (4 mg / L) or a dilution above it [8]. *S. aureus* may present resistance to glycopeptides when it presents a MIC of vancomycin (VAN) of 4–8 mg/L. Furthermore, it is considered resistant with a MIC of NPV ≥ 16 mg/L [10]. The MIC should be determined using the broth microdilution method, according to CLSI.

Due to all those mentioned above, there is a challenge in urgently searching for new antimicrobial approaches to treat bacteria without producing resistance to antibiotics. Several new strategies have been developed, such as metallic nanoparticles, cationic polymers, peptidoglycans, nanocarriers, photothermotherapy and photodynamic therapy (PDT). Due to its demonstrated antitumor activity, PDT has been strongly developed to treat cancer, although not so much in its antimicrobial activity. Some studies have shown that PDT successfully reduces the biological activity of specific virulence factors produced by Gram-negative strains, and therefore, the analysis of the efficacy of this therapy in Gram-positive bacteria is essential [3, 4].

PDT is based on the use of photosensitizer molecules (PS) that produce local cytotoxicity after being activated by light (photo-oxidative stress). PS compounds absorb energy from visible light of a specific wavelength and transfer it to molecular oxygen, producing reactive oxygen species (ROS). **Figure 2** shows the mechanism for ROS production, which could be by electron transfer (e-) to produce superoxide ($O_2^{\bullet -}$) or by energy transfer, which produces highly reactive singlet oxygen ($^1O_2$). ROS production induces nonspecific bacterial death [12].

Very few initiatives have studied the information described to date on PDT antimicrobial therapy against *S. aureus* infections, and a bibliographic exploration of this strategy is relevant. The present review is a bibliographic study of the information available on the application of PDT against strains of *S. aureus* with particular

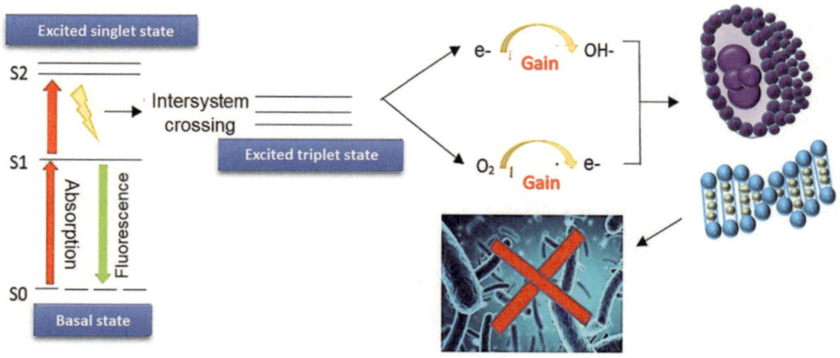

Figure 2.
The extraordinary power of the PSs. The basal state of PS is with two opposite lower energy molecular spin e-. The irradiation must penetrate the tissues deep enough to deliver enough energy to excite an e- to a higher energy orbital. An intersystem crossover can reach the excited state to a triplet state, where the excited e- spin is reversed. Excited triplet can produce two types of reactions: Type I and Type II. Type I: the excited triplet state can gain an e- from a nearby reducing agent, oxidizing it, producing H_2O_2. Type II: the excited triplet state transfers its energy directly to molecular oxygen, forming $^1O_2$. The type II reaction provides most of the photooxidative stress. $^1O_2$ is a ROS that produces concerted addition reactions to groups of alkenes present in organic molecules such as proteins, lipids o nuclear acids leading to nonspecific bacterial death. The generation of $^1O_2$ will be effective, taking into account the PS, where its excited states have a longer half-life. It is essential to improve the probability of interacting with triple oxygen and producing $^1O_2$ [11].

emphasis on *S. aureus* sensitive to multiple drugs (MDSSA); *S. aureus* multi-drug resistant strains (MDRSA); Methicillin-sensitive *S. aureus* (MSSA) and MRSA.

2. Photosensitizers

PS are non-toxic molecules capable of absorbing a specific wavelength's energy and transferring it to oxygen molecules present in biological solutions to produce the activated forms of $O_2^{\bullet -}$ and $^1O_2$. Both forms can produce ROS, which has the ability to promote bacterial cell death through the oxidation of closer organic macromolecules such as membrane components, proteins, lipids, and nucleic acids. In Gram positive bacteria, Pactivated PSs may produce ROS that acts unspecifically on macromolecules present in the envelope, such as lipids and proteins of the plasma membrane, peptidoglycan, and the array of proteins and polysaccharides macromolecules of the matrix (**Figure 1**). A PS has the property of being inert during administration and can be activated by being subjected to a specific wavelength.

2.1 Most used photosensitizer for PDT over *Staphylococcus aureus*

Table 1 summarized some of the more recent efforts to eradicate *S. aureus* by PDT. Porphyrins are an important class of natural macrocyclic molecules found in biological compounds and play an essential role in the metabolism of living organisms. The best known natural porphyrins are the heme group and chlorophyll. The heme group is a porphyrin-iron complex that is part of many active sites of different proteins, such as hemoglobin, myoglobins, and cytochromes. Uroporphyrin and coproporphyrin are the oxidation products of their respective porphyrinogens, which are the proper substrates in the biosynthetic pathway. The basic structure of porphyrin is formed by four pyrrole units interconnected by their alpha carbons linked by methyl bridges. The most commonly used photosensitizer drug in the last decade is porphyrin derivatives, such as the synthetic protoporphyrin Diarginate, T4 Porphyrin, Protoporphyrin IX, Coproporphyrin III, Porphyrin Formulation, among others. However, there are a few studies that have tried to verify whether these natural or synthetic molecules have a photo-oxidative activity with bactericidal action. The vast majority of these studies used porphyrin derivatives under irradiation with the red light of a wavelength range of 618–780 nm. PDT mediated by porphyrin derivatives increased antimicrobial efficacy and significantly reduced bacterial viability [10, 11, 14, 15, 40].

One of the initial studies on this PS was the series by Grinholc *et al.* [13, 16], who evaluated the bactericidal efficacy of PDT mediated by protoporphyrin diarginate over MRSA and MSSA strains in a large number of clinical isolates. They observed a reduction of 0–3 log10 of MRSA strains and 0.2 to 3 log10 for MSSA strains. Although this study's results were not significant, they paved the way for studying and developing PSs [13]. The 5-aminolevulinic acid (5-ALA), a prodrug that becomes protoporphyrin IX (PP IX) in the target cells, was used as a photosensitizer. Compared to other PSs, 5-ALA is only a natural intermediate in the heme biosynthetic pathway and can be removed rapidly from target cells. More importantly, it is small enough to penetrate the matrix and accumulate in target cells with less toxicity. The antimicrobial activity of 5-ALA-PDT was demonstrated on MRSA's planktonic strain in vitro by Huang *et al.* [37]. Their results showed that the number of living cells decreased as the concentration of the compound augmented. In control groups with solely 5-ALA or light, most of the bacterial cells were alive. Consequently, the photodynamic activity of 5-ALA is dose-dependent [37].

Bacteria	PS	Technique	Study	Application	Author and year
MSSA MRSA	PP Diarginate	Red light	In vitro	Clinical isolates	Grinholc et al. [13]
MSSA MRSA	TMP	Red light	In vitro	Biofilm-producing bacteria	Di poto et al. [10]
MRSA	MB and TMP	Red light	Ex vivo	Wound infections	Donelly et al. [14]
MRSA	TMP	Blue light	In vitro	Antibiotic resistant bacteria	Dosselli et al. [15]
MSSA MRSA	PP IX	Red light	In vitro	Antibiotic resistant bacteria	Grinholc et al. [16]
MRSA	HYP	Red light	In vitro In vivo	Biofilm-producing bacteria	Nafee et al. [17]
MDSSA	Hypocrelin B	Blue light LED	In vitro	Bacterial isolates	Yuan Jiang et al. [18]
S. aureus S. epidermidis S. haemolyticus	5-ALA	Red light	In vitro	Wound infections	Barra et al. [19]
MDSSA	HYP with NAC	Yellow light LED	In vitro	Biofilm-producing planktonic bacteria	Kashef et al. [20]
MDSSA	NnPs of gold with MB	Red light LED	In vitro	Skin infections (Impetigo)	Tawfik et al. [21]
MRSA MDRSA	Chlorophyll derivative	Red light LED	In vitro Ex vivo	Clinical isolates	Winkler et al. [22]
S. aureus P. acnes	ZnPc	Red light	In vitro In vivo	Skin infections	Chen et al. [23]
MDSSA	TBO	Red light	In vitro	Bacterial infections	Gandara et al. [24]
MSSA MRSA	TBO	Red light	In vitro	Antibiotic resistant bacteria	Hoorijani et al. [25]
MSSA MRSA	MB and TBO	Red light	In vitro	Biofilm-producing bacteria	Kashef et al. [26]

Bacteria	PS	Technique	Study	Application	Author and year
MDSSA	MB and RB	Red and green light	In vitro	Bacterial isolates	Pérez-Laguna et al. [27]
MDSSA MDRSA	S-PS	Red light	In vivo	Skin infections (burns and wounds)	Mai et al. [28]
MRSA	Cur	Blue light	Ex vivo	Bone tissue infections	Araujo et al. [29]
MDSSA	ZnPc	Red light	In vitro	Biofilm-producing bacteria	Gao et al. [30]
MRSA	ICG	Infrared light LED	In vitro	Skin infections (diabetic foot)	Li et al. [31]
MRSA	Resveratrol	Blue light LED	In vitro In vivo	Bacterial isolates	Dos Santos et al. [32]
MRSA	Silica NnPs conjugated with TBO	Red light LED	In vitro	Biofilm-producing bacteria	Anju et al. [33]
MDSSA	TBO	Red light LED	In vitro	Dental titanium implants	Zhiyu Cai et al. [34]
MDSSA	Iodide IR780	Infrared light	In vitro In vivo	Orthopedic titanium implants	Mu Li et al. [35]
MRSA	TBO	Red light	In vitro	Skin infections (Burns)	Mahmoudi et al. [3]
MRSA	Riboflavin	Blue light LED	In vitro	Bacterial isolates	Makdoumi et al. [36]
MDSSA MDRSA	S-PS	Red light	In vitro	Biofilm-producing planktonic bacteria	Jia et al. [3]
MRSA	5-ALA	Red light	In vitro	Biofilm-producing planktonic bacteria	Huang et al. [37]
MDSSA	NnPs of polydopamine conjugated with ICG	Infrared light	In vitro In vivo	Dental titanium implants	Yuan et al. [38]
P. aeruginosa S. aureus	TBO Conjugated Carbon Nanotubes	Red light	In vitro	Biofilm-producing bacteria	Anju et al. [33]
MRSA	Porphyrin formulation	White light LED	In vitro Ex vivo	Skin infections	Braz et al. [11]

Bacteria	PS	Technique	Study	Application	Author and year
MSSA MRSA	Cur	Blue light LED	In vitro	Biofilm-producing bacteria	Geraldo et al. [39]
MDSSA MDRSA	TBO	Red light	In vitro	Skin and mucous infections (periodontitis, burns and diabetic foot)	Liu et al. [6]
MRSA	CP III	Blue light LED	In vitro	Skin infections	Walter et al. [40]

MSSA: methicillin-sensitive Staphylococcus aureus; *MRSA: Methicillin-resistant* Staphylococcus aureus; *MSSA: methicillin-sensitive* Staphylococcus aureus; *MRSA: Methicillin-resistant* Staphylococcus aureus; *MDSSA: Multi-drug sensitive* Staphylococcus aureus; *MDRSA: Multi-drug resistant* Staphylococcus aureus; *S. aureus:* Staphylococcus aureus; *S. epidermidis:* Staphylococcus epidermidis; *S. haemolyticus: Staphylococcus haemolyticus; P. acnés:* Propionibacterium acnes; *P. aeruginosa:* Pseudomonas aeruginosa; *PS: photosensitizer; PP: protoporphyrin; TMP: porphyrin T4 (meso tetra (N-4-methyl pyridyl)); MB Methylene blue; HYP: Hypericin; NAC: N-acetylcysteine; 5-ALA: aminolevulinic acid; NnPs: nanoparticles; ZnPc: Zinc Phthalocyanine; TBO: Toluidine blue; RB: Bengal rose; S-PS: sinoporphyrin sodium; Cur: Curcumin; ICG: indocyanine green; CP: coproporphyrin; LED: Light-emitting diode.*

Table 1.
List for research and development of S. aureus *PDT.*

The second most prominent PS is Toluidine Blue (TBO), a hydrophilic cationic PS of phenothiazine dyes with a high $^1O_2$ quantum yield and strong absorption bands in the 620–660 nm region. Also, it has a high affinity for bacterial membranes and has been approved for clinical use in PDT, and is considered an effective and membrane-damaging PS [6]. In all studies where TBO act as a PS, irradiation with red LED light in the range of 630–635 nm was used. This combination increased the antibacterial efficacy of PDT and significantly reduced bacterial viability [3, 6, 24, 25, 33, 34]. One of the most prominent studies was carried out by the group of Zhyhyu Cai et al. [19], whose objective was to evaluate how effective the disinfection by combining antiseptics with PDT is in *S. aureus* BF present on the titanium surface is. The results indicate that the administration of antiseptics such as chlorhexidine or H_2O_2 with PDT was the most effective protocol, producing a reduction of approximately 3–4 log10 in the number of adhering bacteria compared to any treatment alone. In addition to bacterial reduction, it was the first study *in vitro* to evaluate the antibacterial effects of the concurrent application of antiseptics with PDT against *S. aureus* BF presented on the surface of Titanium [34].

Several natural PS derived from plants are also highlighted to be used for PDT, such as the sinoporphyrin sodium (S-PS). For example, Mai *et al.* [28], and Jia *et al.* [4], used a similar methodology for activation of S-PS, employing red LED light irradiation. The results indicate that PDT therapy with S-PS has significant antibacterial activity on MDSSA and MDRSA bacteria [4, 28]. Also, the S-PS exceeds the solubility of other PS in a physiological environment and proves to be an ideal PS with low dark toxicity, as well as having high purity and easy extraction. Another natural PS widely used in *in vitro* and *in vivo* studies is hypericin (HYP), polycyclic quinine extracted from *Hypericum perforatum* (commonly known as St. John's wort) and derives its name from the plant. Previous interest in this herb has focused on its antidepressant effects. This plant has been evaluated and tested for its photo-oxidative activity against a series of bacterial and fungal strains in recent years. It has several desirable properties as PS, including a high $^1O_2$ generation quantum yield, a high extinction coefficient close to 600 nm, and relatively low dark toxicity. In studies carried out by the group of Nafee *et al.* [17], the quantity as low as 0.03 M of HYP inhibited *in vitro* 60–120% the growth of BF producing MRSA strains compared to planktonic cells, 55–75%. *In vivo* studies on rats showed higher wound healing potential, better epithelialization, and keratinization of the skin in infected wounds treated with HYP nanoparticles [17]. Finally, hypocrellin B, an active component of traditional Chinese medicine from the herb *Hypocrella bambuase*, was tested for PDT. Numerous studies have shown its antiviral, antibacterial, and antifungal effects and antitumor activity. Interestingly, this PS is also a strong ROS generator when activated by visible light. Yuan Jiang *et al.* [27] observed a significant decrease in the viability of *S. aureus* after LED light irradiation. Remarkable ultrastructural damage was also evidenced in bacterial cells due to the photodynamic action of hypocrellin B [18].

3. Photodynamic therapy in clinical isolates strains

Most of the studies on PDT for *S. aureus* infections found in the literature come from standard bacterial strains acquired from different microbiological laboratories for *in vitro*, *in vivo,* and *ex vivo* studies. The most used certified reference standard bacterial strains came from the American Type Culture Collection (ATCC). ATCC strains are certified microorganisms for quality control in microbiology. Also, their genotypic and phenotypic characteristics guarantee the identity of the microorganism, and by having this documentation, the laboratory will avoid carrying out

Isolations	Unit	Material	Resistance profile
MSSA 26	Surgery room	Respiratory sample	AM, EM, LE, MX, PG
MSSA 27	Surgery room	Lesion swab	–
MSSA 28	Surgery room	Lesion swab	–
MSSA 32	Internal Medicine	Lesion swab	–
MSSA 33	Dermatology	Lesion swab	CM, EM, TC
MSSA 35	Dermatology	Lesion swab	AM, LE, MX, PG
MRSA 36	Surgery room	Lesion swab	CM, EM, LE, MX
MRSA 37	Pneumology	Orin	CM, EM, LE, MX, TM
MRSA 38	Pneumology	Respiratory sample	CM, EM, LE, MX, TM
MRSA 40	Urology	Blood sample	CIP, CM, EM, FM, LE, MX, TC, TM
MRSA 41	Surgery room	Lesion swab	CM, EM, LE, MX, RI, TM
MRSA 42	Surgery room	Blood sample	CIP, CM, EM, LE, MX, TM
MRSA 43	Gynecology	Lesion swab	CM, EM, LE, MX, TM
MRSA 44	Ophthalmology	Lesion swab	CM, EM, LE, MX
MRSA 45	Internal Medicine	Lesion swab	CM, EM, GEM, LE, MX, TC, TM

MSSA: Methicillin-sensitive Staphylococcus aureus; *MRSA: Methicillin-resistant* Staphylococcus aureus; *AM: ampicillin; CIP: ciprofloxacin; CL: chloramphenicol; CM: clindamycin; EM: erythromycin; FM: fosfomycin; GEM gentamicin; LE: levofloxacin; MX: moxifloxacin; PG: penicillin G; RI: rifampicin; TC: Tetracycline; TM: Tobramycin.*

Table 2.
Diversity of the clinical isolates.

additional tests for the identification of the strains, which translates into saving time and resources. However, studies in which clinical isolates of *S. aureus* were used to demonstrate the PDT may be useful for bacteria from active infections.

PDT is an approach that has shown promise in treating skin and soft tissue infections, one of the most recent studies of Mahmoudi *et al.* [3], used clinical isolates of *S. aureus* from samples of burn wounds of 95 patients with symptomatic infection. The viability of *S. aureus* isolates was significantly reduced to 40% after 30 sec of exposure to a LED light, with minimal risk of development of resistance [3]. Another study developed by Tawfik *et al.* [21] was carried out over clinal isolates of *S. aureus* from a population of twenty children aged 3 to 5 years diagnosed with impetigo. The PDT was compared for light-irradiated gold, methylene blue (MB), and gold -MB conjugate nanoparticles. It was shown that the maximum inhibitory effect on *S. aureus* was obtained with the gold nanoparticle-MB conjugate [21]. The 5-ALA has also been used for PDT over clinical isolates of BF of MSSA and MRSA strains of *S. aureus* [41]. The results over isolates from samples of adult patients with chronic rhinosinusitis with or without nasal polyps showed a robust bactericidal effect that increased when the PDT was combined with antibiotics treatment [41]. Finally, one of the most relevant studies carried out by Winkler *et al.* [22] tested the effectiveness of the chlorophyll derivative (Ce6) combined with a red light to eradicate *in vitro* a diverse set of clinical isolates of MSSA and MRSA. Those bacterial isolates, their biological sample, origin, and their susceptibility profiles are listed in **Table 2**, showing the diversity of the strains. The *in vitro* study demonstrated that all clinical isolates of MSSA and MRSA were inactivated by PDT when bacterial cells were previously incubated with ≥128 μM Ce6 [22].

4. Synergism with antibiotics or other drugs

Although PDT presents positive expectations for the treatment of MDRSA, several researchers have wanted to anticipate the generation of resistance, and they began the search for an antimicrobial strategy that generates greater potency and better results. Therefore, a new research sub-field has been opened, combining PDT with antibiotic treatment in *S. aureus*.

Gentamicin (GEN) is one of the most widely used antibiotics for treating various HAIs. The GEN is an aminoglycoside, which inhibits protein synthesis binding to the 30S subunit of the bacterial ribosome and causes protein mistranslation and bacterial death. GEN is a broad-spectrum antibiotic used for clinical treatment, although its frequent use has generated a high resistance level. Several authors have evaluated the synergy of combining the GEN with PDT for the antibacterial treatment of *S. aureus*. Most of these studies use a similar methodology, consisting of pre-treatment of the bacteria in the dark with different tested PS concentrations. This is followed by the transfer of treated bacteria in suspensions to microtiter plates containing different GEN concentrations and irradiated with different doses of light. Finally, the bacterial plaque count is performed in the dark to calculate bacterial viability. In this way, a diminution in the GEN-MIC when combined with PDT is determined [6, 19, 42–44]. One of the most representative and updated studies, developed by the group of Liu *et al.* [6], verified the synergistic effects of PDT by combining TBO with GEN. This combination has a better antibacterial activity on MDSSA compared to MDRSA bacteria. The authors observed a dose-dependent effect with a maximum of 9 μg / mL GEN decreased of up to 1.8 log10 the survival of MDSSA bacteria. However, no bactericidal effect was observed on MDRSA at a GEN concentration of up to 150 μg/mL. Suggesting the MDSSA strains are more sensitive to PDT-GEN therapy than MDRSA [6].

Another widely used antibiotic to treat infections caused by multidrug-resistant bacteria is Linezolid (LN). Linezolid is a bacteriostatic antibiotic that binds to bacterial ribosomal RNA, inhibiting protein translation of Gram-positive bacteria. A large body of evidence shows that PDT significantly increases the effectiveness of LN treatment synergistically for different strains of *S. aureus* [26, 27]. Special mention deserves the study by Kashef *et al.* [31], who observed that the combination of TBO and MB in PDT with LN is useful in eradicating *S. aureus* BF in chronic diabetic foot ulcers. By itself, PDT therapy with MB or TBO did not decrease the bacterial viability of any of the *S. aureus* tested strains. However, the combination of MB-PDT and antibiotics resulted in a 1.2 log10 reduction in viability comparing to the antibiotic treatment alone (0.6 log10 reductions) [31]. The ciprofloxacin (CIP) is an antibiotic agent of the quinolone family, which binds to the DNA gyrase-DNA complex. The DNA gyrase allows the DNA to unwind and rotate freely within the cell; thus, CIP produces bacterial death. PDT studies showed synergism with CIP [45, 46]. For example, Ronqui *et al.* [46] observed a significant antibacterial increase, reducing bacterial survival 5.4 log10 in *S. aureus* BF and approximately 7 log10 for *Escherichia coli* BF combining PDT treatment with MB and CIP [46].

One of the most explored resistance mechanisms in the last two decades has been that of vancomycin-resistant *S. aureus* (VRSA). VAN acts on the synthesis of the bacterial cell-wall, inhibiting the formation of peptidoglycans. Not only the permeability of the cytoplasmic membrane but also the RNA synthesis is altered. Strains of VRSA can transfer their resistance mechanism to other pathogenic bacteria such as *Enterococcus faecalis,* causing a significant number of HAIs outbreaks [47]. For this reason, PDT has been studied as a therapeutic option that enhances the bactericidal action of VAN [10, 41]. Di poto et al. [10], demonstrated that pre-treatment of clinical MSSA and MRSA strains producers of BF with PDT, followed by the addition of NPV, causes disruption of the BF matrix and allows complete elimination of the bacteria. Synergism with PDT improved the antimicrobial activity of VAN with a five-fold decrease in bacterial viability compared to samples treated with PDT alone [10].

The synergism of PDT has also been explored with other drugs such as mucolytics, anticoagulants, antiseptics, and disinfectants. In general, these studies present encouraging results. All showed decreased bacterial viability in combined therapy with these different compounds [11, 20, 31, 34, 35]. For example, Braz *et al.* [11] showed both *in vitro* and *ex vivo* the efficacy of PDT mediated by a formulation based on a non-separate mixture of cationic porphyrins (FORM) in combination with potassium iodide (KI) or povidone-iodine (PVP-I) for photoinactivation of MRSA in the skin. The in vitro results demonstrated that the FORM + KI combination was an effective therapy in a dose-depended manner. Results *ex vivo*, shown a reduction of 3.1 Log10 using FORM + KI or FORM + PVP-I under irradiation [11].

5. Effects of photodynamic therapy on *S. aureus* biofilms

S. aureus is one of the most important etiologic agents of HAIs, in part, due to the ability of *S. aureus* to form BF. The BF provides a microenvironment that protects bacteria from the immune system's action and antibiotics, providing an extended virulence to the strain [10]. The BF formed by *S. aureus* are communities of microorganisms integrated into a matrix of extracellular polymers. The matrix comprises adhesion polysaccharides and extracellular enzymes, which have shown aggressive behavior [48].

Infections by organisms that produce BF are an important challenge in medical practice, leading to new therapeutic strategies. PDT has been a central focus and shows mixed results in the literature. Studies using TBO as PS to eradicate *S. aureus* BF have shown a significant reduction in bacterial viability [33, 34, 48]. Noteworthy Anju *et al.* [25], used silica nanoparticles to enhance the antimicrobial efficacy of TBO. The authors evaluated the anti-BF efficacy of the photoactivated TBO silica nanoparticles against *Pseudomonas aeruginosa* (*P. aeruginosa*) as well as *S. aureus.* The results showed that the PDT reduced the viability in *P. aeruginosa* by 66.39 ± 4.22% and the viability of *S. aureus* by 76.22 ± 3.45%. Regarding the controls, the use of TBO alone resulted in an inhibition of 27.28 ± 1.87 and 48.52 ± 1.91% for BF formation by *P. aeruginosa* and *S. aureus*, respectively [25]. A modification in the encapsulation of TBO for PDT was achieved employing carbon nanotubes, which were useful and showed improved results over BF of *P. aeruginosa* and *S. aureus* [33]. The anti-BF activity of TBO with nanotubes after exposure to light was 69.94% and 75.54% for *P. aeruginosa* and *S. aureus*, respectively. Compared to the study by Anju *et al.* [25], the photoinactivation of bacteria was much higher, and cell viability and exopolysaccharide production were more reduced [33].

Authors using indocyanine green (ICG) as PS observed mixed results [29, 31]. For example, Li *et al.* [31] compared the effect of adding EDTA to ICG for PDT on planktonic and BF bacteria. The results showed that PDT induced by ICG -EDTA combination has a more pronounced antibacterial effect in *S. aureus* and *P. aeruginosa* than PDT with ICG alone. In turn, *P. aeruginosa* was more sensitive to ICG -EDTA PDT than *S. aureus.* Also, PDT combined with antibiotic treatment contributed significantly to eradicating bacteria and disrupting the BF structure. Different results were obtained when combining polydopamine nanoparticles with ICG for PDT of orthopedic titanium implants [29]. Evaluations demonstrated that PDT-mediated ROS and nor hyperthermia were sufficient by themselves to achieve a significant bactericidal effect on *S. aureus* BF. However, both effects, local hyperthermia and ROS production, were synergistic and effectively inhibited most *S. aureus* BF [29].

The photodynamic activity of Curcumin (Cur) by high photooxidation was demonstrated to efficiently abolishing *S. aureus* BF [30, 39]. The group of Geraldo *et al.* [30] established the efficacy of Cur -PDT over MSSA and MRSA BF. The results showed that concentrations as low as 20–40 μM resulted in 1log10 reduction of MSSA BF, but the effect reaches 3log10 inactivation at 80 μM. For MRSA BF, it was observed that at 20 μM of Cur produced a reduction of 1log10, and similarly higher concentrations, 40 and 80 μM, decreased the bacterial survival to 2 log10 in a dose-dependent activity [39]. Hypericin (HYP) is one of the natural derivatives widely used in PDT for the elimination of *S. aureus* BF [17, 20]. However, its bactericidal effect is only achieved in combination with N-acetylcysteine (NAC) [20]. The combination of HYP-NAC in PDT is able to interrupt the preformed BF of *S. aureus* (ATCC 25923), reducing the bacterial viability between 5.2 to 6.3 log10. The treatment for clinical isolates demonstrated similar bactericidal activity, decreasing the viability by 5.5–6.7 log10 [20]. Gao *et al.* [49] showed that zinc phthalocyanine (ZnPc) generates ROS during the PDT treatment of *S. aureus* BF. According to his flow cytometric studies, the bacterial DNA was severely damaged [49]. Finally, combining iodine IR780- PDT with thermal phototherapy (PTT) is effective both *in vitro* and *in vivo* [35]. The authors observed that antibacterial treatment applying only PDT or PTT is not effective in completely eradicating already formed BF [35].

6. Modulation in gene expression by photodynamic therapy

Without considering prophages, plasmids, and transposons, the *S. aureus* genome core is a circular chromosome of approximately 2,800 Kb. The genes that encode virulence factors in *S. aureus* may be contained in the core genome and in accessory elements. Genes encoding virulence factors can be transferred between different staphylococci strains or transferred to bacteria from other species, including Gram-negative bacteria. In *S. aureus*, the expression of virulence genes is controlled by several regulatory genes; the most studied is the *agr* gene (accessory genetic regulator). The *agr* gene has become associated with a quorum-sensing (QS) system. The RNAIII gene is the main effector of the *agr* system. It acts as a small RNA that regulates the expression of many virulence factors, including most of the genes that encode proteins associated with the cell wall and extracellular structures [50]. These factors are also associated with the formation of BF. Given its importance, the *agr* system can be a good therapeutic target for treating acute and chronic infections associated with the formation of BF. [23]. Therefore, the researchers emphasize the use of PDT can interfere with these systems' actions by inhibiting the spread of BF-forming strains [16, 23, 24].

Pourhajibagher *et al.* [50], evaluated in multiple species, including *S. aureus*, the cell viability of bacterial BF subjected to ICG as a photosensitizer. The gene expression of the QS system and the *arg* gene was determined and compared to untreated bacteria. In both *S. aureus* and other bacteria, *agr* gene and QS gene expression levels decreased after PDT. The *agr* gene expression was reduced approximately 3.7 times, as well as the bacterial viability of *S. aureus* decreased between 42 and 82%, revealing an association of the gene with bacterial BF [23]. In another study, Mahmoudi *et al.* [3] determined the ICA operon gene expression changes in bacteria subjected to sub-lethal doses of PDT in clinical isolates from wound infections in patients with burns. The ICA gene regulates *S aureus* BF production. A significant decrease in the expression of the ICA gene was observed in all *S. aureus* isolates after treatment, suggesting that the inactivation of virulence factors through interference in the expression of the ICA gene by PDT may reduce the pathogenesis of *S. aureus* [3].

One of the objectives that PDT seeks is to modulate the virulence of multi-resistant strains by repressing the expression levels of genes involved in bacterial resistance. An example was that of Huang *et al.* [37], who studied the expression response of a specific MRSA gene (*nuc* gene). The *nuc* gene encodes the expression of a thermally stable extracellular nuclease produced by *S. aureus*. The authors observed that this gene's transcription, ordinarily high, was down-regulated after PDT, suggesting the treatment interferes with its expression [37].

7. Discussion

S. aureus is the main pathogenic species of its genus, and a common cause of various superficial and internal infections. Although some of this infection can be quickly resolved, this pathogen's current interest derives from its high frequency in life-threatening diseases such as sepsis, meningitis, or pneumonia by MDR-bacteria. The variability of *S. aureus* and the rapid adaptive response to changes in the environment and its continuous acquisition of antibiotic resistance determinants have made it a habitual resident of the hospital habitat and an important agent of HAIs. Since the main consequence of bacterial resistance is antibiotic therapy failure, the increase in morbidity and mortality, and the increase in medical care costs, it is essential to containing the problem. As MDR-infections with *S. aureus* increases worldwide to dangerous levels, the urgent search for new antimicrobial strategies is required. Complementary therapies and antimicrobial treatment options may help relieve pressure from multidrug-resistant bacteria on healthcare systems. PDT then promises to be very useful to complement antibiotic treatment. The PDT is a noninvasive strategy, which uses inert compounds that need to be activated locally [6].

As we see in **Figure 1**, PDT's mechanism can change the internal and external structural integrity of bacterial cells and cause unspecific cell death. This process is closely related to the formation of ROS, without the generation of resistance. **Table 1**, shows the most widely used and explored SP are those derived from porphyrins since these present a high decrease in bacterial viability when irradiated. It should be noted that the irradiation to activate the photo-oxidative effect of PS is essential since the effectiveness of the treatment depends on this. The wavelength in the ranges of 620 to 700 nm is considered the most efficient technique as the red light manages to penetrate deep enough into the target tissue to produce its activity.

The BFs are important to point considering the pathogenicity of *S. aureus*. The PDT achieved the eradication of the BF in most investigations, but this disruption capacity was variable and is highly dependent on the technique used (the type of PS, type of irradiation, combination with antibiotics, among others). The decrease in bacterial survival in BF after PDT was much lower than observed for planktonic bacteria. The difference may radicate in the cell wall composition and growth rate, and the matrix components that hinder the photosensitizer absorption and light penetration.

The synergy with antimicrobials in combination therapy effectively increases microorganisms' sensitivity to the antibiotics of choice. In addition to avoiding a large amount of antibiotic use, this strategy minimizes the spread of resistance. On the other hand, a lower drug concentration can be used during combined therapy to reduce the side effects.

Genetics plays an important role, and PDT showed that it might generate a modulation in the genes associated with virulence. Promoting the silencing of gene expression, the PDT significantly decreases bacterial viability. In turn, the *agr* gene has been assigned a central role in the pathogenesis of *S. aureus*. Its down-regulation may affect colonization factors, components of the microbial surface, and the formation of BF that are regulated by *agr* gene.

8. Conclusions

Based on the above, we can conclude that PDT treatment is highly recommended to strengthen antibacterial therapies. The PDT generates unspecific photo-oxidative effects that improve an effective elimination of *S. aureus* strains without generation of resistance. The information presented here could help develop standardized protocols for managing infections caused by *S. aureus*, particularly those with antimicrobial resistance. We believe it is necessary to expand future studies of this therapy *in vivo,* including clinical trials since, according to what has been presented, there are several *in vitro*, *in vivo,* and *ex vivo* evidence that proves that PDT is secure and its bactericidal effect does not produce resistance.

Conflict of interest

The authors declare no conflict of interest.

DOI: http://dx.doi.org/10.5772/intechopen.95455

Author details

Christian Erick Palavecino[1]*, Camila Pérez[2] and Tania Zuñiga[2]

1 Laboratory of Cellular Microbiology, Institute for Research and Innovation in Health, Faculty of Health Sciences, Central University of Chile, Lord Cochrane, Santiago, Chile

2 School of Medical Technology, Faculty of Health Sciences, Central University of Chile, Chile

*Address all correspondence to: christian.palavecino@ucentral.cl

References

[1] Harris LG, Foster SJ, Richards RG. An introduction to Staphylococcus aureus, and techniques for identifying and quantifying S. aureus adhesins in relation to adhesion to biomaterials: review. Eur Cell Mater. 2002;4:39-60.

[2] Hodille E, Rose W, Diep BA, Goutelle S, Lina G, Dumitrescu O. The Role of Antibiotics in Modulating Virulence in Staphylococcus aureus. Clin Microbiol Rev. 2017;30(4):887-917.

[3] Mahmoudi H, Pourhajibagher M, Alikhani MY, Bahador A. The effect of antimicrobial photodynamic therapy on the expression of biofilm associated genes in Staphylococcus aureus strains isolated from wound infections in burn patients. Photodiagnosis Photodyn Ther. 2019;25:406-413.

[4] Jia M, Mai B, Liu S, Li Z, Liu Q, Wang P. Antibacterial effect of S-Porphin sodium photodynamic therapy on Staphylococcus aureus and multiple drug resistance Staphylococcus aureus. Photodiagnosis and photodynamic therapy. 2019;28:80-87.

[5] Li S, Dong S, Xu W, Tu S, Yan L, Zhao C, et al. Antibacterial Hydrogels. Advanced Science. 2018;5(5):1700527.

[6] Liu S, Mai B, Jia M, Lin D, Zhang J, Liu Q, et al. Synergistic antimicrobial effects of photodynamic antimicrobial chemotherapy and gentamicin on Staphylococcus aureus and multidrug-resistant Staphylococcus aureus. Photodiagnosis and photodynamic therapy. 2020:101703.

[7] Willyard C. The drug-resistant bacteria that pose the greatest health threats. Nature. 2017; 543(7643):15.

[8] Morosini MI, Cercenado E, Ardanuy C, Torres C. [Phenotypic detection of resistance mechanisms in gram-positive bacteria]. Enferm Infecc Microbiol Clin. 2012;30(6):325-332.

[9] Wong TW, Liao SZ, Ko WC, Wu CJ, Wu SB, Chuang YC, et al. Indocyanine Green-Mediated Photodynamic Therapy Reduces Methicillin-Resistant Staphylococcus aureus Drug Resistance. Journal of clinical medicine. 2019;8(3).

[10] Di Poto A, Sbarra MS, Provenza G, Visai L, Speziale P. The effect of photodynamic treatment combined with antibiotic action or host defence mechanisms on Staphylococcus aureus biofilms. Biomaterials. 2009;30(18):3158-3166.

[11] Braz M, Salvador D, Gomes A, Mesquita MQ, Faustino MAF, Neves M, et al. Photodynamic inactivation of methicillin-resistant Staphylococcus aureus on skin using a porphyrinic formulation. Photodiagnosis and photodynamic therapy. 2020:101754.

[12] Valenzuela-Valderrama M, Bustamante V, Carrasco N, Gonzalez IA, Dreyse P, Palavecino CE. Photodynamic treatment with cationic Ir(III) complexes induces a synergistic antimicrobial effect with imipenem over carbapenem-resistant Klebsiella pneumoniae. Photodiagnosis Photodyn Ther. 2020;30:101662.

[13] Grinholc M, Szramka B, Kurlenda J, Graczyk A, Bielawski KP. Bactericidal effect of photodynamic inactivation against methicillin-resistant and methicillin-susceptible Staphylococcus aureus is strain-dependent. Journal of photochemistry and photobiology B, Biology. 2008;90(1):57-63.

[14] Donnelly RF, Cassidy CM, Loughlin RG, Brown A, Tunney MM, Jenkins MG, et al. Delivery of Methylene Blue and meso-tetra (N-methyl-4-pyridyl) porphine tetra tosylate from cross-linked poly(vinyl alcohol) hydrogels: a potential means of photodynamic therapy of infected wounds. Journal of photochemistry

and photobiology B, Biology. 2009;96(3):223-231.

[15] Dosselli R, Millioni R, Puricelli L, Tessari P, Arrigoni G, Franchin C, et al. Molecular targets of antimicrobial photodynamic therapy identified by a proteomic approach. Journal of proteomics. 2012;77:329-343.

[16] Grinholc M, Nakonieczna J, Negri A, Rapacka-Zdonczyk A, Motyka A, Fila G, et al. The agr function and polymorphism: impact on Staphylococcus aureus susceptibility to photoinactivation. Journal of photochemistry and photobiology B, Biology. 2013;129:100-107.

[17] N. Nafee, A. Youssef, H. El-Gowelli, H. Asem, S. Kandil, Antibiotic-free nanotherapeutics: hypericin nanoparticles thereof for improved in vitro and in vivo antimicrobial photodynamic therapy and wound healing, International journal of pharmaceutics 454(1) (2013) 249-58. doi: 10.1016/j.ijpharm.2013.06.067

[18] Y. Jiang, A.W. Leung, X. Wang, H. Zhang, C. Xu, Inactivation of Staphylococcus aureus by photodynamic action of hypocrellin B, Photodiagnosis and photodynamic therapy 10(4) (2013) 600-6. doi: 10.1016/j.pdpdt.2013.06.004

[19] F. Barra, E. Roscetto, A.A. Soriano, A. Vollaro, I. Postiglione, G.M. Pierantoni, G. Palumbo, M.R. Catania, Photodynamic and Antibiotic Therapy in Combination to Fight Biofilms and Resistant Surface Bacterial Infections, Int J Mol Sci 16(9) (2015) 20417-30. doi: 10.3390/ijms160920417

[20] N. Kashef, S. Karami, G.E. Djavid, Phototoxic effect of hypericin alone and in combination with acetylcysteine on Staphylococcus aureus biofilms, Photodiagnosis and photodynamic therapy 12(2) (2015) 186-92. doi: 10.1016/j.pdpdt.2015.04.001

[21] A.A. Tawfik, J. Alsharnoubi, M. Morsy, Photodynamic antibacterial enhanced effect of methylene blue-gold nanoparticles conjugate on Staphylococcal aureus isolated from impetigo lesions in vitro study, Photodiagnosis and photodynamic therapy 12(2) (2015) 215-20. doi: 10.1016/j.pdpdt.2015.03.003

[22] K. Winkler, C. Simon, M. Finke, K. Bleses, M. Birke, N. Szentmary, D. Huttenberger, T. Eppig, T. Stachon, A. Langenbucher, H.J. Foth, M. Herrmann, B. Seitz, M. Bischoff, Photodynamic inactivation of multidrug-resistant Staphylococcus aureus by chlorin e6 and red light (lambda=670nm), Journal of photochemistry and photobiology. B, Biology 162 (2016) 340-347. doi: 10.1016/j.jphotobiol.2016.07.007

[23] Z. Chen, Y. Zhang, D. Wang, L. Li, S. Zhou, J.H. Huang, J. Chen, P. Hu, M. Huang, Photodynamic antimicrobial chemotherapy using zinc phthalocyanine derivatives in treatment of bacterial skin infection, J Biomed Opt 21(1) (2016) 18001. doi: 10.1117/1.JBO.21.1.018001

[24] Gandara L, Mamone L, Dotto C, Buzzola F, Casas A. Sae regulator factor impairs the response to photodynamic inactivation mediated by Toluidine blue in Staphylococcus aureus. Photodiagnosis and photodynamic therapy. 2016;16:136-141.

[25] M.N. Hoorijani, H. Rostami, M. Pourhajibagher, N. Chiniforush, M. Heidari, B. Pourakbari, H. Kazemian, K. Davari, V. Amini, R. Raoofian, A. Bahador, The effect of antimicrobial photodynamic therapy on the expression of novel methicillin resistance markers determined using cDNA-AFLP approach in Staphylococcus aureus, Photodiagnosis and photodynamic therapy 19 (2017) 249-255. doi: 10.1016/j.pdpdt.2017.06.012

[26] N. Kashef, M. Akbarizare, M.R. Razzaghi, In vitro Activity of Linezolid in Combination with Photodynamic Inactivation Against Staphylococcus aureus Biofilms, Avicenna journal of medical biotechnology 9(1) (2017) 44-48. doi:

[27] V. Pérez-Laguna, L. Pérez-Artiaga, V. Lampaya-Pérez, I. García-Luque, S. Ballesta, S. Nonell, M.P. Paz-Cristobal, Y. Gilaberte, A. Rezusta, Bactericidal Effect of Photodynamic Therapy, Alone or in Combination with Mupirocin or Linezolid, on Staphylococcus aureus, Frontiers in Microbiology 8 (2017) doi: 10.3389/fmicb.2017.01002

[28] B. Mai, Y. Gao, M. Li, X. Wang, K. Zhang, Q. Liu, C. Xu, P. Wang, Photodynamic antimicrobial chemotherapy for *Staphylococcus aureus* and multidrug-resistant bacterial burn infection in vitro and in vivo, Int J Nanomedicine 12 (2017) 5915-5931. doi: 10.2147/IJN.S138185

[29] T.S.D. Araujo, P.L.F. Rodrigues, M.S. Santos, J.M. de Oliveira, L.P. Rosa, V.S. Bagnato, K.C. Blanco, F.C. da Silva, Reduced methicillin-resistant Staphylococcus aureus biofilm formation in bone cavities by photodynamic therapy, Photodiagnosis and photodynamic therapy 21 (2018) 219-223. doi: 10.1016/j.pdpdt.2017.12.011

[30] Y. Gao, B. Mai, A. Wang, M. Li, X. Wang, K. Zhang, Q. Liu, S. Wei, P. Wang, Antimicrobial properties of a new type of photosensitizer derived from phthalocyanine against planktonic and biofilm forms of Staphylococcus aureus, Photodiagnosis and photodynamic therapy 21 (2018) 316-326. doi: 10.1016/j.pdpdt.2018.01.003

[31] X. Li, W. Huang, X. Zheng, S. Chang, C. Liu, Q. Cheng, S. Zhu, Synergistic in vitro effects of indocyanine green and ethylenediamine tetraacetate-mediated antimicrobial photodynamic therapy combined with antibiotics for resistant bacterial biofilms in diabetic foot infection, Photodiagnosis and Photodynamic Therapy 25 (2019) 300-308. doi: 10.1016/j.pdpdt.2019.01.010

[32] D.P. Dos Santos, D.P. Soares Lopes, R.C.J. de Moraes, C. Vieira Goncalves, L. Pereira Rosa, F.C. da Silva Rosa, R.A.A. da Silva, Photoactivated resveratrol against Staphylococcus aureus infection in mice, Photodiagnosis and photodynamic therapy 25 (2019) 227-236. doi: 10.1016/j.pdpdt.2019.01.005

[33] V.T. Anju, P. Paramanantham, B.S. S, A. Sharan, A. Syed, N.A. Bahkali, M.H. Alsaedi, K. K, S. Busi, Antimicrobial photodynamic activity of toluidine blue-carbon nanotube conjugate against Pseudomonas aeruginosa and Staphylococcus aureus - Understanding the mechanism of action, Photodiagnosis and photodynamic therapy 27 (2019) 305-316. doi: 10.1016/j.pdpdt.2019.06.014

[34] Cai Z, Li Y, Wang Y, Chen S, Jiang S, Ge H, et al. Antimicrobial effects of photodynamic therapy with antiseptics on Staphylococcus aureus biofilm on titanium surface. Photodiagnosis and photodynamic therapy. 2019;25:382-388.

[35] M. Li, L. Li, K. Su, X. Liu, T. Zhang, Y. Liang, D. Jing, X. Yang, D. Zheng, Z. Cui, Z. Li, S. Zhu, K.W.K. Yeung, Y. Zheng, X. Wang, S. Wu, Highly Effective and Noninvasive Near-Infrared Eradication of a Staphylococcus aureus Biofilm on Implants by a Photoresponsive Coating within 20 Min, Adv Sci (Weinh) 6(17) (2019) 1900599. doi: 10.1002/advs.201900599

[36] K. Makdoumi, M. Hedin, A. Backman, Different photodynamic effects of blue light with and without riboflavin on methicillin-resistant Staphylococcus aureus (MRSA) and human keratinocytes in vitro, Lasers in medical science 34(9) (2019) 1799-1805. doi: 10.1007/s10103-019-02774-9

[37] Huang J, Guo M, Jin S, Wu M, Yang C, Zhang G, et al. Antibacterial photodynamic therapy mediated by 5-aminolevulinic acid on methicillin-resistant Staphylococcus aureus. Photodiagnosis and photodynamic therapy. 2019;28:330-337.

[38] Z. Yuan, B. Tao, Y. He, C. Mu, G. Liu, J. Zhang, Q. Liao, P. Liu, K. Cai, Remote eradication of biofilm on titanium implant via near-infrared light triggered photothermal/photodynamic therapy strategy, Biomaterials 223 (2019) 119479. doi: 10.1016/j.biomaterials.2019.119479

[39] C.G. de Souza Teixeira, P.V. Sanita, A.P. Dias Ribeiro, L.M. Dias, J.H. Jorge, A.C. Pavarina, Antimicrobial photodynamic therapy effectiveness against susceptible and methicillin-resistant Staphylococcus aureus biofilms, Photodiagnosis and photodynamic therapy (2020) 101760. doi: 10.1016/j.pdpdt.2020.101760

[40] Walter AB, Simpson J, Jenkins JL, Skaar EP, Jansen ED. Optimization of optical parameters for improved photodynamic therapy of Staphylococcus aureus using endogenous coproporphyrin III. Photodiagnosis and photodynamic therapy. 2020;29:101624.

[41] M. Hamblin, Q.-Z. Zhang, K.-Q. Zhao, Y. Wu, X.-H. Li, C. Yang, L.-M. Guo, C.-H. Liu, D. Qu, C.-Q. Zheng, 5-aminolevulinic acid-mediated photodynamic therapy and its strain-dependent combined effect with antibiotics on Staphylococcus aureus biofilm, Plos One 12(3) (2017) e0174627. doi: 10.1371/journal.pone.0174627

[42] M. Adibhesami, M. Ahmadi, A.A. Farshid, F. Sarrafzadeh-Rezaei, B. Dalir-Naghadeh, Effects of silver nanoparticles on Staphylococcus aureus contaminated open wounds healing in mice: An experimental study, Veterinary research forum : an international quarterly journal 8(1) (2017) 23-28. doi:

[43] X. Lu, R. Chen, J. Lv, W. Xu, H. Chen, Z. Ma, S. Huang, S. Li, H. Liu, J. Hu, L. Nie, High-resolution bimodal imaging and potent antibiotic/photodynamic synergistic therapy for osteomyelitis with a bacterial inflammation-specific versatile agent, Acta biomaterialia 99 (2019) 363-372. doi: 10.1016/j.actbio.2019.08.043

[44] V. Perez-Laguna, I. Garcia-Luque, S. Ballesta, L. Perez-Artiaga, V. Lampaya-Perez, S. Samper, P. Soria-Lozano, A. Rezusta, Y. Gilaberte, Antimicrobial photodynamic activity of Rose Bengal, alone or in combination with Gentamicin, against planktonic and biofilm Staphylococcus aureus, Photodiagnosis and photodynamic therapy 21 (2018) 211-216. doi: 10.1016/j.pdpdt.2017.11.012

[45] P.L. Paez, C.M. Bazan, M.E. Bongiovanni, J. Toneatto, I. Albesa, M.C. Becerra, G.A. Arguello, Oxidative stress and antimicrobial activity of chromium(III) and ruthenium(II) complexes on *Staphylococcus aureus* and *Escherichia coli*, BioMed research international 2013 (2013) 906912. doi: 10.1155/2013/906912

[46] M.R. Ronqui, T.M. de Aguiar Coletti, L.M. de Freitas, E.T. Miranda, C.R. Fontana, Synergistic antimicrobial effect of photodynamic therapy and ciprofloxacin, Journal of photochemistry and photobiology. B, Biology 158 (2016) 122-9. doi: 10.1016/j.jphotobiol.2016.02.036

[47] C. Pigrau, [Oxazolidinones and glycopeptides], Enfermedades infecciosas y microbiologia clinica 21(3) (2003) 157-64; quiz 165, 169. doi: 10.1016/s0213-005x(03)72907-3

[48] L.P. Rosa, F.C. da Silva, S.A. Nader, G.A. Meira, M.S. Viana, Antimicrobial photodynamic inactivation of Staphylococcus aureus biofilms in bone specimens using methylene blue, toluidine blue ortho and malachite

green: An in vitro study, Archives of oral biology 60(5) (2015) 675-80. doi: 10.1016/j.archoralbio.2015.02.010

[49] J. Gong, D. Li, J. Yan, Y. Liu, D. Li, J. Dong, Y. Gao, T. Sun, G. Yang, The accessory gene regulator (agr) controls Staphylococcus aureus virulence in a murine intracranial abscesses model, The Brazilian journal of infectious diseases : an official publication of the Brazilian Society of Infectious Diseases 18(5) (2014) 501-6. doi: 10.1016/j.bjid.2014.03.005

[50] M. Pourhajibagher, H. Mahmoudi, L. Rezaei-Soufi, M.Y. Alikhani, A. Bahador, Potentiation effects of antimicrobial photodynamic therapy on quorum sensing genes expression: A promising treatment for multi-species bacterial biofilms in burn wound infections, Photodiagnosis and photodynamic therapy (2020) 101717. doi: 10.1016/j.pdpdt.2020.101717

Chapter 9

Cell Death after Photodynamic Therapy Treatment in Unicellular Protozoan Parasite *Tritrichomonas foetus*

Newton Soares da Silva, Aline Margraf Ferreira, Carolina Weigert Galvão, Rafael Mazer Etto and Cristina Pacheco Soares

Abstract

Programmed cell death in *T. foetus* does not seem to make sense at first sight; however, different mechanisms of cellular death in this unicellular organism have been observed. This review summarizes the available data related to programmed cell death already published for the cattle parasite *T. foetus* and attempts to clarify some crucial points to understand this mechanism found in non-mitochondriates parasites, as well as assist in future research. Important results with different treatments showed that the *T. foetus* can choose among different pathways how to initiate cell death. Thus, a major challenge for cellular death research remains the identification of the molecular cell death machinery of this protist, such as caspases pathway, nuclear abnormalities, morphology cell changes, cellular death in this parasite and the prospects in the future research. Although, the possibility of the existence of different pathways to cell death in trichomonads is discussed and a model for possible executioners pathways during *T. foetus* cell death is proposed.

Keywords: cell death mechanism, amitochondrial protozoan, photodynamic therapy, apoptosis, necrosis

1. Introduction

The cell death mechanisms used by the parasite *Tritrichomonas foetus* is a matter of an ongoing debate. Many mechanisms have been studied in different treatments, but much remains to be elucidated with respect to the protein machinery developed by these organisms with regard to death pathways. This review summarizes the current knowledge about cell death of *T. foetus* by showing all models. The aim is to show, on the one hand, that there is too much data requiring one or more explanatory model (s), but, the authors proposed specific models, on the other hand that the present data is not sufficient to definitely proof programmed cell death for this organism. Furthermore, we would like to point out perspectives on the proteomic of programmed cell death in this protist.

Besides the significance of the parasite as an etiologic agent, *T. foetus* has been used as a model for the study of drug carriers such as graphene oxide and carbon nanotube oxide (GCN-O) composite. It is still considered fascinating to study the mode of cell death since they do not have mitochondria but possess an unusual anaerobic membrane-bound organelle named the hydrogenosome [1–3].

Cell death has been studied in many organisms: in mitochondriate organisms there are multiple forms of cell death, including the "programmed cellular death" (PCD) types, that will be described below, and depends or not on the presence of family of proteins, which control the mitochondrial membrane permeabilization and the release of some mitochondrial proteins to cytosol, like observed mainly in apoptosis [4]. Besides, other types of programmed death accompanied by changes in morphological and biochemical features like autophagic cell death, for exemple, have been studied. The amitochondriate organisms, like *T. foetus*, do not have a known usual programmed death machinery [5].

Despite apoptosis has been shown to be the major mechanisms of death observed in *T. foetus* [6], different studies suggest the existence of more than one mechanism of cell death and, it's the type of stimuli and/or the degree of stimuli that determines the mechanism of death chosen by this cell.

Photodynamic Therapy (PDT) and drugs administration used for cancer chemotherapy results in DNA damage in some cells. A variety of injurious stimuli such as heat, radiation, hypoxia and cytotoxic anticancer drugs can induce apoptosis in low doses or result in necrosis at higher doses [7]. It has been assumed that the machinery of PCD is absent in amitochondrial organism, like trichomonads, however, recent studies show that *T. foetus* have the capacity of choose which way will take among many forms of cell death caspases dependent or independent, depending on the stimuli of this parasite, once individuals in the same culture can take different pathways, either inside of the parasite can occur more than one mechanism of cellular death [4]. It has become increasingly apparent that the mechanisms of cell death

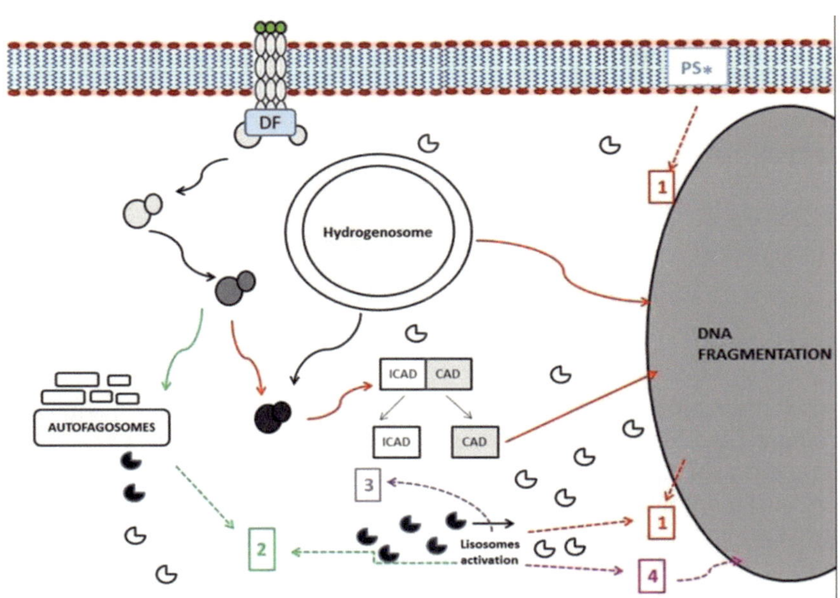

Figure 1.
Proposed model for possible executioners pathways during T. foetus *cell death, which includes the presence of possible apoptosis, autophagy, paraptosis and necrosis. Abbreviations: 1 = apoptosis, 2 = autophagy, 3 = necrosis, 4 = Paraptosis, DF = death receptor, PS * = phosphatidylserine exposure, CAD = caspase-activated DNase, ICAD = inhibitor of CAD.*

show a large diversity of phenotypes and cellular mechanisms, and, apparently, a modulation mechanism of cell death may lead to another [8]. Besides, the conservation of the molecular mechanism is relevant to the functional role of PCD process in the biology of protozoa since studies confirm the existence of this process in unicellular eukaryotes of different phylogenetic origins [9]. Hypotheses of alternative pathways of trichomonads cell death are suggested in **Figure 1**.

Other types of cell death may also be considered to be forms of PCD, because they require gene activation and function in an energy dependent manner. PCD is a genetically regulated physiological process, fundamental for multicellular organism development and homeostasis. Studies show that depending on the damage infringed, the cells seem to "choose" how to die [8, 10].

2. Trichomonad hydrogenosomes

According to Müller (1988) [11], *Entamoeba histolytica*, *Giardia lamblia*, *Trichomonas vaginalis*, *Tritrichomonas foetus* and rumen ciliates, they have hydrogenosomes instead of mitochondria. Hydrogenosomes of trichomonads are involved by two membrane layers, as mitochondria, and are organelles related to oxidation of pyruvate and the synthesis of ATP, as well as the storage of Ca^{2+} [12, 13]. As shown previously [14], Succinyl-coenzyme A synthetase (SCS) catalyzes the formation of ATP via substrate-level phosphorylation in hydrogenosome as it does, in mitochondria. Both organelles, mitochondria and hydrogenosome, use pyruvate as a major substrate and form acetyl-CoA (**Figure 2a, b**). Hydrogenosomes convert pyruvate quantitatively to acetate, malate, CO_2, and H_2, with acetate as the major product. The electrons from pyruvate:ferredoxin oxidoreductase (PFO) pass through ferredoxin and are transferred to NAD or NADP by ferredoxin:NAD(P) oxidoreductase. This process is accompanied by the phosphorylation of ADP to ATP in presence of

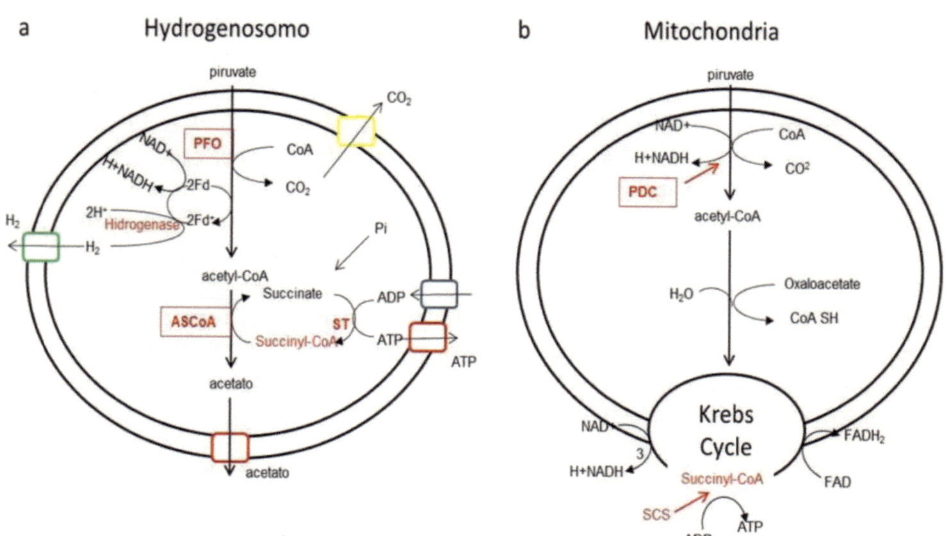

Figure 2.
Comparison of oxidation metabolism of pyruvate between hydrogenosome and mitochondria. (a) In T. foetus *and probably in all other trichomonad flagellates acetate is formed by the sucessive action of ASCoA (reaction acetyl-CoA+succinate = acetate + succinyl-CoA) and ST (reaction succinyl-CoA+ADP+Pi = succinate + ATP). ASCoA = acetate:succinate CoA transferase; PFO = pyruvate:ferredoxin oxidoreductase; ST = succinate thiokinase. (b) Piruvate oxidation in mitochondria precedes the Krebs cycle. PDC = pyruvate dehydrogenase. SCS = succinyl CoA sintetase.*

succinate and acetate:succinate CoA-tranferase. The production of H_2 is catalyzed by a hydrogenase which transfers electrons to protons H^+, a process not available to organisms without hidrogenosomo (**Figure 2a**) [11].

Evidences indicate that hydrogenosomes are anaerobic forms of mitochondria [15] or a specialized form of mitochondria useful in lower O_2 environments [16]. According to Martin (2005) [16] hydrogenosomes and mitochondria are, respectively, anaerobic and aerobic manifestations of the same organelle. Although, unlike mitochondria, the hydrogenosomes lack the DNA [15].

Trichomonad hydrogenosomes possess many proteins in common with mitochondria [15]. Translocation studies using hydrogenosomal ADP/ATP carrier of *T. vaginalis* revealed compatibility in membrane protein import between mitochondria and hydrogenosomes. These hydrogenosomal ADP/ATP carriers utilize the same translocation pathway for translocation into mitochondrial inner membrane [17]. Hydrogenosomes also contain heat-shock proteins which are known to participate in protein translocation and folding in mitochondria [17].

The most accept hypothesis for the origin of hydrogenosomes and mitochondria is that both organelles share a common ancestral. Phylogenetic studies demonstrated the existence of a typical Hsp 70 gene in the *T. vaginalis* genome DNA that in other eukaryotes codes for a protein located in mitochondria. This suggests that trichomonads have had mitochondria in their early history, and this nuclear sequence could be the result of an ancient gene transfer from mitochondria to nucleus [18]. Many components of classical mitochondria are absent in hydrogenosomes, and they generate molecular hydrogen instead of consume oxygen. It is interesting to study whether hydrogenosomes are involved in the cell death at all [1].

During hydrogenosome formation, they have different forms, and then acquire a spherical structure, which can be changed in stress conditions [19]. Studies proposed that *T. foetus* under treatment with hydroxyurea, zinc or under serum deprivation present endoplasmic reticulum cisternae surrounded by abnormal hydrogenosomes, which have bigger size enlarged peripheral vesicles, and sometimes presenting a degraded aspect [20, 21].

Hydrogenosomes also exhibited altered size and shape and they were randomly distributed within parasites cells after lycorine treatment [2]. The sequence of alterations during the degradation of hydrogenosomes after treatment with lycorine included: matrix swelling, rupture of outer membrane, appearance of flocculent densities, and fragmentation of all membranous structures except the peripheral vesicle [20]. *T. foetus* treated with taxol, nocodazole or colchicine showed modifications in size, shape and distribution of the hydrogenosomes [22]. The presence of hydrogenosomes with altered morphologies was also observed in parasites incubated with different concentrations of thiabendazole [23]. Recent studies showed that alterations in lysosomes and hydrogenosomes were also observed in *T. foetus* after proteossome inhibitors treatment [24]. Other studies suggest that tetracycline disrupts hydrogenosomal function since it reduced the hydrogenosomal energy metabolism efficiency in *T. vaginalis* [25].

3. Morphological features to define programmed cellular death

PCD is not confined to apoptosis but that cells use different pathways for active self-destruction: condensation prominent or apoptosis; autophagy prominent, etc. [26, 27]. Although, there is some resistance to the exclusive use of the term PCD to specifically describe apoptosis [7]. PCD It now generally refers to any cell death that is mediated by the intracellular death program, no matter what triggers it and whether or not it displays all of the characteristic features of apoptosis It has become increasingly apparent that cell death mechanisms include a highly diverse array of phenotypes and molecular mechanisms. Because other types of cell death may require gene activation and function in an energy dependent manner, they are also considered to be forms of PCD. There is evidence of other forms of non-apoptotic programmed cell death that should also be considered since they may lead to new insights into cell death programs and reveal their potentially unique roles in development, homeostasis, neoplasia and degeneration. It is probable that all normal cell deaths, as well as many pathological cell deaths, utilize this evolutionarily conserved death program [28].

Apoptosis, autophagy and necrosis was previously named as 'type I, II and III cell death', respectively [29, 30]. Although, several critiques are related to this clear-cut distinction [31, 32]. According to morphological criteria, the cell death modalities during tissue development and homeostasis can be defined with three distinct routes of cellular catabolism.

3.1 Apoptosis

APOPTOSIS is characterized by specific morphological and biochemical changes of dying cells, including cell shrinkage, nuclear condensation and fragmentation, dynamic membrane blebbing and loss of adhesion to neighbors or to extracellular matrix. The biochemical changes include chromosomal DNA cleavage into internucleosomal fragments, phosphatidylserine externalization and a number of intracellular substrate cleavages by specific proteolysis [33].

3.2 Autophagic

AUTOPHAGIC is characterized by the sequestration of cytoplasm and organelles in double or multimembrane vesicles and delivery to the cells own lysosomes for subsequent degradation, exhibits extensive degradation of Golgi apparatus, polyribosomes and endoplasmatic reticulum, which precedes nuclear destruction [27, 34]. Later, swelling of cavities was observed and the dying cells were ultimately fragmented and were phagocytosed by the neighboring cells. The process of autophagy depends on both continuous protein synthesis and the continuous presence of ATP. The molecular mechanisms have been extensively studied in yeast and mammalian orthologues continue to be elucidated [35, 36]. In PDT treatments, a process employing UV-light and photosensitizes to kill cancer cells, as well as accumulation of lysosomotropic agents within the organelle, a process also triggers the lysosomal pathway of cell death [37, 38].

3.3 Citoplasmatic death or programmed necrosis

CITOPLASMATIC DEATH or PROGRAMMED NECROSIS is characterized by the swelling of cavities with a membrane border, such as mitochondria, followed by extensive fragmentation of the cells into fragments so small that cell debris can no longer be observed. This type of cell death occurred without the lysosomal system taking part and with recognizable reaction of the neighboring cells and was observed in regions of vacuolated cartilage during mineralization [27].

There is evidence that modulation of one form of cell death may lead to another [7]. Under some circumstances, apoptosis and autophagy can exert synergetic effects, whereas in other situations autophagy can be triggered only when apoptosis is suppressed [33].

4. Biochimical and morphological features to define cell death in parasite trichomonas

4.1 Caspases pathway

Caspases are essential proteins involved in cellular death that exist in cytosol of most cells in its inactive form as a polypeptide. They are, activated by cleavage, and apoptosis is considered a consequence of their activation cascade [39].

In some cases caspases can induce cellular death and in others they seem to be irrelevant in decision between death and life. In both situations, caspases participate in morphology of apoptosis [39]. According to Mariante et al. [4], caspases dependent cell death in trichomonads can occur through different known mechanisms, either by death receptors pathway, or through unknown signaling pathways, like the release of hydrogenosomes molecules, which may have analogous functions of mitochondrial proteins.

Although it is stablished that the apoptosis regulated by caspases are an important form of PCD, in many instances, PCD is caspase independent and non-apoptotic. Necrosis-like might or might not require caspases to activate cell death, while paraptosis and autophagic/vacuolar cell death traditionally do not call for the participation of caspases [10, 40]. Despite, some studies in mammalian cells indicate that caspases can regulate both apoptotic and nonapoptotic cell death, as autophagy [41].

In eukaryotic organisms, it is known that the caspases possess a fundamental role during the process of cellular death, especially on apoptosis, being the primary site of interaction with Bcl-2 proteins family. However, despite of the lack of mitochondria in trichomonads, Mariante et al. [42] confirm the participation of proteases of the Caspase-3 family in *T. foetus* cellular death, after treatment with H_2O_2. They showed that hydrogen peroxide may have degenerative effects. Studies suggest that progressive destabilization of the membranes of intracellular organelles, which would be caused for short-term exposure to low concentrations of H_2O_2 may induce lysosomal rupture indirectly by activation of phospholipases [43]. PDT treatment also leads to the release of lysosomes enzymes in *T. foetus* citoplasm, which by the increase of reactive oxygen species (ROS) activate procaspases that in turn active caspases inducing the occurrence of the cell death process [44].

4.2 Nuclear abnormalities

Trichomonads treated with different concentrations of H_2O_2 showed severe nuclear changes like unusual DNA condensation. Peripheral heterochromatin masses and nuclear DNA fragmentation can be observed in the nucleus of some cells, probably due to the activation of different endonucleases. One the other hand, in mammals the same treatment lead a different nuclear organization [42]. Nuclear changes was observed in *T. foetus* after treatment with H_2O_2 and griseofulvine, which may be related to the presence of activated molecules through caspases pathway, and/or, molecules released from hydrogenosomes [5]. After treatment of *T. foetus* with $AlPcS_4$, cellular disorder such as nucleus fragmentation was observed in several cells [6]. *T. foetus* PDT treatment associated with the same photosensitizer ($AlPcS_4$) showed a "ladder pattern" of DNA fragments of *T. foetus* in electrophoresis assay which can be a hallmark of apoptosis. Comet Assay testes confirmed DNA fragmentation in this condition as longer tails was observed (unpublished data). However, taxol and nocodazole induced the formation of multinucleated cells, abnormal distribution of the nuclear contents and, sometimes, nuclear fragmentation [22]. In recent studies utilizing tetracycline, it was observed DNA fragmentation in *T. vaginalis* [25].

4.3 Morphology cell changes

T. foetus has a simple life cycle that consists of only a trophozoitic form, which is characterized by a pear-shaped (PS) body, three anterior flagella and one recurrent flagellum [24, 45]. The trophozoite undergoes profound morphological alterations and takes on an endoflagellar form (EFF), also known as pseudocyst, under unfavorable environmental conditions, such as abrupt changes in temperature or in the presence of drugs, e.g. colchicine [22]. In *T. foetus* treated with $AlPcS_4$, the internalized flagella and fragmented axostyle-pelta complex was seen, whereas changes in the elongated shape were not observed after 24 h. Although, after 48 h of treatment was observed changes in the shape of parasites. The same changes were observed in *T. foetus* after treatment with PDT [6]. However, after treatment with H_2O_2, the parasites exhibit a change in their morphology, changing from elongated shape to spherical one [42]. After treatment with taxol, nocodazole or colchicine, a large number of cellular changes and drastic effects were observed such as the loss of the cells original shape, the flagella were gradually internalized and the cells assumed the pseudocyst form. During treatment with taxol cell size was increased, and giant, multinucleate and abnormal cells were observed, as well as the presence of zoids and membrane blebbing formation [22]. In *T. vaginalis* tetracycline-treatment the cell exhibited a round shape, a not disrupted plasma membrane, and a rough cell surface [25]. However, the parasites treated with mepoxomicin and bortezomib showed the appearance of wrinkled or rounded cells with externalized flagella, membrane blebbing, cell lysis, intense cytosolic and nuclear vacuolization, cytoplasmic disintegration and abnormal Golgi reduction [24]. The flagella were internalized after treatment of *T. foetus* with thiabendazole, and about 70% of the parasites were observed as giant form. Furthermore, after treatment with mebendazole, more than 90% of these parasites presented drastically altered morphologies [23]. The EFF occurs in living cells able to undertake nuclear division to form multinucleated cells and able to provoke damage to host cell. It is a reversible form of parasite and can have the ecto-phosphatase activities responsible to signaling this process [45, 46].

5. Possible cell death modalities in trichomonas

The biochemical basis for alternative forms of cell death morphologically distinct from PCD continues unknown. Understanding the mechanisms for these forms has implications for the understanding of evolutionary aspects of cell death programs, developmental cell death, neurodegeneration, and cancer therapeutics and for the design of novel therapeutic agents for diseases featuring these alternative forms of cell death [30].

Death of *T. foetus* was observed after higher concentrations of hydroxyurea or zinc, or longer times of serum deprivation [12, 21]. Recent studies show that the molecular events governing tetracyclines induced cell death in trichomonads provided via activating of several specific pathways and genes families [25] which leads to a programmed type of death.

The parasite *T. foetus* submitted to treatment with H_2O_2 and griseofulvine, demonstrated the induction of mechanisms of a second pathway of cellular death related to autophagy machinery with formation of autophagosomes [4]. When subjected to different treatments such as griseofulvine and PDT, the parasite cytoplasm either shows the formation of autophagic vacuoles, which can be related to the mechanism of autophagic cell death [4, 6]. The process of autophagy is suggested also after treatment of *T. vaginalis* with lycorine, owing to fragments of

	Apoptosis	Paraptosis	Autophagy	Treatment	Presence	References
Nuclear Fragmentation	YES	YES	YES (lack of chromatin condensation)	H_2O_2 PDT Griseofulvine $AlPcS_4$ Taxol Nocodazole Tetracycline (*T. vaginalis*)	YES	[42] [6] [4] [6] [22] [22] [25]
Caspases Activation	YES	*	YES	H_2O_2 Griseofulvine	YES NO	[42] [4]
PS Externalization	YES	NO		Licorine (*T. vaginalis*)	NO	[2]
Citoplasmic vacuolization	NO	YES	YES	H_2O_2 PDT Licorine (*T. vaginalis*) Proteassome inhibitors Mepoxomicin and Bertezomid	YES	[42] [6] [2] [24] [24] [23]
Cellular shapped changes	YES			H_2O_2 PDT Licorine (*T. vaginalis*) Mepoxomicin and Bertezomid Mebendazole	YES	[42] [6] [2] [24] [23]
Lysossomal enzime release	YES		YES	PDT	YES	[44]
Flagelar internalization	*	*	*	$AlPcS_4$ Taxol, Nacodazole and Colchicine Thiabendazole	YES	[6] [20] [23]
Plasmatic Membrane Projections (Blebs)	YES	NO	NO	H_2O_2 Licorine (*T. vaginalis*) Taxol, Nacodazole and Colchicine	YES NO YES	[42] [2] [20]

	Apoptosis	Paraptosis	Autophagy	Treatment	Presence	References
Hydrogenosomes shaped changes	*	*	*	H_2O_2 PDT Hidroxiuréia Zinc Serum deprivation Taxol, Nacodazole and Colchicine Licorine (*T. vginalis*) Lactacystin Mebendazole	YES	[42] [6] [21] [20] [20] [20] [2] [24] [23]
Citoplasmatic components degradetion	YES (Fragmention of citoplasm)	YES	YES	Licorine (*T. vginalis*) Mepoxomicin and Bertezomid	YES	[2] [24]

Major structural changes and pathways in cell death of the parasite T. foetus.
Unreferenced data.

Table 1.
Ultrastructural changes leading to cell death pathways on T. foetus.

endoplasmic reticulum seen in close contact with abnormal hydrogenosomes [2]. Furthermore, parasites treated with proteossome inhibitors exhibit the appearance of an uncommon enlarged endoplasmic reticulum and concentric membrane whorls, which resembled autophagic vacuoles [24]. The round-shaped mebendazole-treated parasites presented an intense cytoplasmic vacuolization, and profiles of endoplasmic reticulum were frequently seen in association with abnormal hydrogenosomes and vacuoles [23]. Another autophagy way can be necessary for caspases activation and induction of apoptosis in trichomonads. However, cellular death induced by griseofulvine in trichomonad seems to not involve the path of caspases autophagy way. Since both the mechanisms, apoptosis and autophagy, can lead to release of lysosomal components after treatment of *T. foetus* with PDT [44], it is not known which of these mechanisms the parasite is using in different treatments.

The absence of apoptotic bodies and the characterization of a non-apoptotic-like cell death which fails to fulfill the criteria for apoptosis suggest paraptosis mechanism, once the cell death features shown by lycorine treatment in *T. vaginalis* differ from the apoptosis-like characteristics reported for this protist [2]. Although *T. foetus* presents some morphological aspects similar to apoptosis such as nuclear fragmentation and chromatin condensation, it also features aspects of paraptosis such as cytoplasmic vacuolization and chromatin condensation [6]. The main feature of paraptosis consists of extensive cytoplasmic vacuolation without significant cell membrane blebbing, nuclear shrinkage, or pyknosis. To date the most defining feature that differentiates it from autophagic cell death is the absence of autophagic vacuoles in paraptosis (**Table 1**) [29, 30, 42, 47].

Although, recent studies showed the "ladder pattern" compatible internucleosomic genomic DNA fragmentation characteristic of apoptosis, in *T foetus* submitted to PDT treatment (unpublished data).

The different treatments and the different results obtained with *T. foetus* suggest the existence of more than one mechanism of cell demise in these parasites (**Figure 1**).

6. Implications and future directions

The evidence of that alternative, non-apoptotic, PCD in unicellular organisms has important implications for understanding cell dynamics. The environmental stimuli can produce different types of cell death depending on the intensity of stimulus, and that classic apoptosis and necrosis may represent only two extremes of a continuum intermediate form of cell death, applicable to also unicellular organisms [10]. Comparatives analyses of proteome maps from parasites exhibiting such pathogenic characteristics may provide valuable data to understand the pathogenic mechanisms involved in urogenital trichomoniasis. Besides, the metabolic pathways that are different from those of their mammal hosts, given that Trichomonads possesses a hydrogenosomal/cytosolic compartmentalization of metabolism and metabolic pathway, the identification of proteins involved in such metabolic pathways could reveal good targets for drugs development [1, 48].

Several laboratories have contributed to understand the protein expression of Trichomonads, but despite numerous research and efforts to unravel the mechanisms of cell death, detailed description of the molecular mechanisms is still unknown. Identification of proteins related to the machinery of death of these cells should be the main focus of studies in the coming years. Studies related to molecular biology and biochemistry are still needed because little is known about the overall proteomic expression profiling of this parasite.

Acknowledgements

We gratefully acknowledge the Brazilian agency FAPESP (São Paulo Research Foundation) (2013/20054-8) for financial support.

Author details

Newton Soares da Silva[1*], Aline Margraf Ferreira[1], Carolina Weigert Galvão[2], Rafael Mazer Etto[3] and Cristina Pacheco Soares[1]

1 Institute of Research and Development, UNIVAP, São José dos Campos, SP, Brazil

2 Department of Structural and Molecular Biology and Genetics, UEPG, Ponta Grossa, PR, Brasil

3 Department of Chemistry, UEPG - Ponta Grossa PR, Brasil

*Address all correspondence to: nsoares@univap.br

References

[1] Deponte, M., 2008. Programmed cell death in protists. Biochim. Bioph ys. Acta 1783, 1396-405. doi:10.1016/j.bbamcr.2008.01.018

[2] Giordani, R.B., De Brum Vieira, P., Weizenmann, M., Rosemberg, D.B., Souza, A.P., Bonorino, C., De Carli, G.A., Bogo, M.R., Zuanazzi, J.A., Tasca, T., 2011. Lycorine induces cell death in the amitochondriate parasite, *Trichomonas vaginalis*, via an alternative non-apoptotic death pathway. Phytochemistry 72, 645-650. doi:10.1016/j.phytochem.2011.01.023

[3] Zanin, H., Margraf-Ferreira, A., Da Silva, N.S., Marciano, F.R., Corat, E.J., Lobo, A.O., 2014. Graphene and carbon nanotube composite enabling a new prospective treatment for trichomoniasis disease. Mater. Sci. Eng. C 41, 65-69. doi:10.1016/j.msec.2014.04.020

[4] Mariante, R.M., Vancini, R.G., Benchimol, M., 2006. Cell death in trichomonads: New insights. Histochem. Cell Biol. 125, 545-556. doi:10.1007/s00418-005-0098-5

[5] Chose, O., Sarde, C.O., Gerbod, D., Viscogliosi, E., Roseto, A., 2003. Programmed cell death in parasitic protozoans that lack mitochondria. Trends Parasitol. 19, 559-564. doi:10.1016/j.pt.2003.09.016

[6] Da Silva, N.S., Ribeiro, C. de M., Machado, A.H.A., Pacheco-Soares, C., 2007. Ultrastructural changes in *Tritrichomonas foetus* after treatments with AlPcS4 and photodynamic therapy. Vet. Parasitol. 146, 175-181. doi:10.1016/j.vetpar.2007.02.006

[7] Elmore, S., 2007. Apoptosis: a review of programmed cell death. Toxicol. Pathol. 35, 495-516. doi:10.1080/01926230701320337

[8] Dal Canto, M.C., Gurney, M.E., 1994. Development of central nervous system pathology in a murine transgenic model of human amyotrophic lateral sclerosis. Am. J. Pathol. 145, 1271-1279.

[9] Da Silva, N.S. 2011. Basic biological aspects of *Tritrichomonas foetus* of re-levance to the treatment of bovines suffering of tricho-moniasis. Open J. Anim. Sci. 01, 112-120. doi:10.4236/ojas.2011.13015

[10] Jiménez, C., Capasso, J.M., Edelstein, C.L., Rivard, C.J., Lucia, S., Breusegem, S., Berl, T., Segovia, M., 2009. Different ways to die: Cell death modes of the unicellular chlorophyte Dunaliella viridis exposed to various environmental stresses are mediated by the caspase-like activity DEVDase. J. Exp. Bot. 60, 815-828. doi:10.1093/jxb/ern330

[11] Müller, M., 1988. Energy metabolism of protozoa without mitochondria. Annu. Rev. Microbiol. 42, 465-488. doi:10.1146/annurev.micro.42.1.465

[12] Almeida, J.C.A., Benchimol, M., De Souza, W., Okorokov, L.A., 2003. Ca^{2+} sequestering in the early-branching amitochondriate protozoan *Tritrichomonas foetus:* An important role of the Golgi complex and its Ca^{2+}-ATPase. Biochim. Biophys. Acta - Biomembr. 1615, 60-68. doi:10.1016/S0005-2736(03)00192-5

[13] Benchimol, M., Elias, C.A., De Souza, W., 1982. *Tritrichomonas foetus:* Ultrastructural localisation of calcium in the plasma membrane and in the hydrogenosome 54, 277-284.

[14] Lahti, C.J., Bradley, P.J., Johnson, P.J., 1994. Molecular characterization of the α-subunit of *Trichomonas vaginalis* hydrogenosomal

succinyl CoA synthetase. Mol. Biochem. Parasitol. 66, 309-318. doi:10.1016/0166-6851(94)90157-0

[15] Rotte, C., Henze, K., Müller, M., Martin, W., n.d. Origins of hydrogenosomes and mitochondria Commentary. Curr. Opin. Microbiol. 481-486. doi:Doi 10.1016/S1369-5274(00)00126-0

[16] Martin, W., 2005. The missing link between hydrogenosomes and mitochondria. Trends Microbiol. 13, 457-459. doi:10.1016/j.tim.2005.08.005

[17] Dyall, S.D., Johnson, P.J., 2000. Origins of hydrogenosomes and mitochondria: Evolution and organelle biogenesis. Curr. Opin. Microbiol. 3, 404-411. doi:10.1016/S1369-5274(00)00112-0

[18] Germot, A., Philippe, H., Le Guyader, H., 1996. Presence of a mitochondrial-type 70-kDa heat shock protein in *Trichomonas vaginalis* suggests a very early mitochondrial endosymbiosis in eukaryotes. Proc. Natl. Acad. Sci. U. S. A. 93, 14614-14617. doi:10.1073/pnas.93.25.14614

[19] Benchimol, M., Almeida, J.C.A., De Souza, W., 1996. Further studies on the organization of the hydrogenosome in *Tritrichomonas foetus*. Tissue Cell 28, 287-299. doi:10.1016/S0040-8166(96)80016-4

[20] Benchimol, M., 1999. Hydrogenosome autophagy: an ultrastructural and cytochemical study. Biol. Cell 91, 165-74.

[21] Ribeiro, K.C., Mariante, R.M., Coutinho, L.L., Benchimol, M., 2002. Nucleus behavior during the closed mitosis of *Tritrichomonas foetus*. Biol. Cell 94, 289-301. doi:10.1016/S0248-4900(02)01206-6

[22] Madeiro Da Costa, R.F., Benchimol, M., 2004. The effect of drugs on cell structure of *Tritrichomonas foetus*. Parasitol. Res. 92, 159-170. doi:10.1007/s00436-003-1023-2

[23] Carvalho, K.P., Gadelha, A.P.R., 2007. Effects of three benzimidazoles on growth, general morphology and ultrastructure of *Tritrichomonas foetus*. FEMS Microbiol. Lett. 275, 292-300. doi:10.1111/j.1574-6968.2007.00897.x

[24] Pereira-Neves, A., Gonzaga, L., Menna-Barreto, R.F.S., Benchimol, M., 2015. Characterisation of 20S Proteasome in *Tritrichomonas foetus* and Its Role during the Cell Cycle and Transformation into Endoflagellar Form. PLoS One 10, e0129165. doi:10.1371/journal.pone.0129165

[25] Huang, K.Y., Ku, F.M., Cheng, W.H., Lee, C.C., Huang, P.J., Chu, L.J., Cheng, C.C., Fang, Y.K., Wu, H.H., Tang, P., 2015. Novel insights into the molecular events linking to cell death induced by tetracycline in the amitochondriate protozoan *Trichomonas vaginalis*. Antimicrob. Agents Chemother. 59, 6891-6903. doi:10.1128/AAC.01779-15

[26] Bursch, W., 2001. The autophagosomal-lysosomal compartment in programmed cell death. Cell Death Differ. 8, 569-581. doi:10.1038/sj.cdd.4400852

[27] Bursch, W., Hochegger, K., Torok, L., Marian, B., Ellinger, A., Hermann, R.S., 2000. Autophagic and apoptotic types of programmed cell death exhibit different fates of cytoskeletal filaments. J. Cell Sci. 113, 1189-1198.

[28] Jacobson, M., Weil, M., Raff, M., 1997. Programmed cell death in animal development. Cell 88, 347-354. doi:10.1016/S0092-8674(00)81873-5

[29] Sperandio, S., Poksay, K., de Belle, I., Lafuente, M.J., Liu, B., Nasir, J., Bredesen, D.E., 2004. Paraptosis: mediation by MAP kinases and

inhibition by AIP-1/Alix. Cell Death Differ. 11, 1066-1075. doi:10.1038/sj.cdd.4401465

[30] Sperandio, S., de Belle, I., Bredesen, D.E., 2000. An alternative, nonapoptotic form of programmed cell death. Proc. Natl. Acad. Sci. 97, 14376-14381. doi:10.1073/pnas.97.26.14376

[31] Galluzzi, L., Vitale, I., Abrams, J.M., Alnemri, E.S., Baehrecke, E.H., Blagosklonny, M. V, Dawson, T.M., Dawson, V.L., El-Deiry, W.S., Fulda, S., Gottlieb, E., Green, D.R., Hengartner, M.O., Kepp, O., Knight, R.A., Kumar, S., Lipton, S.A., Lu, X., Madeo, F., Malorni, W., Mehlen, P., Nuñez, G., Peter, M.E., Piacentini, M., Rubinsztein, D.C., Shi, Y., Simon, H.-U., Vandenabeele, P., White, E., Yuan, J., Zhivotovsky, B., Melino, G., Kroemer, G., 2012. Molecular definitions of cell death subroutines: recommendations of the Nomenclature Committee on Cell Death 2012. Cell Death Differ. 19, 107-120. doi:10.1038/cdd.2011.96

[32] Kroemer, G., Galluzzi, L., Vandenabeele, P., Abrams, J., Alnemri, E.S., Baehrecke, E.H., Blagosklonny, M. V, El-Deiry, W.S., Golstein, P., Green, D.R., Hengartner, M., Knight, R.A., Kumar, S., Lipton, S.A., Malorni, W., Nuñez, G., Peter, M.E., Tschopp, J., Yuan, J., Piacentini, M., Zhivotovsky, B., Melino, G., 2009. Classification of cell death: recommendations of the Nomenclature Committee on Cell Death 2009. Cell Death Differ. 16, 3-11. doi:10.1038/cdd.2008.150

[33] Ouyang, L., Shi, Z., Zhao, S., Wang, F.T., Zhou, T.T., Liu, B., Bao, J.K., 2012. Programmed cell death pathways in cancer: A review of apoptosis, autophagy and programmed necrosis. Cell Prolif. 45, 487-498. doi:10.1111/j.1365-2184.2012.00845.x

[34] Noda, T., Suzuki, K., Ohsumi, Y., 2002. Yeast autophagosomes: De novo formation of a membrane structure. Trends Cell Biol. 12, 231-235. doi:10.1016/S0962-8924(02)02278-X

[35] Huang, W.-P., Klionsky, D.J., 2002. Autophagy in yeast: a review of the molecular machinery. Cell Struct. Funct. 27, 409-420. doi:10.1247/csf.27.409

[36] Ohsumi, Y., 2001. Molecular dissection of autophagy: two ubiquitin-like systems. Nat. Rev. Mol. Cell Biol. 2, 211-216. doi:10.1038/35056522

[37] Boya, P., Andreau, K., Poncet, D., Zamzami, N., Perfettini, J.-L., Metivier, D., Ojcius, D.M., Jäättelä, M., Kroemer, G., 2003. Lysosomal membrane permeabilization induces cell death in a mitochondrion-dependent fashion. J. Exp. Med. 197, 1323-34. doi:10.1084/jem.20021952

[38] Cirman, T., Orešić, K., Mazovec, G.D., Turk, V., Reed, J.C., Myers, R.M., Salvesen, G.S., Turk, B., 2004. Selective Disruption of Lysosomes in HeLa Cells Triggers Apoptosis Mediated by Cleavage of Bid by Multiple Papain-like Lysosomal Cathepsins. J. Biol. Chem. 279, 3578-3587. doi:10.1074/jbc.M308347200

[39] Green, D., Kroemer, G., 1998. The central executioners of apoptosis: Caspases or mitochondria? Trends Cell Biol. 8, 267-271. doi:10.1016/S0962-8924(98)01273-2

[40] Wang, W., Scali, M., Vignani, R., Spadafora, A., Sensi, E., Mazzuca, S., Cresti, M., 2003. Protein extraction for two-dimensional electrophoresis from olive leaf, a plant tissue containing high levels of interfering compounds. Electrophoresis 24, 2369-2375. doi:10.1002/elps.200305500

[41] Yu, L., Alva, A., Su, H., Dutt, P., Freundt, E., Welsh, S., Baehrecke, E.H., Lenardo, M.J., 2004. Regulation of an ATG7-beclin 1 program of autophagic cell death by caspase-8. Science

(80-.). 304, 1500-1502. doi:10.1126/science.1096645\r1096645 [pii]

[42] Mariante, R.M., Guimar??es, C.A., Linden, R., Benchimol, M., 2003. Hydrogen peroxide induces caspase activation and programmed cell death in the amitochondrial *Tritrichomonas foetus*. Histochem. Cell Biol. 120, 129-141. doi:10.1007/s00418-003-0548-x

[43] Zhao, Baozhong; He, Y.Y., 2010. Recent advances in the prevention and treatment of skin cancer using photodynamic therapy. Expert Rev Anticancer Ther. 10, 1797-1809. doi:10.1586/era.10.154.Recent

[44] Machado, S.M., Pacheco-Soares, C., Marciano, F.R., Lobo, A.O., Da Silva, N.S., 2014. Photodynamic therapy in the cattle protozoan *Tritrichomonas foetus* cultivated on superhydrophilic carbon nanotube. Mater. Sci. Eng. C 36, 180-186. doi:10.1016/j.msec.2013.12.004

[45] de Andrade Rosa, I., de Souza, W., Benchimol, M., 2015. Changes in the structural organization of the cytoskeleton of *Tritrichomonas foetus* during trophozoite-pseudocyst transformation. Micron 73, 28-35. doi:10.1016/j.micron.2015.03.008

[46] Pereira-Neves, A., Rosales-Encina, J.L., Meyer-Fernandes, J.R., Benchimol, M., 2014. *Tritrichomonas foetus:* Characterisation of ecto-phosphatase activities in the endoflagelar form and their possible participation on the parasite's transformation and cytotoxicity. Exp. Parasitol. 142, 67-82. doi:10.1016/j.exppara.2014.04.007

[47] Sperandio, S., Poksay, K.S., Schilling, B., Crippen, D., Gibson, B.W., Bredesen, D.E., 2010. Identification of new modulators and protein alterations in non-apoptotic programmed cell death. J. Cell. Biochem. 111, 1401-1412. doi:10.1002/jcb.22870

[48] De Jesus, J.B., Cuervo, P., Junqueira, M., Britto, C., Silva-Filho, F.C., Sabóia-Vahia, L., González, L.J., Barbosa Domont, G., 2007. Application of two-dimensional electrophoresis and matrix-assisted laser desorption/ionization time-of-flight mass spectrometry for proteomic analysis of the sexually transmitted parasite*Trichomonas vaginalis*. J. Mass Spectrom. 42, 1463-1473. doi:10.1002/jms.1286

Chapter 10

Evaluation of the Antimicrobial Efficacy of Different Types of Photodynamic Therapy on the Main Pathogenic Bacteria of Peri-Implantitis

Dragana Gabrić, Ana Budimir, Ivona Bago, Luka Marković, Verica Pavlić and Bleron Azizi

Abstract

Every year, with the increasing number of dental implants placed, there is an increase in the incidence of peri-implantitis. The treatment of peri-implantitis is very complex and among other things includes mechanical and chemical decontamination of the implant surfaces, which is very challenging and often not predictable due to the surface properties of the implants. Photodynamic therapy recently has emerged as a potential treatment alternative or adjuvant treatment to peri-implantitis. Its potential to decontaminate implant surfaces without damaging the surface and the implants surrounding tissues has generated much interest in the scientific community. The possibilities of photodynamic therapy in treatment of peri-implantitis are opening new challenges in establishing optimal conditions for the clinical application of aPDT. Due to its non-invasiveness and ease of use this method can be effective when applied alone or as an adjunct therapy to conventional methods for treating peri-implantitis.

Keywords: photodynamic therapy, implants, peri-implanitits, titanium, zirconia

1. Introduction

Antimicrobial photodynamic therapy (aPDT) is becoming a treatment option in dental medicine in different areas such as the diagnosis of malignant transformation of oral lesions, the treatment of head and neck cancer, as well as the treatment of bacterial and fungal infections [1, 2].

In periodontology, the conventional therapeutic approach for treating periodontal diseases consists of mechanical cleaning combined with chemical decontamination, or the use of antimicrobial therapy which can be applied systemically or locally. The mechanical debridement has its own limitations in removing all the infections, such as the difficulties in reaching deep pockets and, as a result, the etiological factors continue to damage the periodontal ligament. Also, when mechanical debridement is used frequently, it can cause damage of the root surface [3].

The limitations of the conventional periodontal therapy have shifted the focus towards aPDT, as an effective alternative treatment for periodontal diseases [4–8]. aPDT is having many advantages over conventional therapy. The main advantage is the fact that photosensitizer can be placed directly into the periodontal pocket and then activated with an optical fiber tip in order to kill microbial cells, without damaging the host tissues. This makes aPDT a safe procedure against periodontal microbiota [9, 10].

Many studies have demonstrated potential improvements after the use of aPDT in conjunction with mechanical debridement [11–13]. However, there are several studies that report different results [5, 14–16]. Atieh suggested as a result of his meta-analysis, potential improvements after aPDT combined with scaling and root planning in probing periodontal pocket depth (PPD) reduction and greater clinical attachment level (CAL) gain [13]. Similarly, in their study Sgolastra et al. reported that the combination of aPDT and conventional treatment provides additional benefits by reducing the PPD and increasing the CAL [11].

In endodontics, aPDT is used for the disinfection of the root canal. Conventional endodontic treatment consists of a combination of mechanical cleaning and shaping of the canals, the use of disinfecting solutions for irrigation and the placement of medicaments in between appointments. Sometimes, due to the root canal anatomy it is difficult to completely disinfect the canals by using only mechanical and chemical decontamination methods [17, 18]. aPDT demonstrated promising results as an adjunct therapy for the root canal disinfection in many studies. Raymond et al. [17] evaluated the efficacy of the combination of conventional treatment with photodynamic therapy *in vitro*. Their results showed that the combination of both therapies is more effective than the use of traditional treatment alone. Rios et al. [19] in their study used a combination of light-emitting diode (LED) as a light source and toluidine blue O dye as a photosensitizer. They suggested that photodynamic therapy can be used as an adjunctive antimicrobial procedure in endodontics. Similarly in their clinical study, Bago et al. [20] demonstrated that aPDT when used as an addition to the conventional mechanical and chemical root canal cleaning, can lead to significantly more reduction of the bacteria and in some samples the total elimination of the bacteria.

Photodynamic therapy is used also in oral and maxillofacial surgery due to its potential to be used as an anti-cancer treatment and its antimicrobial potential. Oral squamous cell carcinomas (SCC) are the most frequent tumors in the oral cavity [21]. Up to date the traditional methods for treating SCC have not been very successful in increasing the 5-year survival rate. Furthermore they cause different side effects such as mouth sore, jaw pain and difficulties in chewing or swallowing [22].

One of the developing factors of oral SCC are considered to be the pre-malignant lesions such as erythroplakias and dysplastic leukoplakias. Around half of oral SCC cases are associated with leukoplakias [23]. The potential therapeutic possibilities of photodynamic therapy are not limited only for oral SCC and other head and neck cancers, but also against pre-malignant, primary, recurrent and metastatic lesions [24, 25]. PDT when compared to conventional treatments of these lesions, has an advantage due to its selective tumor destruction and minimal invasiveness without affecting the healthy tissues. In addition, it can combined with conventional therapy to increase the overall treatment success [26].

The PDT antimicrobial potential in oral and maxillofacial surgery, is mostly used for the disinfection of soft tissue or bone during surgical interventions, as a preventive measure. In a study done by Neugebauer et al. [27] it was demonstrated that use of aPDT caused significantly lower incidence of alveolar ostitis. In a another study it was concluded that the effect of photodynamic therapy is almost the same as the effect of 2.5% NaOCl without causing adverse effects on surrounding tissues on periapical lesion model *in vitro* [28]. Batinjan et al. [29] showed that aPDT causes reduced postoperative wound swelling and decreased wound temperature after the removal of the impacted third mandibular molar.

PDT has recently also been used as an adjuvant therapy for the treatment of medication-related osteonecrosis of jaws (MRONJ), that is highly related to bisphosphonate-related osteonecrosis of the jaw (BRONJ). In a study done by Minamisako et al. [30], it was suggested that both low level laser therapy (LLLT) and PDT are beneficial in the clinical management of the MRONJ. Similarly, Rugani et al. [31] concluded that photodynamic therapy can be used as treatment option in the early stages of BRONJ or as an adjunct therapy when surgical intervention is indicated.

1.1 Peri-implant diseases and aPDT

In 1978. Brånemark presented two-stage threaded titanium implants in a root-form [32]. The concept of osseointegration of the implants was first brought during the 1950s and 1960s after observing bone growth in contact with titanium. Brånemark defined osseointegration as: "A direct connection between living bone and a load-carrying endosseous implant at the light microscopic level." [33]. Since then, dental implants have become a long-term reliable treatment option for replacing missing teeth [34]. An ideal implant should have the following properties: biocompatibility, adequate toughness, strength, corrosion resistance, facture and wear resistance [35–37].

The "gold standard" of dental implants are considered to be the implants produced from titanium and its alloys. Titanium has excellent biocompatibility and it was shown that long term surgical rates of titanium implants are excellent [38, 39]. However, due to their dark gray color sometimes the implants can reflect through the peri-implant soft tissue. This poses an esthetic challenge especially when a thin biotype of gingiva is present or when there is a resorption of the buccal lamina [39, 40]. Due to these reasons, many scientists have shifted their focus into producing ceramic implants [41].

The infection around dental implants can be presented as peri-implant mucositis or peri-implantitis. Peri-implant mucositis is a reversible inflammatory process and it affects only the soft tissues around the dental implant. This is followed by reddening, swelling and bleeding on probing [42]. Peri-implantitis on the other hand affects both soft and hard tissues around the implant and as a result loss of supporting bone occurs [43]. The microbial etiology of peri-implantitis is well documented in literature [44]. The microorganisms found in peri-implantits are very similar to those found in advanced periodontitis [45, 46]. Most of them are spirochetes and non-motile anaerobic Gram-negative bacteria such as: *Porphyromonas gingivalis, Aggregatibacter actinomycetemcomitans,, Prevotella intermedia, Tannarella forsythia, Treponema denticola* etc. [47]. In the oral cavity the implant surfaces are colonized very rapidly by the bacteria, which leads to the formation of a bacterial biofilm on the implant surface. When peri-implanitits is in its early stages, there are no significant symptoms and most of the time it is diagnosed during routine dental check-up. It is of great importance to diagnose peri-implanitits in its early stages in order to prevent the progression of the disease and increase the chances for good osseointegration [48].

According to Teughels et al. [49], the quantity and quality of plaque formation and bacterial adhesion on implant surfaces is influenced by the chemical composition, and the surface roughness of the implant. Rough surfaces and those with greater surface free energy, accumulate more plaque. Furthermore, initial bacterial adhesion is attracted more to surfaces with high wettability and pits and grooves in the roughened surfaces. The formation of bacterial plaque in these surfaces is difficult to remove.

To date, many treatment methods have been proposed for treating peri-implantitis. They can be grouped in two categories: resective and regenerative therapies [50].

The main goal of resective treatments is to eliminate the etiological factors of peri-implanittis and maintain optimal conditions. These treatments are mainly done by cleaning and decontaminating implant surfaces. Regenerative treatments aim to reconstruct the pre-existing hard and soft tissues by using bone substitute grafts, membranes and growth factors [50, 51]. Resective treatment of peri-implanitits is similar to the treatment of periodontitis and it consists of mechanical cleaning of the biofilm from the implant surface. This is of the utmost importance when treating peri-implanitits. During resective treatment, plastic curettes, air-powder abrasive or ablative lasers and ultrasonic scalers are used [52]. The main objective is to clean the surface which can stop the progression of the disease and increase the chances for re-osseointegration of the implant. However, due to the implant surface roughness, the bacterial adhesion and colonization is very difficult to remove and sometimes mechanical debridement alone is not very effective [53]. It has been suggested by some authors that the mechanical elimination of the implant threads and then smoothing the implant surface (implantoplasty) should be done, in order to improve the decontamination of the implant surface. In addition this procedure allows better maintenance and oral hygiene when threads are exposed to the oral environment [54]. When decontaminating the implant surface, the use of metallic curettes is not recommended due to the fact that they can alter the surface roughness of the implant and favor bacterial colonization. As an alternative, plastic curettes should be used because they do very little damage or none at all [55, 56].

Recently, as a treatment alternative, many scientists have shifted their focus towards the laser decontamination of the implant surfaces. In a study done by Kreisler et al. [57] the mechanical effects of Nd:YAG (Neodymium: yttrium-aluminum-garnet), Ho:YAG (Holmium: yttrium-aluminum-garnet), Er:YAG (Erbium: yttrium-aluminum-garnet), CO2 (Carbon dioxide) and GaAlAs (Gallium-Aluminum-Arsenide) lasers were evaluated, on different types of implant surfaces.. According to their results, Nd:YAG and Ho:YAG lasers cause significant damage to the implant surfaces, while CO2 and Er:YAG lasers when used in specific power settings do not cause any damage. GaAlAs laser did not damage the implant surface in any power settings. As an adjunct therapy to mechanical methods for treating peri-implantitis, the use of chemical decontamination and antibiotic therapy are being used with the aim of improving the treatment outcome. The most commonly used antimicrobial solutions are chlorhexidine, hydrogen peroxide, tetracycline or minocycline, citric acid, and phosphoric acid [58].

Recently aPDT has emerged as a new treatment option or adjuvant treatment to the conventional treatment of peri-implantitis. Its potential to decontaminate the implant surfaces without any damage to the implant or the surrounding tissues has generated a lot of interest in the scientific community. In addition aPDT is more effective than the use of lasers alone [53]. In their study, Hayek et al. [59] demonstrated that aPDT is both effective and non-invasive method when compared to traditional therapy during surgical treatment of peri-implantitis with elevated mucoperiosteal mucosal flaps. These beneficial characteristics of aPDT make it as promising novel and non-invasive method which can be used alone or as an adjunct therapy of peri-implantitis [2].

2. The efficacy of photodynamic therapy in *in vitro* conditions

There are many *in vitro* studies evaluating the efficacy of photodynamic therapy against causative bacteria of peri-implantitis. The aim of our research was to evaluate the efficacy of aPDT on titanium and zirconia dental implants. For this purpose three different devices in combination with photosensitive dye were used.

In addition, our aim was to evaluate if aPDT causes damage and alteration to the implant surfaces which would interfere with the re-osseoinegration of the implants in the clinical conditions.

The study sample consisted of 144 sterile dental implants (72 titanium dental implants and 72 zirconia dental implants) (Bredent®, Senden, Germany). Both, titanium and zirconia dental implants were with a diameter of 4.0 mm and 12 mm of length, with sandblasted and acid etched surface. Each of the implants was in an unopened sterile packaging.

2.1 Bacterial contamination of dental implants

A bacterial suspension was prepared from three bacteria species: *Prevotella intermedia, Aggregatibacter actinomycetemcomitans*, and *Porphyromonas gingivalis*. These bacteria are commonly found in peri-implant diseases.

The bacteria were cultivated separately in Columbia Agar for 72 hours and then, using thioglycolate broth, a bacterial suspension was prepared for each of the bacteria. The suspension of each of the bacteria was then mixed together in a joint suspension.

In a single use tubes 300 μl of the bacterial suspension was put and then each implant was put separately in single use tubes (**Figure 1**). The tubes were incubated in anaerobic conditions for 72 hours.

After the incubation period, the implants were taken out of anaerobic conditions and they were randomly divided into four study groups and two control groups, each group containing twelve implants (n = 12).

2.2 Group 1. LaserHF (PDT1)

The implants were treated with a diode laser (Laser HF®, Hager Werken, Duisburg, Germany) and a toluidine blue-based dye (155 μg/ml, LaserHF® Paro-PDT solution). The laser parameters are presented in **Table 1**.

2.3 Group 2. Helbo laser (PDT2)

A combination of a diode laser (Helbo® Therapielaser, Helbo Photodynamic Systems GmbH & Co KG, Grieskirchen, Austria) and a phenothiazine chloride dye (Helbo® Blue photosensitizer) was used for the treatment of the implants belonging to this group. The laser parameters are presented in **Table 2**.

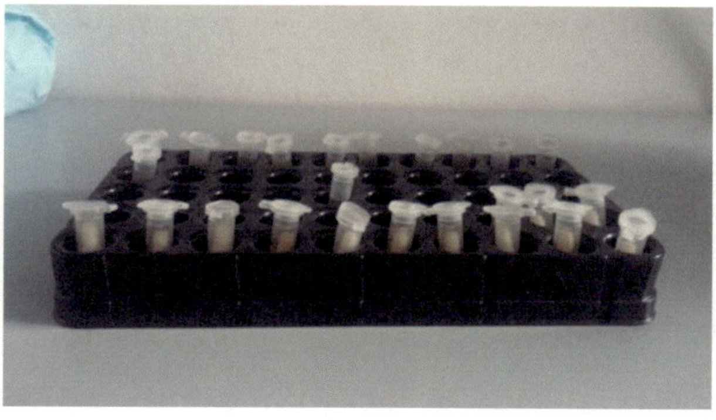

Figure 1.
Implants placed in Eppendorf tubes containing bacterial suspension. Implants covered in their entire length by the bacterial suspension.

Wavelength: 660 nm
Fiber tip: 320 μm optical fiber tip
Power output: 100 mW
Power density: 124.3 W/cm^2
Irradiation Time: 60 seconds
Distance from the implant: 5 mm

Table 1.
PDT1 treatment parameters.

Wavelength: 660 nm
Fiber tip: 3D pocket probe
Power output: 100 mW
Power density: 35.37 W/cm^2
Irradiation Time: 60 seconds
Distance from the implant: 5 mm

Table 2.
PDT2 treatment parameters.

2.4 Group 3. Light-emitting diode treatment group (PDT3)

The implants belonging to this group, were treated with LED curing light (Optilight Ld®, Gnatus, Brazil). A red LED light, (Ledengin,Inc.®, San Jose, USA) was used in combination with a toluidine blue solution (Biognost®, Zagreb, Croatia). The laser parameters are presented in **Table 3**.

2.5 PDT1, PDT2 and PDT3 decontamination steps

The first step was coating the implants with the respective photosensitive dye according to the treatment group. After 60 seconds the implants were rinsed with sterile saline solution. For standardization of the treatment protocols for every treatment group, the implants, were placed in a rotating electric motor (Shenzhen Powerful Electronics, Shajing, China), with a rotating speed of 10 rpm.

The treatment time was 60 seconds for every group from a distance of 5 mm from the implant. The treatment procedures for titanium and zirconia implants are shown in **Figures 2** and **3**.

2.6 Group 4. Treatment with toluidine blue only (TB)

The implants belonging to this group were placed in photosensitive dye (toluidine blue; Biognost®, Zagreb, Croatia) solution (1 mg/ml) for 60 seconds. Then they were rinsed with sterile saline solution.

2.7 Control groups

Two control groups were included. The negative control group (NC) did not receive any treatment. After removing the implants from the bacterial suspension and keeping them in room conditions for 60 seconds, microbiologycal analysis followed.

Wavelength: 660 nm
Fiber tip: 6 mm LED composite curing tip
Power output: 200 mW
Power density: 0.71 W/cm^2
Irradiation Time: 60 seconds
Distance from the implant: 5 mm

Table 3.
PDT3 treatment parameters.

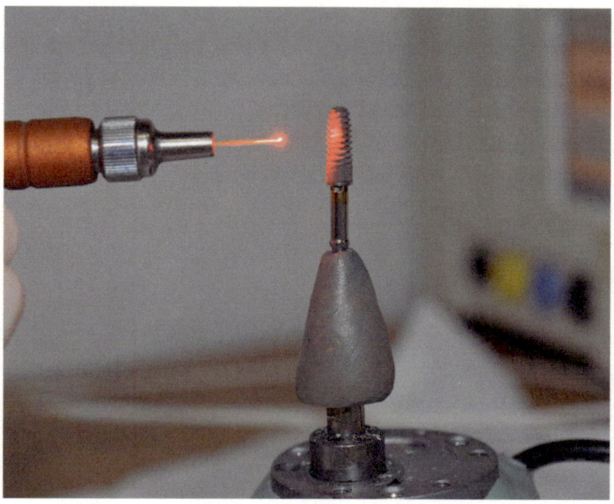

Figure 2.
A titanium implant treated from a distance of 5 mm for 60 seconds while rotating on the electric motor.

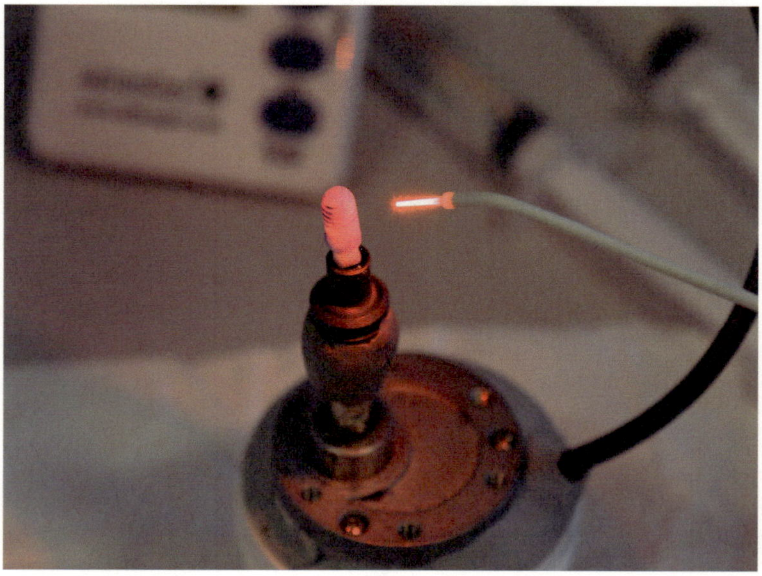

Figure 3.
A zirconia dental implant placed in a rotational motor and treated with PDT2 for 60 seconds.

The implants belonging to the positive control group (PC) were put in 0.2% chlorhexidine gluconate solution (Curasept ADS® Curaden International AG, Kriens, Switzerland) for a duration of 60 seconds. After their removal from the chlorhexidine solution, the implants were only rinsed with sterile saline to remove the remaining solution.

2.8 Microbiological analysis

After treatment procedures each implant was placed in a tube containing 500 μl of phosphate buffered saline (PBS). The tubes were vortexed for 60 seconds (Vortex, Genius 3, IKA, Germany). This was done to remove the remaining bacterial cells from the implant surfaces.

From each tube, 100 μl were taken and using a 96-well microtiter plates a ten-fold dilution was performed and 30 μl of suspension from each well was then inoculated to Brucella agar plates.

The plates were placed in anaerobic conditions and after 72 hours and the colony forming units per milliliter (CFU/ml) were counted (**Figure 4**). MALDI Biotyper (Bruker Daltonics, Germany) was used to macroscopically differentiate distinctive colonies.

2.9 Scanning electron microscopy analysis

Scanning electron microscopy (SEM) was performed on one randomly selected implant from each of the treatment groups and one sterile non-treated implant. The implants for SEM analysis were stored for 2 hours in 2% paraformaldehyde and, later on dehydrated in increasing concentrations of ethanol (60%, 75% and 95%), for 30 minutes in each and dried overnight. The surfaces of the prepared implants

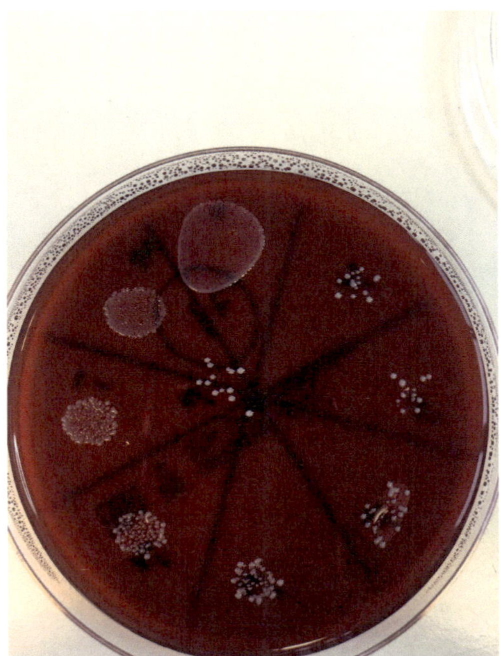

Figure 4.
Visible colonies of bacteria on Brucella agar plate.

were analyzed by SEM (Vega TS5136MM, Tescan, Brno, Czech Republic). The SEM images were taken at 1:250 magnifications under high vacuum (HiVac) with a high voltage (HV) of 30 kV. All the images were taken between the fourth and the fifth thread of the implants. As for the zirconia implants, they are non-conducting material and in order to make the samples conductive and avoid charging of the sample surface, the implants were coated with gold and palladium sputter (SC7620 Mini Sputter Coater, Quorum Technologies Ltd., UK).

2.10 Statistical analysis

The differences between the groups for each bacterial species separately and for the total count of bacteria, were compared by analysis of variance test (ANOVA) and Tukey test, as a post hoc. The level of significance was set at 5%. The statistical package SAS system for Windows (Release 8.02, SAS Institute Inc., Cary, NC, USA) was used.

3. Results

To determine the difference among the groups and between the two types of implants, multivariate analysis of variance test was applied.

The comparison between the two types of implants: titanium and zirconia, regardless of the study groups, showed that there was a significantly lower number of bacteria on zirconia implants for all three types of bacteria separately, as well as for the total number of bacteria (**Table 4**).

For the comparison among the study groups regardless of the type of implant, Tukey test was applied. Regarding the total number of bacteria, the least bacteria were found in PDT1 and PDT2. These two groups were followed by PDT3 and PC without significant difference among them. The negative control group (NC) as expected, had the largest number of bacteria compared to the other groups. The same results were obtained for the number of each bacteria separately.

The total number of bacteria for every group and both implant types are shown in **Figure 5** in schematic form. The difference between zirconia implants and titanium implants was not the same for all groups. The smallest difference between both types of implants in the number of bacteria was for the control group. The impact was almost the same for PDT1, PDT2, PC and TB, while the largest difference between titanium and zirconia implants were in the PDT3 group. The results for each of the bacteria separately are shown in **Figures 6–8**.

3.1 Titanium implants

There were statistically significant differences among the groups for each of the bacteria separately and also for the total number of bacteria ($p = 0.0022$). These results are presented in **Table 5** in logarithmic form. Regarding the total number of bacteria, the largest reduction was observed in the PDT1 (98.3%) and PDT2 (97.8%) groups. These two groups had statistically significant difference when compared to NC ($p < 0.05$). In the PDT3 group there was a 68.7% bacterial reduction, without statistically significant difference when compared to NC (**Table 5**).

When each bacteria was compared separately, the PDT1 and PDT2 groups also showed the largest bacterial reduction. PDT1 group, was significantly more effective in the eliminating *A. actinomycetemcomitans* and *P. gingivalis* ($p < 0.05$).

	Aggregatibacter actynomycetemcomitans					Porphyromonas gingivalis				
Factor	N	mean	st.d.		p*	N	mean	st.d.		p*
Implants										
Zirconia	72	1.9	(2.1)		**<0.0001**	72	1.6	(2.1)		**<0.0001**
Titanium	72	4.9	(2.5)			72	4.9	(2.6)		
Group										
PDT1	24	1.9	(2.2)	b	**<0.0001**	24	2.0	(2.5)	b	**<0.0001**
PDT2	24	1.8	(2.0)	b		24	1.6	(2.1)	b	
PDT3	24	3.1	(2.9)	ab		24	2.9	(2.8)	ab	
TB	24	4.3	(2.7)	a		24	4.0	(2.7)	a	
PC	24	2.9	(2.7)	ab		24	2.8	(2.6)	ab	
NC	24	6.2	(1.3)			24	6.2	(1.6)		
	Prevotella intermedia					**Total**				
Factor	N	mean	st.d.		p*	N	mean	st.d.		p*
Implants										
Zirconia	72	2.0	(2.1)		**<0.0001**	72	2.3	(2.3)		**<0.0001**
Titanium	72	5.3	(2.7)			72	5.8	(2.5)		
Group										
PDT1	24	2.6	(2.5)	b	**<0.0001**	24	2.8	(2.6)	b	**<0.0001**
PDT2	24	2.0	(2.3)	b		24	2.3	(2.4)	b	
PDT3	24	3.1	(3.2)	ab		24	3.6	(3.2)	ab	
TB	24	4.5	(2.9)	a		24	5.0	(2.7)	a	
PC	24	3.2	(2.7)	ab		24	3.6	(2.7)	ab	
NC	24	6.4	(1.8)			24	7.1	(1.5)		

**p-value for MANOVA test.*
abc - result of post-hoc comparison (Tukey test). Having the same letter means that there is no statistically significant difference.

Table 4.
Number of bacteria by implant type and treatment groups in logarithmic form.

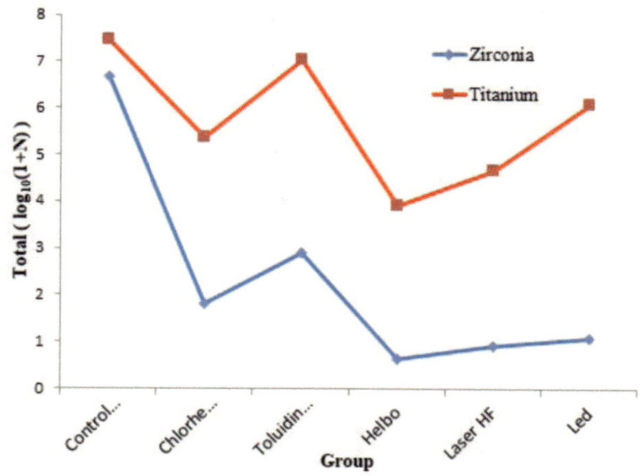

Figure 5.
The total number of bacteria in logarithmic form, for both types of implants and for each study groups.

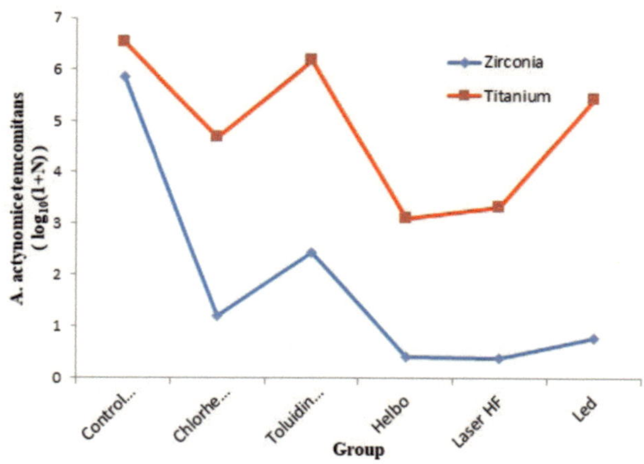

Figure 6.
The number of A. actinymycetemcomitans in logarithmic form for both types of implants and the study groups.

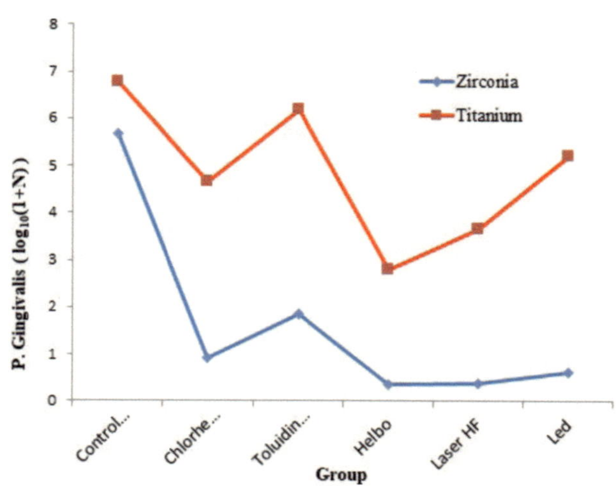

Figure 7.
The number of P. gingivalis in logarithmic form for both types of implants and the study groups.

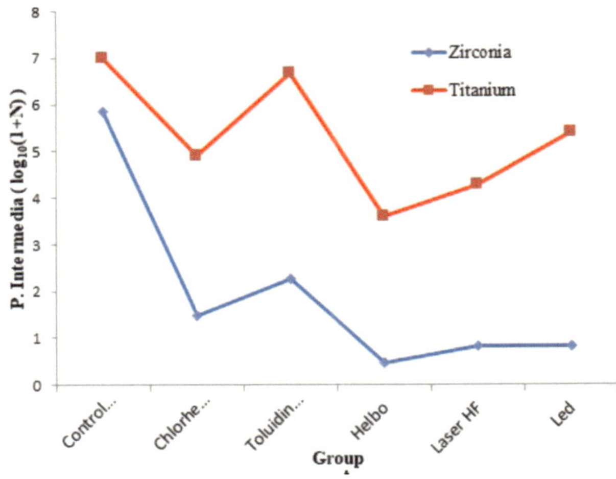

Figure 8.
The number of P. intermedia in logarithmic form for both types of implants and the study groups.

As for *P.intermedia* the PDT1 group showed no significant difference compared to NC group. On the other hand the PDT2 group was significantly more effective in the elimination of each of the bacteria separately when compared to the NC group ($p < 0.05$).

The least effective among the groups, when compared to the NC group, was the TB group (62.4%). Compared to NC there was no significant difference neither for the total number nor for each bacteria separately.

3.2 Zirconia implants

Statistically significant difference was observed among the groups. This was the case for both the total number of bacteria and each bacteria separately ($p < 0.0001$). Every group showed vast bacterial reduction with statistically significant difference when compared to the negative control (NC). These results are shown in **Table 6** in logarithmic form.

The PDT1, PDT2 and PDT3 had the largest bacterial reduction for each bacterium separately, as well as for the total count of bacteria. There was a reduction of more than 99% in comparison to NC. However, between these three groups the differences in bacterial reduction were not statistically significant difference neither for each of the bacteria separately nor for the total number of bacteria ($p > 0.05$).

The lowest bacterial reduction for each bacteria separately and also for the total number of bacteria was observed in the TB group. The PC group had lower bacterial reduction compared to PDT1, PDT2 and PDT3 without statistically significant differences among them. It also did not differ significantly compared to the TB in terms of the total bacterial count, *P. gingivalis* and *P. intermedia*. It had a significant difference compared to the TB only for *A. actinomycetemcomitans*.

3.3 Scanning electron microscope analysis

The SEM images from the PDT1, PDT2, and PDT3 groups did not show any surface alterations, cracks, or damage when compared to the images obtained for the sterile implants. Visually, their surface appeared to be very similar to the surface of the sterile implant, for both titanium and zirconia implants (**Figures 9–12**).

	Aggregatibacter actynomycetemcomitans					Porphyromonas gingivalis					Wilks' lambda
Group	N	mean	st.d.		p*	N	mean	st.d.		p*	p
PDT1	12	3.3	2.2	b	**0.0006**	12	3.7	2.5	bc	**0.0003**	**0.0026**
PDT2	12	3.1	2.0	b		12	2.8	2.4	c		
PDT3	12	5.4	2.3	ab		12	5.2	2.2	abc		
TB	12	6.2	2.3	a		12	6.2	2.0	ab		
PC	12	4.7	2.7	ab		12	4.7	2.3	abc		
NC	12	6.5	1.7	a		12	6.8	1.9	a		
	Prevotella intermedia					**Total number of bacteria**					Wilks' lambda
Group	N	mean	st.d.		p*	N	mean	st.d.		p*	p
PDT1	12	4.3	2.4	ab	**0.0096**	12	4.7	2.3	bc	**0.0022**	**0.0026**
PDT2	12	3.6	2.4	b		12	3.9	2.3	c		
PDT3	12	5.4	3.1	ab		12	6.1	2.5	abc		
TB	12	6.7	2.4	a		12	7.0	2.2	ab		
PC	12	4.9	2.7	ab		12	5.4	2.6	abc		
NC	12	7.0	2.2	a		12	7.4	1.8	a		

**p-value for ANOVA test.*
abc - result of post-hoc comparison (Tukey test). Having the same letter means that there is no statistically significant difference.

Table 5.
Results of ANOVA and Tukey's post hoc test for the titanium implants.

	Aggregatibacter actynomycetemcomitans					Porphyromonas gingivalis					Wilks' lambda
Group	N	mean	st.d.		p^*	N	mean	st.d.		p^*	p
PDT1	12	0.4	0.8	a	**0.0001**	12	0.4	0.8	b	**0.0001**	**0.0001**
PDT2	12	0.4	0.6	a		12	0.3	0.5	b		
PDT3	12	0.8	1.1	a		12	0.6	0.7	b		
TB	12	2.4	1.3			12	1.9	1.1	a		
PC	12	1.2	1.0	a		12	0.9	1.2	ab		
NC	12	5.9	0.7			12	5.7	1.0			
	Prevotella intermedia					**Total number of bacteria**					Wilks' lambda
Group	N	mean	st.d.		p^*	N	mean	st.d.		p^*	p
PDT1	12	0.8	0.9	b	**0.0001**	12	0.9	1.0	b	**0.0001**	**0.0001**
PDT2	12	0.5	0.7	b		12	0.7	0.8	b		
PDT3	12	0.8	0.9	b		12	1.1	1.2	b		
TB	12	2.3	1.2	a		12	2.9	1.2	a		
PC	12	1.5	1.5	ab		12	1.8	1.5	ab		
NC	12	5.9	1.3			12	6.7	0.9			

**p-value for ANOVA test.*
abc - result of post-hoc comparison (Tukey test). Having the same letter means that there is no statistically significant difference.

Table 6.
Results of ANOVA and Tukey's post hoc test for the zirconia implants.

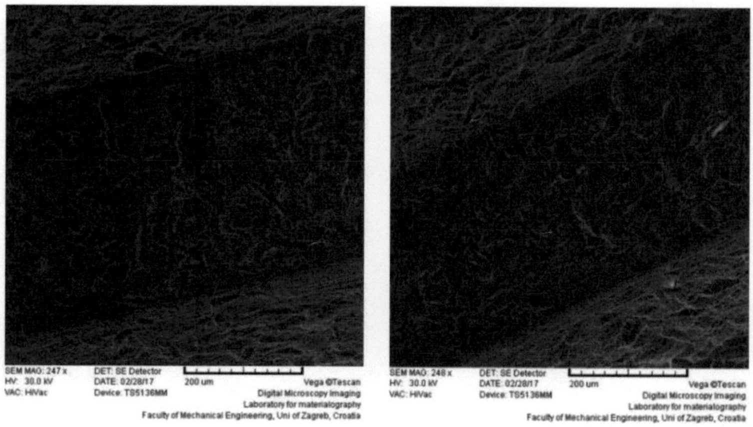

Figure 9.
Sterile titanium implant; magnification 1:250 (left). Titanium implant treated with PDT1; magnification 1:250 (right).

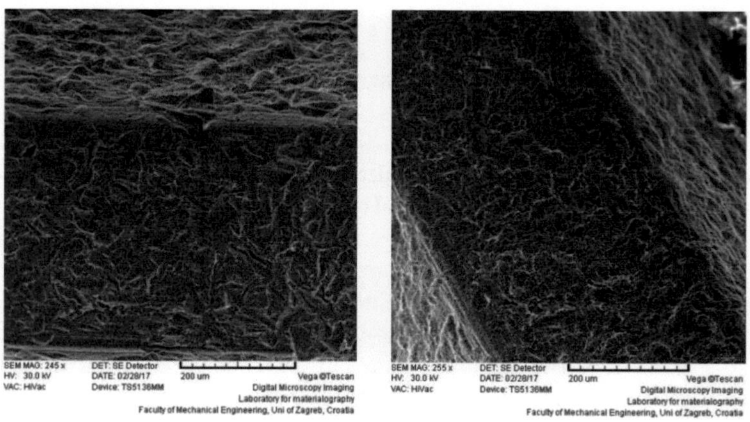

Figure 10.
Titanium implant treated with PDT2; magnification 1:250 (left). Titanium implant treated with PDT3; magnification 1:250 (right).

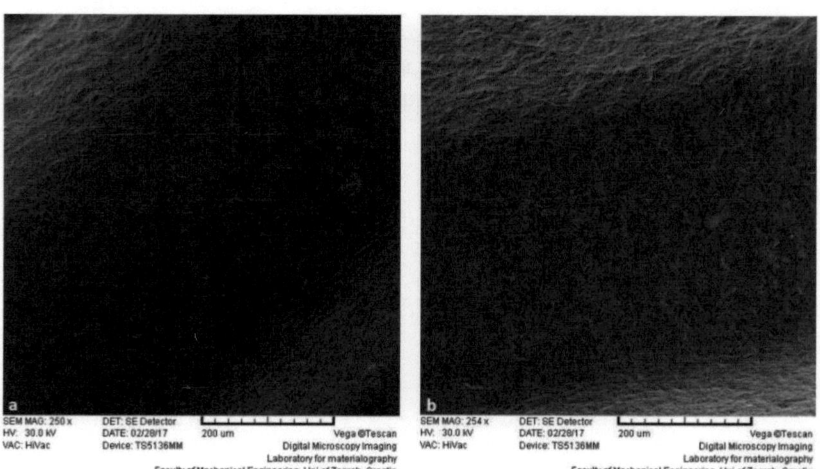

Figure 11.
Sterile zirconia implant; magnification 1:250 (left). Zirconia implant treated with PDT1; magnification 1:250 (right).

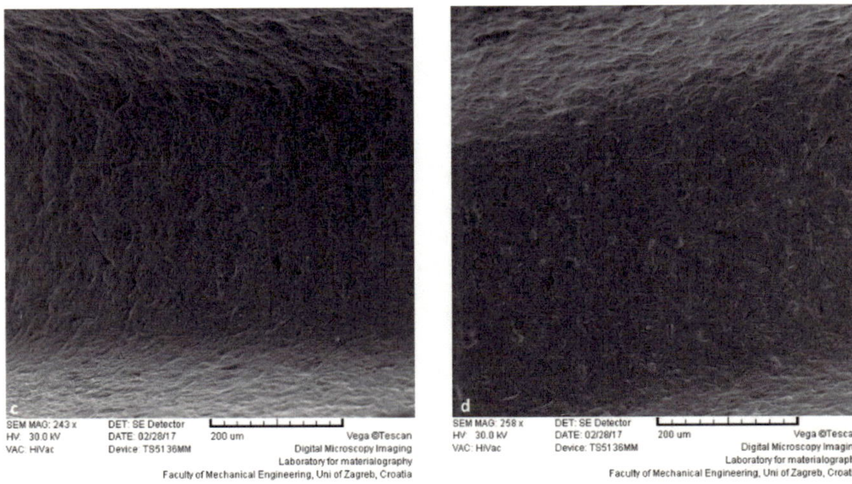

Figure 12.
Zirconia implant treated with PDT2; magnification 1:250 (left). Zirconia implant treated with PDT3; magnification 1:250 (right).

4. Clinical application of photodynamic therapy

The clinical efficacy of PDT against peri-implantitis has been demonstrated in several clinical studies. In a randomized controlled trial study by Wang et al. [60] it was shown that PDT combined with mechanical debridement significantly improved pocket depth, clinical attachment loss, plaque index and sulcus bleeding index compared with baseline and the control groups in participants with peri-implantitis. Similar results were obtained in a 3 months randomized clinical trial done by Rakasevic et al. [61].

Since the main goal when treating peri-implantitis is to eliminate the bacteria from the soft tissues and the implant surface, in order to create conditions for grafting and re-osseointegration, the use of photodynamic therapy is mostly used as an adjunct therapy during the treatment of peri-implanitits with the purpose of eliminating bacteria from the rough surfaces of the implants. The treatment of peri-implantitis can be non-surgical and surgical. During the non-surgical treatment of peri-implantitis the photosensitive dye is applied on the pocket around the infected implant and the light source is applied. This procedure is shown in **Figure 13**.

However, photodynamic therapy is mostly used in conjunction with surgical treatment of peri-implantitis as an adjunct therapy after implantoplasty, mechanical debridement and chemical decontamination of the implant surface. The surgical approach is presented in **Figures 14–17**.

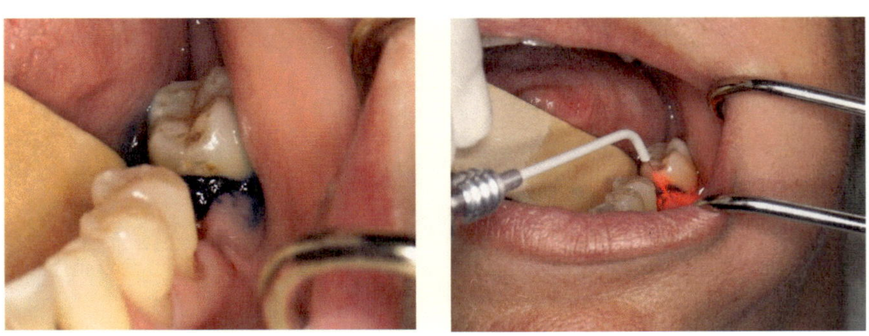

Figure 13.
(Left) application of the dye. (Right) application of the light source.

DOI: http://dx.doi.org/10.5772/intechopen.94268

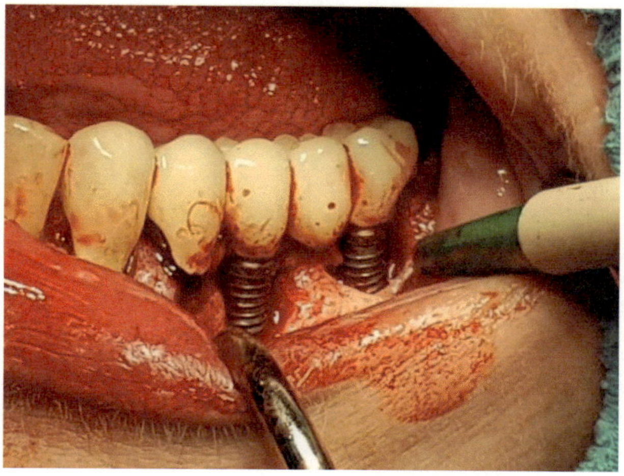

Figure 14.
Surgical treatment of peri-implantitis. Visible bone resorption around the implants.

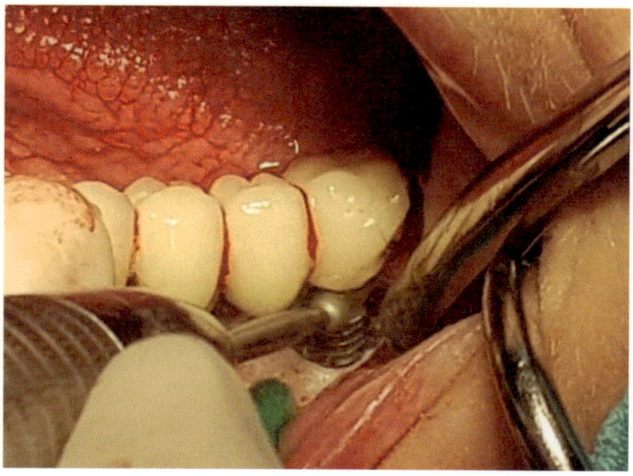

Figure 15.
Implantoplasty procedure.

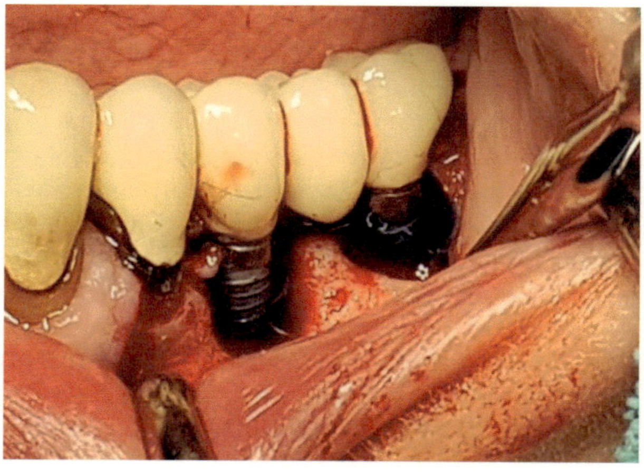

Figure 16.
Application of the photosensitive dye.

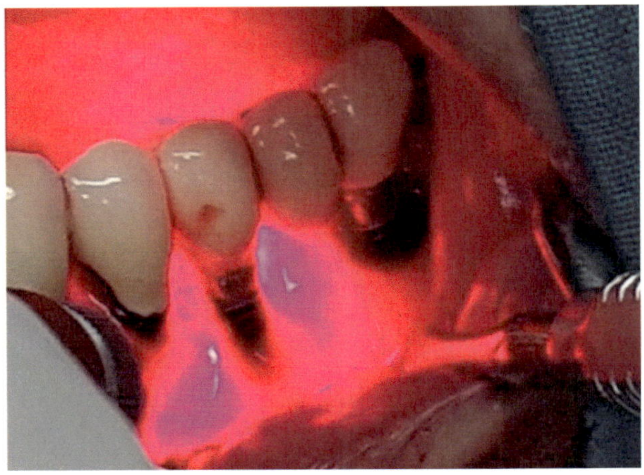

Figure 17.
Application of the light source.

5. Discussion

One of the main reasons of implant failure is peri-implantitis. The prevalence rates of peri-implantitis differs among different studies and this is due to the different reporting methods and characteristics [62–64]. Van Velzen et al. [65] in their 10 years prospective cohort study reported a prevalence of 7%. Meijer et al. [66] reported that after 10 years 29.7% of patients were affected by peri-implantitis. Fardal et al. [67] report a rate of 53.5% at the patient level and 31.1% at the implant level, which is much higher than the data from other studies.

The treatment of peri-implantitis is complex and it often includes combination of conventional therapy with the addition of antimicrobials. However, use of antimicrobials does not have a long term effects and it can lead to antimicrobial resistance and development of superinfections [68]. Therefore, alternative antimicrobial approaches for achieving implant disinfection have been sought.

Photodynamic therapy is a promising alternative when treating periodontal diseases and peri- implant diseases. Up to date there have been many *in vitro* [69–71] and clinical studies [60, 61] evaluating the effect of photodynamic therapy in treating peri-implantitis.

Regarding the *in vitro* evaluation, the present study aimed to evaluate the efficacy of photodynamic therapy on dental implants contaminated under *in vitro* conditions. The implants were contaminated in order to try to recreate the adhesion stage of biofilm formation on the implant surface. Many *in vitro* studies have used similar methodology to achieve titanium implant contamination [62, 63, 71].

The main focus of our study was to evaluate if photodynamic therapy is efficient in eradicating the bacteria from the implant surface when compared to the negative control group (NC) and to the conventional treatment with chlorhexidine solution (PC). Furthermore, the focus was to evaluate different types of devices and with different parameters and photosensitizers and the reaction of different bacteria to aPDT.

The results from our study showed that PDT1 and PDT2 groups were more eliminated 98.3% and 97.8% of the total number of bacteria when compared to NC group. These groups were the most effective among the study groups. Both PDT1 and PDT2 groups were a combination of a diode laser with a wavelength of 660 nm and a photosensitizer.

The results of this study are similar to other *in vitro*, *in vivo* and clinical studies [64, 71, 72]. Marotti et al. [71] in their study demonstrated that aPDT is effective against the bacteria present in peri-implantitis. The irradiation time did not influence the results. Similar results were obtained from both the groups (3 minute and 5 minutes irradiation time) and there was no significant difference between them. The effect of aPDT did not differ significantly from the disinfection with 0.12% chlorhexidine solution. Our results were similar to this study and even though we used a higher concentration of chlorhexidine (0.2%), both PDT1 and PDT2 had no significant difference when compared to PC.

In a study done by Haas et al. [64] it was demonstrated that 60 seconds of light exposure in combination with photosensitizer can effectively eradicate *A. actinomycetemcomitans, P. gingivalis* and *P. intermedia*. One of the goals of the present study was to evaluate aPDT against each bacteria separately. The results obtained for *A. actinomycetemcomitans* and *P. gingivalis* were similar to the results obtained for the total bacterial count. Both PDT1 and PDT2 had significant difference when compared to the NC. However, the results of *P. intermedia* showed that PDT2 was more effective against this bacteria when compared to the other groups.

The least effective treatment group was PDT3 without statistically significant difference compared to NC or PC groups regarding the total bacterial count. It must be noted that for the PDT3 group we used a modified dental LED light and not a diode laser. This was done to evaluate and compare the LED light against diode lasers as a light source.

The efficacy of LED lights as a light source in photodynamic therapy has been tested in many studies however, only a few studies have tested its efficacy on titanium implant surfaces. The results from these studies are conflicting since the study design and light source parameters differ greatly. In a study conducted by Cho et al. [73] the efficacy of a green LED light was tested. The LED light was combined with erythrosine dye and was evaluated against *A. actinomycetemcomitans*. Their results showed that this combination is effective and reduces the bacteria attached titanium surfaces up to 92.4%. The irradiation time in this study was 60 seconds and the treatment was done on only one surface of titanium discs. This provides uniform distribution of the light source. In contrast, in the present study we applied the light source in a rotating motion in order to emulate clinical application of aPDT around a contaminated implant. This might be the reason why our results showed differ with the aforementioned study [73].

In contrast to the *in vitro* study by Cho et al. [73], in a clinical study done by De Angelis et al. [74] the use of LED light showed no significant difference after 4 months of follow up when compared to mechanical debridement and scaling.

In our study we evaluated the efficacy of aPDT on two types of implants: titanium and zirconia dental implants. The efficacy of aPDT on zirconia implant surfaces has not been evaluated in other studies up to date.

The results obtained from our study showed that each test group was very effective in eliminating the bacteria from the zirconia surface and all had significantly lower bacterial count when compared to NC. However, in between the groups there was no significant difference. The higher efficacy of aPDT against zirconia surfaces when compared to titanium surfaces might be due to the surface properties of zirconia which might lead to a lower affinity of the bacteria to be attached to zirconia surfaces. Zirconia surfaces are smoother, have a lower surface roughness and lower surface free energy [75, 76]. In a study done by Scarano et al. [75] titanium and zirconia oxide discs were placed in the mouths of patients in order to evaluate in which surface the bacteria adhere less. After 24 h it was shown that there were significantly less bacteria on the zirconium oxide surfaces. Al-Radha et al. [76] showed similar results. In their study titanium blasted with zirconia and the zirconia material showed better results when compared to the titanium surface regarding the adhesion of bacteria after coating the surfaces with saliva pellicle.

PDT1, PDT2 and PDT3 in addition to the significant difference compared to NC, they also had significant difference from the TB group. The results of the

PDT3 group for the zirconia dental implants were comparable to PDT1 and PDT2. This can suggest that LED light with additional improvements in light distribution and parameters can have an antimicrobial effect. As mentioned before there are conflicting results regarding the antimicrobial effect of using LED. Several studies reported beneficial results following use of LED lights, as a light source [77, 78]. On the other hand, several studies reported insignificant improvement in the treatment outcomes using LED light for PDT [74]. However, it is difficult to compare the results of present study with the previous ones, mainly due to the differences in the study protocols and lack of studies conducted on zirconia implant surfaces.

The use of diode lasers in many studies has been shown to be safe in regard to the implant surface, compared to Nd:YAG, Er:YAG, CO2 and Ho:YAG lasers, which can damage the implant surfaces [57]. Castro et al. [79] concluded that 980 nm diode laser irradiation does not damage titanium implant surfaces and seems to be safe irrespective of power output used.

In the present research, no structural changes on the implant surfaces following therapy was observed. PDT1, PDT2 and PDT3, did not cause visible damage on titanium or zirconia implant surface at a magnification of 1:250.

Regarding the clinical use of PDT, several studies reported conflicting results. Many studies demonstrated improvement in clinical outcomes of patients with peri-implantitis when aPDT was combined with mechanical debridement [60, 80, 81]. Romeo et al. [82] suggested that PDT is a useful adjunct therapy but it could not replace the mechanical and surgical treatment of peri-implantitis. Similarly other studies suggest that the PDT improves the outcomes of peri-implantitis [60, 83, 84].

On the other hand, there are several studies that report no added benefit from using PDT when compared to conventional treatment modalities for peri-implantitis [85, 86].

The results of this *in vitro* study should be considered preliminary, since it cannot be generalized to *in vivo* and clinical conditions. The biggest concern related to future *in vivo* and clinical applications is stability of achieved *in vitro* results (short term beneficial effects in reducing the number of periopathogens). Also, the presence of plaque formation on implants, degree of salivation and host-immune response is very important.

6. Conclusion

It is of utmost importance that further clinical trials be conducted in order to clarify the potential efficacy of PDT as an adjunct therapy to peri-implantitis and clear and effective treatment protocols should be established in order to benefit the most from the properties of PDT.

Conflict of interest

The authors declare no conflicts of interest.

Author details

Dragana Gabrić[1*], Ana Budimir[2], Ivona Bago[3], Luka Marković[4], Verica Pavlić[5] and Bleron Azizi[6]

1 Department of Oral Surgery, School of Dental Medicine, University of Zagreb, University Hospital Center Zagreb, Zagreb, Croatia

2 Department of Clinical and Molecular Microbiology, University Hospital Centre Zagreb, School of Dental Medicine, University of Zagreb, Zagreb, Croatia

3 Department of Endodontics and Restorative Dentistry, School of Dental Medicine, University of Zagreb, Zagreb, Croatia

4 Department of Periodontology, School of Dental Medicine, University of Zagreb, Zagreb, Croatia

5 Department of Periodontology and Oral Medicine, Faculty of Medicine, University of Banja Luka, Banja Luka, Bosnia and Herzegovina

6 Faculty of Dentistry, AAB College, Prishtina, Kosovo

*Address all correspondence to: dgabric@sfzg.hr

References

[1] Konopka K, Goslinski T. Photodynamic therapy in dentistry. J Dent Res. 2007;86(8): 694-707.

[2] Gursoy H, Ozcakir-Tomruk C, Tanalp J, Yilmaz S. Photodynamic therapy in dentistry: a literature review. Clin Oral Investig. 2013;17(4):1113-25.

[3] Schmidlin PR, Beuchat M, Busslinger A, Lehmann B, Lutz F. Tooth substance loss resulting from mechanical, sonic and ultrasonic root instrumentation assessed by liquid scintillation. J Clin Periodontol. 2001;28(11):1058-66.

[4] de Almeida JM, Theodoro LH, Bosco AF, Nagata MJ, Bonfante S, Garcia VG. Treatment of experimental periodontal disease by photodynamic therapy in rats with diabetes. J Periodontol. 2008;79(11):2156-65.

[5] Braun A, Dehn C, Krause F, Jepsen S. Short-term clinical effects of adjunctive antimicrobial photodynamic therapy in periodontal treatment: a randomized clinical trial. J Clin Periodontol. 2008;35(10):877-84.

[6] Meisel P, Kocher T. Photodynamic therapy for periodontal diseases: state of the art. J Photochem Photobiol B. 2005;79(2):159-70.

[7] Wilson M. Photolysis of oral bacteria and its potential use in the treatment of caries and periodontal disease. J Appl Bacteriol. 1993;75(4):299-306.

[8] Hamblin MR, Hasan T. Photodynamic therapy: a new antimicrobial approach to infectious disease? Photochem Photobiol Sci. 2004;3(5):436-50.

[9] Qin YL, Luan XL, Bi LJ, Sheng YQ, Zhou CN, Zhang ZG. Comparison of toluidine blue-mediated photodynamic therapy and conventional scaling treatment for periodontitis in rats. J Periodontal Res. 2008;43(2):162-7.

[10] Maisch T. Anti-microbial photodynamic therapy: useful in the future? Lasers Med Sci. 2007;22(2):83-91.

[11] Sgolastra F, Petrucci A, Severino M, Graziani F, Gatto R, Monaco A. Adjunctive photodynamic therapy to non-surgical treatment of chronic periodontitis: a systematic review and meta-analysis. J Clin Periodontol. 2013;40(5):514-26.

[12] Smiley CJ, Tracy SL, Abt E, Michalowicz BS, John MT, Gunsolley J, et al. Systematic review and meta-analysis on the nonsurgical treatment of chronic periodontitis by means of scaling and root planing with or without adjuncts. J Am Dent Assoc. 2015;146(7):508-24.

[13] Atieh MA. Photodynamic therapy as an adjunctive treatment for chronic periodontitis: a meta-analysis. Lasers Med Sci. 2010;25(4):605-13.

[14] Betsy J, Prasanth CS, Baiju KV, Prasanthila J, Subhash N. Efficacy of antimicrobial photodynamic therapy in the management of chronic periodontitis: a randomized controlled clinical trial. J Clin Periodontol. 2014;41(6):573-81.

[15] Christodoulides N, Nikolidakis D, Chondros P, Becker J, Schwarz F, Rössler R, et al. Photodynamic therapy as an adjunct to non-surgical periodontal treatment: a randomized, controlled clinical trial. J Periodontol. 2008;79(9):1638-44.

[16] Chondros P, Nikolidakis D, Christodoulides N, Rössler R, Gutknecht N, Sculean A. Photodynamic therapy as adjunct to non-surgical periodontal treatment in patients on periodontal maintenance: a randomized

controlled clinical trial. Lasers Med Sci. 2009;24(5):681-8.

[17] Ng R, Singh F, Papamanou DA, Song X, Patel C, Holewa C, et al. Endodontic photodynamic therapy ex vivo. J Endod. 2011;37(2):217-22.

[18] Saleh IM, Ruyter IE, Haapasalo M, Ørstavik D. Survival of *Enterococcus faecalis* in infected dentinal tubules after root canal filling with different root canal sealers in vitro. Int Endod J. 2004;37(3):193-8.

[19] Rios A, He J, Glickman GN, Spears R, Schneiderman ED, Honeyman AL. Evaluation of photodynamic therapy using a light-emitting diode lamp against *Enterococcus faecalis* in extracted human teeth. J Endod. 2011;37(6):856-9.

[20] Bago I, Plečko V, Gabrić Pandurić D, Schauperl Z, Baraba A, Anić I. Antimicrobial efficacy of a high-power diode laser, photo-activated disinfection, conventional and sonic activated irrigation during root canal treatment. Int Endod J. 2013;46(4):339-47.

[21] Massano J, Regateiro FS, Januário G, Ferreira A. Oral squamous cell carcinoma: review of prognostic and predictive factors. Oral Surg Oral Med Oral Pathol Oral Radiol Endo. 2006;102(1):67-76.

[22] Silverman S Jr. Oral cancer: complications of therapy. Oral Surg Oral Med Oral Pathol Oral Radiol Endod. 1999;88(2):122-6.

[23] Van der Waal I, Axéll T. Oral leukoplakia: a proposal for uniform reporting. Oral Oncol. 2002;38(6):521-6.

[24] Sieroń A, Adamek M, Kawczyk-Krupka A, Mazur S, Ilewicz L. Photodynamic therapy (PDT) using topically applied delta-aminolevulinic acid (ALA) for the treatment of oral leukoplakia. J Oral Pathol Med. 2003;32(6):330-6.

[25] Selvam NP, Sadaksharam J, Singaravelu G, Ramu R. Treatment of oral leukoplakia with photodynamic therapy: A pilot study. J Cancer Res Ther. 2015;11(2):464-7.

[26] Biel MA. Photodynamic therapy in head and neck cancer. Curr Oncol Rep. 2002;4(1):87-96.

[27] Neugebauer J, Jozsa M, Kübler A. Die antimikrobielle photodynamische Therapie zur Prävention der alveolären Ostitis und des Dolor post extractionem. [Antimicrobial photodynamic therapy for prevention of alveolar ostitis and post-extraction pain] Mund Kiefer Gesichtschir. 2004;8(6):350-5.

[28] Nagayoshi M, Nishihara T, Nakashima K, Iwaki S, Chen KK, Terashita M, et al. Bactericidal effects of diode laser irradiation on *Enterococcus faecalis* using periapical lesion defect model. ISRN Dent. 2011;2011:870364

[29] Batinjan G, Zore Z, Čelebić A, Papić M, Gabrić Pandurić D, Filipović Zore I. Thermographic monitoring of wound healing and oral health-related quality of life in patients treated with laser (aPDT) after impacted mandibular third molar removal. Int J Oral Maxillofac Surg. 2014;43(12):1503-8.

[30] Minamisako MC, Ribeiro GH, Lisboa ML, Mariela Rodríguez Cordeiro M, Grando LJ. Medication-related osteonecrosis of jaws: a low-level laser therapy and antimicrobial photodynamic therapy case approach. Case Rep Dent. 2016;2016:6267406.

[31] Rugani P, Truschnegg A, Acham S, Kirnbauer B, Jakse N. Use of photodynamic therapy in treatment of bisphosphonate-related osteonecrosis of the jaws: literature review and case series. J Anal Bioanal Tech. 2013;S1:006.

[32] Abraham CM. A brief historical perspective on dental implants, their

surface coatings and treatments. Open Dent J. 2014;8:50-5.

[33] Brånemark P, Chien S, Gröndahl H, Robinson K, Brånemark BK. The Osseointegration book: from calvarium to calcaneus. Hanover Park Quintessence Publ Co, Inc, USA,. 2005;5548-59.

[34] Saini M, Singh Y, Arora P, Jain K. Implant biomaterials: a comprehensive review. World J Clin Cases. 2015;3(1):52-7.

[35] Sykaras N, Iacopino AM, Marker VA, Triplett RG, Woody RD. Implant materials, designs, and surface topographies: their effect on osseointegration. A literature review. Int J Oral Maxillofac Implants. 2000;15(5):675-90.

[36] Misch C. Contemporary implant dentistry, 2nd edn. CV Mosby, St Louis. 1999;76-194.

[37] Lemons JE. Dental implant biomaterials. J Am Dent Assoc. 1990;121(6):716-9.

[38] Leonhardt A, Gröndahl K, Bergström C, Lekholm U. Long-term follow-up of osseointegrated titanium implants using clinical, radiographic and microbiological parameters. Clin Oral Implants Res. 2002;13(2):127-32.

[39] Özkurt Z, Kazazoğlu E. Zirconia dental implants: a literature review. J Oral Implantol. 2011;37(3):367-76.

[40] Gahlert M, Röhling S, Wieland M, Eichhorn S, Küchenhoff H, Kniha H. A comparison study of the osseointegration of zirconia and titanium dental implants. A biomechanical vvaluation in the maxilla of pigs. Clin Implant Dent Relat Res. 2010;12(4):297-305.

[41] Kohal RJ, Klaus G. A zirconia implant-crown system: a case report. Int J Periodontics Restorative Dent. 2004;24(2):147-53.

[42] Mombelli A, Müller N, Cionca N. The epidemiology of peri-implantitis. Clin Oral Implants Res. 2012;23 Suppl 6:67-76.

[43] Mombelli A, Lang NP. The diagnosis and treatment of peri-implantitis. Periodontol 2000. 1998;17(1):63-76.

[44] Heitz-Mayfield LJ, Lang NP. Antimicrobial treatment of peri-implant diseases. Int J Oral Maxillofac Implants. 2004;19 Suppl:128-39.

[45] Becker W, Becker BE, Newman MG, Nyman S. Clinical and microbiologic findings that may contribute to dental implant failure. Int J Oral Maxillofac Implants. 1990;5(1):31-8.

[46] Salvi GE, Aglietta M, Eick S, Sculean A, Lang NP, Ramseier CA. Reversibility of experimental peri-implant mucositis compared with experimental gingivitis in humans. Clin Oral Implants Res. 2012;23(2):182-90.

[47] Hultin M, Gustafsson A, Hallström H, Johansson L, Ekfeldt A, Klinge B. Microbiological findings and host response in patients with peri-implantitis. Clin Oral Implants Res. 2002;13(4):349-58.

[48] Salvi GE, Persson GR, Heitz-Mayfield LJ, Frei M, Lang NP. Adjunctive local antibiotic therapy in the treatment of peri-implantitis II: clinical and radiographic outcomes. Clin Oral Implants Res. 2007;18(3):281-5.

[49] Teughels W, Van Assche N, Sliepen I, Quirynen M. Effect of material characteristics and/ or surface topography on biofilm development. Clin Oral Implants Res. 2006;17 Suppl 2:68-81.

[50] Mahato N, Wu X, Wang L. Management of peri-implantitis: a

systematic review, 2010-2015. Springerplus. 2016;5:105.

[51] Smeets R, Henningsen A, Jung O, Heiland M, Hammächer C, Stein JM. Definition, etiology, prevention and treatment of peri-implantitis – a review. Head Face Med. 2014;10:34.

[52] Faggion CM Jr, Schmitter M. Using the best available evidence to support clinical decisions in implant dentistry. Int J Oral Maxillofac Implants. 2010;25(5):960-9.

[53] Mellado-Valero A, Buitrago-Vera P, Solá-Ruiz MF, Ferrer-García JC. Decontamination of dental implant surface in peri-implantitis treatment: A literature review. Med Oral Patol Oral Cir Bucal. 2013;18(6):e869-e876.

[54] Romeo E, Ghisolfi M, Murgolo N, Chiapasco M, Lops D, Vogel G. Therapy of peri-implantitis with resective surgery. A 3-year clinical trial on rough screw-shaped oral implants. Part I: clinical outcome. Clin Oral Implants Res. 2005;16(1):9-18.

[55] Mengel R, Meer C, Flores-de-Jacoby L. The treatment of uncoated and titanium nitride-coated abutments with different instruments. Int J Oral Maxillofac Implants. 2004;19(2):232-8.

[56] Duarte PM, Reis AF, de Freitas PM, Ota-Tsuzuki C. Bacterial adhesion on smooth and rough titanium surfaces after treatment with different instruments. J Periodontol. 2009;80(11):1824-32.

[57] Kreisler M, Götz H, Duschner H. Effect of Nd:YAG, Ho:YAG, Er:YAG, CO2, and GaAIAs laser irradiation on surface properties of endosseous dental implants. Int J Oral Maxillofac Implants. 2002;17(2):202-11.

[58] Subramani K, Wismeijer D. Decontamination of titanium implant surface and re-osseointegration to treat peri-implantitis: a literature review. Int J Oral Maxillofac Implants. 2012;27(5):1043-54.

[59] Hayek RR, Araújo NS, Gioso MA, Ferreira J, Baptista-Sobrinho C, Yamada AM, et al. Comparative study between the effects of photodynamic therapy and conventional therapy on microbial reduction in ligature-induced peri-implantitis in dogs. J Periodontol. 2005;76(8):1275-81.

[60] Wang H, Li W, Zhang D, Li W, Wang Z. Adjunctive photodynamic therapy improves the outcomes of peri-implantitis: a randomized controlled trial. Aust Dent J. 2019; 64(3):256-62.

[61] Rakašević D, Lazić Z, Rakonjac B, Soldatović I, Janković S, Magić M, et al. Efficiency of photodynamic therapy in the treatment of peri-implantitis - A three-month randomized controlled clinical trial. Srp Arh Celok Lek. 2016; 144(9-10):478-84

[62] Dörtbudak O, Haas R, Bernhart T, Mailath-Pokorny G. Lethal photosensitization for decontamination of implant surfaces in the treatment of peri-implantitis. Clin Oral Implants Res. 2001;12(2):104-8.

[63] Takasaki AA, Aoki A, Mizutani K, Schwarz F, Sculean A, Wang CY, et al. Applicationofantimicrobialphotodynamic therapy in periodontal and peri-implant diseases. Periodontol 2000. 2009;51(1):109-40.

[64] Haas R, Dörtbudak O, Mensdorff-Pouilly N, Mailath G. Elimination of bacteria on different implant surfaces through photosensitization and soft laser. An in vitro study. Clin Oral Implants Res. 1997;8(4):249-54.

[65] van Velzen FJ, Ofec R, Schulten EA, ten Bruggenkate CM. 10-year survival rate and the incidence of peri-implant disease of 374 titanium dental implants

with a SLA surface: a prospective cohort study in 177 fully and partially edentulous patients. Clin Oral Implants Res. 2015; 26(10):1121-8.

[66] Meijer HJ, Raghoebar GM, de Waal YC, Vissink A. Incidence of peri-implant mucositis and peri-implantitis in edentulous patients with an implant-retained mandibular overdenture during a 10-year follow-up period. J Clin Periodontol. 2014; 41(12):1178-83.

[67] Fardal Ø, Grytten J. A comparison of teeth and implants during maintenance therapy in terms of the number of disease-free years and costs - an in vivo internal control study. J Clin Periodontol. 2013; 40(6):645-51.

[68] Mizutani K, Aoki A, Coluzzi D, Yukna R, Wang CY, Pavlic V, et al. Lasers in minimally invasive periodontal and peri-implant therapy. Periodontology 2000. 2016;71(1):185-212.

[69] Azizi B, Budimir A, Bago I, Mehmeti B, Jakovljević S, Kelmendi J, et al. Antimicrobial efficacy of photodynamic therapy and light-activated disinfection on contaminated zirconia implants: An in vitro study. Photodiagnosis Photodyn Ther. 2018; ;21:328-33.

[70] Azizi B, Budimir A, Mehmeti B, Jakovljević S, Bago I, Gjorgievska E, et al. Antimicrobial efficacy of photodynamic therapy and light-activated disinfection against bacterial species on titanium dental implants. Int J Oral Maxillofac Implants. 2018;33(4):831-7.

[71] Marotti J, Tortamano P, Cai S, Ribeiro MS, Franco JE, de Campos TT. Decontamination of dental implant surfaces by means of photodynamic therapy. Lasers Med Sci. 2013;28(1):303-9.

[72] Shibli JA, Martins MC, Theodoro LH, Lotufo RF, Garcia VG, Marcantonio EJ. Lethal photosensitization in microbiological treatment of ligature-induced peri-implantitis: a preliminary study in dogs. J Oral Sci. 2003;45(1):17-23.

[73] Cho K, Lee SY, Chang BS, Um HS, Lee JK. The effect of photodynamic therapy on Aggregatibacter actinomycetemcomitans attached to surface-modified titanium. J Periodontal Implant Sci. 2015;45(2):38-45.

[74] De Angelis N, Felice P, Grusovin MG, Camurati A, Esposito M. The effectiveness of adjunctive light-activated disinfection (LAD) in the treatment of periimplantitis: 4-month results from a multicentre pragmatic randomised controlled trial. Eur J Oral Implantol. 2012;5(4):321-31.

[75] Scarano A, Piattelli M, Caputi S, Favero GA, Piattelli A. Bacterial adhesion on commercially pure titanium and zirconium oxide disks: an in vivo human study. J Periodontol. 2004;75(2):292-6.

[76] Al-Radha AS, Dymock D, Younes C, O'Sullivan D. Surface properties of titanium and zirconia dental implant materials and their effect on bacterial adhesion. J Dent. 2012;40(2):146-53.

[77] Nielsen HK, Garcia J, Væth M, Schlafer S. Comparison of riboflavin and toluidine blue O as photosensitizers for photoactivated disinfection on endodontic and periodontal pathogens in vitro. PLoS One. 2015;10(10):e0140720.

[78] Umeda M, Tsuno A, Okagami Y, Tsuchiya F, Izumi Y, Ishikawa I. Bactericidal effects of a high-power, red light-emitting diode on two periodontopathic bacteria in antimicrobial photodynamic therapy in vitro. J Investig Clin Dent. 2011;2(4):268-74.

[79] Castro GL, Gallas M, Núñez IR, Borrajo JL, Álvarez JC, Varela LG.

Scanning electron microscopic analysis of diode laser-treated titanium implant surfaces. Photomed Laser Surg. 2007;25(2):124-8.

[80] Karimi MR, Hasani A, Khosroshahian S. Efficacy of antimicrobial photodynamic therapy as an adjunctive to mechanical debridement in the treatment of peri-implant diseases: a randomized controlled clinical trial. J Lasers Med Sci. 2016;7(3):139-45.

[81] Bassetti M, Schär D, Wicki B, Eick S, Ramseier CA, Arweiler NB, et al. Anti-infective therapy of peri-implantitis with adjunctive local drug delivery or photodynamic therapy: 12-month outcomes of a randomized controlled clinical trial. Clin Oral Implants Res. 2014; 25(3):279-87.

[82] Romeo U, Nardi GM, Libotte F, Sabatini S, Palaia G, Grassi FR. The antimicrobial photodynamic therapy in the treatment of peri-implantitis. Int J Dent. 2016;2016:7692387.

[83] Sivaramakrishnan G, Sridharan K. Photodynamic therapy for the treatment of peri-implant diseases: a network meta-analysis of randomized controlled trials. Photodiagnosis Photodyn Ther. 2018;21:1-9.

[84] Al Habashneh R, Asa'ad FA, Khader Y. Photodynamic therapy in periodontal and peri-implant diseases. Quintessence Int. 2015; 46(8):677-90.

[85] Vohra F, Al-Rifaiy MQ, Lillywhite G, Abu Hassan MI, Javed F. Efficacy of mechanical debridement with adjunct antimicrobial photodynamic therapy for the management of peri-implant diseases: a systematic review. Photochem Photobiol Sci. 2014;13(8):1160-8.

[86] Albaker AM, ArRejaie AS, Alrabiah M, Abduljabbar T. Effect of photodynamic and laser therapy in the treatment of peri-implant mucositis: a systematic review. Photodiagnosis Photodyn Ther. 2018;21:147-52.

Chapter 11

Antimicrobial Photodynamic Therapy of the Respiratory Tract: From the Proof of Principles to Clinical Application

Natalia M. Inada, Lucas D. Dias, Kate C. Blanco, Giulia Kassab, Hilde H. Buzzá and Vanderlei S. Bagnato

Abstract

Antimicrobial resistance (AMR) and its relevant health consequences have been explicitly framed as a shared global problem and are estimated to be one of the largest causes of death worldwide by 2050. Antimicrobial photodynamic therapy (aPDT) proposes an alternative treatment for localized infections in response to AMR's ever-growing problem. This technique combines molecular oxygen, a non-toxic photoactivatable photosensitizer (PS), and light of appropriate wavelength, leading to the formation of cytotoxic reactive oxygen species. Besides the ability to inactivate resistant pathogens via a non-selective approach (multiple targets), a relevant advantage of aPDT resides in the fact that no evidence of microorganism resistance has ever been reported to it. In this chapter, we address some efforts to use this technology to kill bacteria in the respiratory tract, from *in vitro* to clinical applications. We put forward three focuses: pharyngotonsillitis, pneumonia, and preventing secondary infections during the use of a photosensitizer-functionalized endotracheal tube. The results here presented offer a foundation for what may become a much larger clinical approach to treat respiratory tract infections.

Keywords: antimicrobial resistance, antimicrobial photodynamic therapy, photochemotherapy, infections of the respiratory tract, endotracheal tube

1. Introduction

The increasing use of antibiotics has an important impact on human health by introducing the emergence of resistant bacterial strains, both in humans treated in an indiscriminate manner, and in two other situations as worrying as, which are the presence of these molecules in drinking water and abusive use in agriculture. This has all resulted in the phenomenon of antimicrobial resistance (AMR) [1].

Each year worldwide, 700,000 deaths occur, approximately, due to diseases that had antimicrobial resistance as responsible for the deaths. By 2050, these deaths could reach the terrifying 10 million mark [1].

One of the biggest barriers to antibiotic-resistant infections is that they add significant costs to the any nation's already overburdened health system [2].

Thus, the paths have been opened for other ways to fight infections and photodynamic therapy (PDT) has stood out with the aim of inactivating not only bacteria, but also fungi, protozoa, and viruses. It is a promising technique, including the treatment of diseases that already have antimicrobial resistance.

In this chapter we will address the theme of advances in research involving microbiological control with photodynamic action, more specifically in the treatment or prevention of diseases of the respiratory tract.

1.1 Antimicrobial resistance

The bacteria have developed several mechanisms to fight against antibiotics action. An important molecular mechanism involves the horizontal transfer of genes from the efflux pumps when the organism acquires a gene that confers the ability to eliminate antibiotics from the intracellular environment [3]. A well-known example is the acquisition of the β-lactamase gene from antibiotic inactivating enzymes, which inactivates β-lactam antibiotics, such as penicillin and cephalosporins [3], where bacteria acquire the ability to inactivate antibiotics through an enzymatic mechanism.

Two interesting aspects are related to cell wall morphology and the ability of bacterial colonies to form biofilms, and interestingly, these aspects are directly related to the cell wall structure of Gram-positive bacteria. The cell-wall glycopolymers from Gram-positive bacteria present an essential role in host-cell adhesion, the first step towards forming a bacterial biofilm. In contrast to Gram-negative, Gram-positive bacteria have a thicker cell wall structure with multiple layers of peptidoglycan. In addition, many Gram-positive bacteria have protective surface structures, typically with glycopolymers bound to peptidoglycan or membrane lipids. These structures include glycopolymers of teicoic acids and branched mycobacterial polymers [4]. Infections caused by Gram-positive bacteria are important for human health and it is worrying that these bacteria are becoming increasingly resistant to existing antibiotics. The teicoic acids wall has multiple functional roles in Gram-positive bacteria including resistance to cationic antimicrobial peptides, such as the vancomycin, a glycopeptide antibiotic. Other cellular processes influenced by this wall include autolysis, cell division, the location of penicillin-binding protein, survival at higher temperatures, biofilm formation and epithelial cell adhesion [5].

Biofilms have an important impact on bacterial infections and also on bacterial resistance. Organisms structured in biofilms exhibit up to 1,000 times more resistance to antibiotics than planktonic cells.

1.2 Mechanisms of antibiotic resistance

Pathogenic bacteria resistant to antibiotics are prevalent in different populations of the environment such as from the soil and water containing encode genes with resistance mechanisms [6], which can be mobilized for new hosts, including humans [7] and, depending on genic expression, may result in significant public health problems [8]. If the microbial mutations are for its benefice, such as antibiotic resistance, they are predominant in the species and transmitted for subsequent generations, making the bacteria predominant antibiotic-resistant [9]. The mechanisms of an antimicrobial resistance may be intrinsic to the microorganisms or even acquired through the transmission of the genetic material or by mutation (which may occur during replication) during the bacterial evolution, whether induced or spontaneous, by mutation mechanisms in a chromosome or transfer genes loci, which can encode inactivate enzymes in antibiotics or even reducing their permeability in cells [10]. The bacterial mutations that can occur are replacement (transition and transversion); deletion (macrodelection and microdeletion); insertion (macroinsertion and microinsection) and inversion, with exchange of pyrimidine or purine, removal of nucleotides, the inclusion of nucleotides, and removal or insertion of DNA, respectively.

Strains resistant to antibiotics can be transmitted between patients in healthcare units, often through healthcare professionals' contaminated hands, medical-surgical equipment, or inanimate objects from the hospital environment [11]. This type of spread is generally clonal, involving the transmission of a single resistant strain. Outbreaks caused by the clonal spread of an antibiotic-resistant organism have been commonly reported in *S. aureus* MRSA strains [12]. Patients' transmission can be clonal in multiple species of strains with different prevalence according to the geographic region [13].

1.3 The worldwide impact of antimicrobial resistance

Infectious diseases are a major cause of human deaths. According to the World Health Organization (WHO), on the top ten global causes of death (2016), chronic obstructive pulmonary disease and lower respiratory infections are occupying the third and fourth places, respectively, behind ischemic heart disease and stroke [14]. It is relevant to note that infectious diseases outperform all types of cancer in terms of mortality, according to WHO data. Figures reported in 2016 indicate that there were 3.190 million deaths due to respiratory infections, with a mortality rate of 43/100,000. Analyzing again the top ten global causes of death but now, in low-income countries (2016), lower respiratory infections were among the leading causes of death across all income groups [14].

It is essential to discover and invest in the development of new antibiotic molecules, following the growing global need. But just as importantly, research into new non-antibiotic approaches for the prevention and protection against infectious diseases is needed and should be encouraged and a high priority research and development project [15].

In the US, the Centers for Disease Control and Prevention (CDC) estimated that antibiotic-resistant infections are responsible for $20 billion a year in additional health care costs, and $35 billion a due to loss of productivity [16]. Thus, a deeper understanding of the mechanisms of resistance to antibiotics is relevant in terms of human health, that is, it saves human lives, but it also reduces an important economic burden for public and private health systems.

Penicillin, discovered by Fleming in 1928, was first tested for the treatment of infectious diseases in the 1930s and became a widespread drug in the 1940s. β-lactam antibiotics, the group to which penicillin belongs, are effectively drugs of choice for the treatment of community-based respiratory diseases, for example, which are usually caused by Gram-positive bacteria, such as *Staphylococcus* and *Streptococcus*.

The introduction of new antibiotics in clinical use was quickly followed by the clinical observation of resistant strains and the time between clinical use and resistance has become shorter and shorter. For example, sulfonamides were introduced for clinical use in 1930 and resistant strains appeared in the 1940s. Vancomycin was introduced in 1956 and resistant strains were first reported in 1988. However, for newer antibiotics, such as daptomycin, fidaxomycin and linezolid, resistance was observed in the same year in which clinical use began [17].

2. Antimicrobial photodynamic therapy (aPDT)

The mechanisms of aPDT are basically the same of PDT for tumors, based on the combined action of three elements: a photosensitizer (PS), a light source at appropriate wavelength to excite the PS and molecular oxygen (O_2) in the target tissue.

The photodynamic process inactivating microorganisms occurs through the action of reactive oxygen species (ROS) that destroy vital constituents of fungi, bacteria, viruses and protozoa. In 1933 Jablonski published his article explaining the electronic states of a molecule and the transitions between them [18]. In this famous "Jablonski's diagram", we understand how a photosensitizer in the singlet ground state, moves to the excited singlet state after absorbing photons from a light source. And through the process named "intersystem crossing", a spin inversion occurs and then, this molecule goes to the excited triplet state, giving it conditions to transfer energy (type II mechanism) or electron (type I mechanism) to O_2, generating ROS.

For antimicrobial purposes, the photodynamic action will take place within the cells or at the extracellular matrix of the microbial biofilm where the photosensitizer molecules are present, the main sites being the outer membrane or cell wall, membrane lipids and lipopolysaccharides. The singlet oxygen produced has a very small radius of action, less than 0.02 μm, so the damage produced by PDT will only be in the presence of the photosensitizer and under photoactivation. As a result, cell death is caused by cell wall or membrane lysis and/or inactivation of proteins or enzymes essential for microbial metabolism [19].

3. aPDT of respiratory tract diseases

3.1 Pharyngotonsillitis

Sore throat is a frequent complaint in outpatient medical consultations and emergencies. Acute pharyngotonsillitis represents a significant source of social disorders in the child population, such as missed classes repeated use of antimicrobials, and can cause complications such as peritonsillar or retropharyngeal abscess, otitis, sinusitis, pneumonia, rheumatic fever, and post-streptococcal glomerulonephritis [20]. Bacterial infections of the respiratory system can be located in the pharynx (pharyngotonsillitis). Viruses cause around 90% of pharyngitis, and 10% are caused by bacteria that have the vast majority associated with *Streptococcus pyogenes* or Beta-hemolytics of Lancefield group A (EBHGA) [21] however, other bacteria can cause pharyngotonsillitis such as *Streptococcus mutans and Streptococcus pyogenes, Staphylococcus aureus, Moraxella catarrhalis, Haemophilus influenzae, Prevotella* sp., *Bacteroids fragilis, and Fusobacterium* sp.

The diagnosis of EBHGA infection should preferably be confirmed microbiologically by rapid antigens detection tests and through oropharyngeal secretion culture. The gold standard for diagnosing oropharyngeal infections by EBHGA is culture [22], which should be done before starting treatment with antibiotics [23]. Clinical samples should be seeded on blood agar plates, which allows a preliminary screening of β-hemolytic colonies. Subsequent confirmation of suspected colonies such as EBHGA can be obtained by several laboratory tests, which are easily and quickly performed and which are still widely applied in clinical microbiology, despite the increasing use of automatic identification systems. EBHGA can be an oropharyngeal colonizing agent and thus, the microbiological investigation must be guided by clinical and epidemiological factors: patient's age, clinical signs and symptoms, season, and personal exposure to EBHGA [24].

According to the World Health Organization (WHO), approximately 600 million new pharyngotonsillitis cases due to EBHGA occur annually, and of these, 500 thousand may progress with rheumatic fever and about 300 thousand with rheumatic carditis [25]. In developing countries, the occurrence is three times higher than in developed countries. The preliminary diagnosis and treatment of tonsillitis and pharyngitis is a common cause of inappropriate use of antibiotics.

Penicillin is the drug of choice for *S. pyogenes* infections' empirical treatment, despite more than 60 years of use. S. pyogenes remains sensitive to penicillin, and resistance tests for penicillins or other beta-lactams approved for its treatment are unnecessary. However, more than 10% of patients report an allergy to penicillin, which leads to the use of cephalosporins, clindamycin, or macrolides as alternative treatments [26]. As rates of resistance to macrolides among isolated *S. pyogenes* have been increasing in North America and Europe, resistance tests for these substances may be indicated. Sore throat is a symptom that leading people to seek medical attention, and although it spontaneously remits, primary care doctors usually prescribe antibiotics for it. In a systematic review, Spinks and collaborators concluded that antibiotics confer relative benefits in the treatment of sore throat. However, the absolute benefits are modest [27].

The research carried out at Santa Casa Hospital of São Carlos city (São Paulo, Brazil) by the CEPOF - Optics and Photonics Research Center" from University of São Paulo - São Carlos is composed of a clinical trial - "Turmeric and LED in the treatment of sore throat" with objectives as assessing the therapeutic efficacy of PDT with curcumin as an adjunct in the treatment of acute pharyngotonsillitis in adults in the municipality of São Carlos [28]. The photosensitizer used in this study was curcumin (0.75 mg/ml), using two minutes of illumination with a blue light (LED) at 450 nm. The clinical trial is randomized and controlled with adults aged 18 to 45 years diagnosed with acute pharyngotonsillitis. Participants are undergoing a rapid test for the detection of group A beta-hemolytic streptococcus (EBHGA). Participants with streptococcal pharyngotonsillitis are divided into Antibiotic therapy comparison groups in conjunction with photodynamic therapy; and Antibiotic Therapy Group in conjunction with a photodynamic therapy placebo, and the therapeutic response will be evaluated in terms of clinical symptoms (sore throat and fever) and microbiological response, mainly considering the presence of EBHGA in the clinical response.

3.2 Designing antimicrobial-coating for endotracheal tube to prevent ventilator-associated respiratory tract infections

Mechanical ventilation (endotracheal intubation) is an effective intervention performed for breathing support in patients admitted in the intensive care unit, but it is also identified as one of the highest risk factors for developing ventilator-associated pneumonia (VAP) [29]. VAP is a type of nosocomial infection that results in a higher mortality (increase from 20–75%) and morbidity rate, prolonged lengths of hospitalization, and also increased hospitalization costs ($10,000 to $25,000) [30–32]. Furthermore, each year, approximately 50 million patients in the intensive care unit are intubated with an endotracheal tube (ETT) for breathing support worldwide [33].

Most cases of VAP are caused by the aspiration of infected (bacteria and/or virus) secretions from the oropharynx, although a small number of cases can result from direct bloodstream infection [34]. Moreover, there is a growing concern associated with the ETT as the primary target related to VAP by biofilm formation on its surface [35]. Biofilms are characterized by its resistance to commercial antibiotics that favor resistant microorganisms' proliferation and make them inaccessible to antimicrobials [36].

Regarding VAP occur by ETT, aspiration occurs when there is distal migration of microorganisms present in the secretions accumulated above the ETT cuff. Moreover, biofilm is formed and attached in the lumen of ETT facilitating the transfer to the sterile bronchial tree [37], as presented in **Figure 1**.

Currently, there are methods used to prevent VAP based on its pathogenesis such as prevent aspiration of secretions and bacterial colonization of aerodigestive tract. Lastly, strategies include measures to minimize the risk of contaminated equipment but these methods show some practical limitations. In this regard, the development of strategies and new medical devices to avoid VAP is urgently need.

New medical devices based on the development of antimicrobial coated for ETT surface should be considered if they have been able to prevent VAP in well-designed clinical studies and be cost-effective [38]. Along the years, different strategies and antimicrobial coated for ETT surface (e.g. metal/antiseptics, metal/zeolites/d--tyrosine, nanorough/fructose, antimicrobial peptides, antibiotics/antiseptics, photo-based therapy, micropatterned surfaces, nanorough surfaces, and hydrophobic/hydrophilic) have been evaluated aiming to prevent the biofilm formation and VAP [38] (**Figure 2**).

These antimicrobial coated are functionalized on ETT surface via covalently or ionic bonding or creating a matrix on a polymer (e.g. polyvinyl chloride (PVC)) depending on the molecular structure of both antimicrobial and type of polymer-based ETT and the presence of additives on ETT constitution [39].

As a selected example, in 2020, the Optics and Photonics Research Center from University of São Paulo developed a photo-based antimicrobial coating for ETT *via* functionalization of a natural product (curcumin) photosensitizer on PVC-based ETT surface [40] (**Figure 3**).

This therapeutic approach is based on the photoactivation of curcumin-functionalized endotracheal tube using an optical fiber followed by the production of reactive oxygen species and $^1O_2$ able to destroy biofilm and preventing its formation in the lumen of ETT. In this regard, the authors observed a photoelimination of bacteria biofilm such as *E. coli* (72%), *S. aureus* (95%), and *P. aeruginosa* (73%) previously formed on the ETT surface using a light dose of 50 J/cm^2. Moreover,

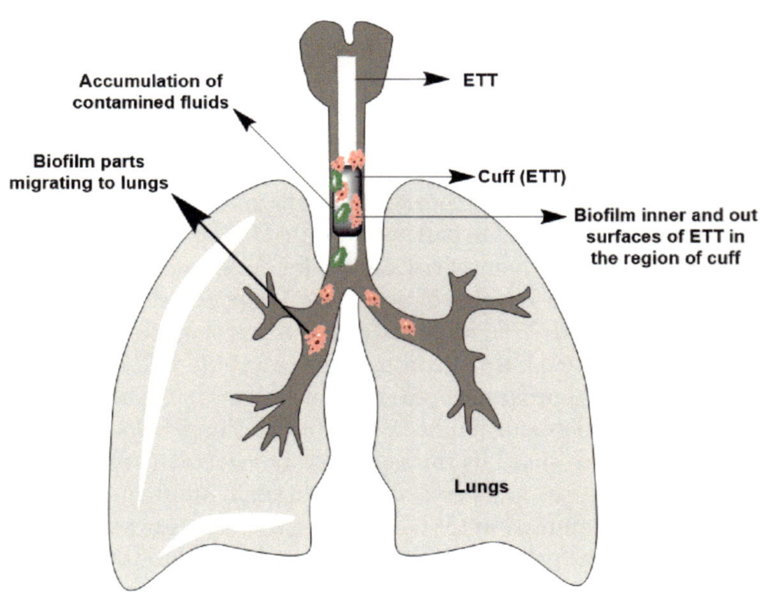

Figure 1.
Pathogenesis of ventilator-associated pneumonia (VAP). Copyright (2020) National Academy of Sciences.

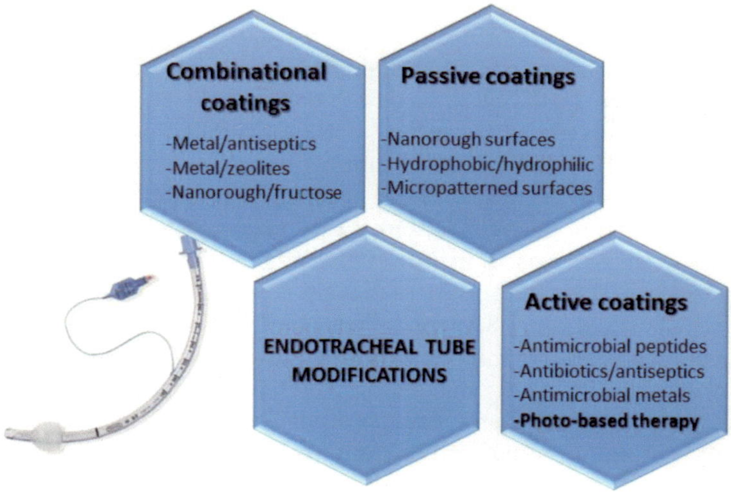

Figure 2.
Antimicrobial coatings for ETT.

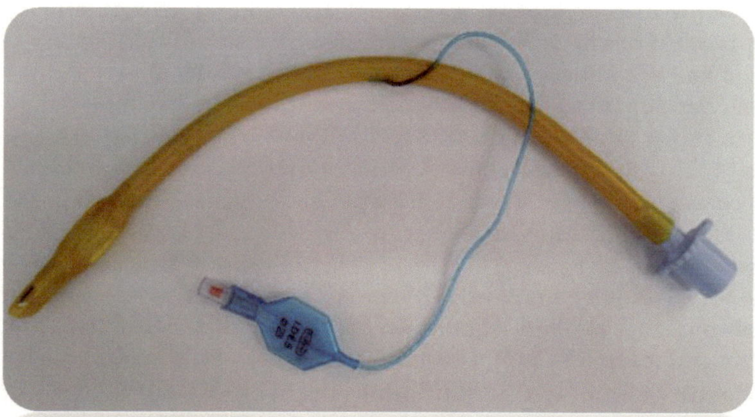

Figure 3.
Curcumin-functionalized endotracheal tube. Copyright (2020) National Academy of Sciences.

a prevention on formation of *S. aureus* bacteria biofilm in the lumen of curcumin-functionalized endotracheal tube was observed when it was under illumination (at 450 nm, 35 mW/cm^2) [39]. Furthermore, no degradation and leaching for curcumin-functionalized endotracheal tube under different pH values (2.0, 4.5, 7.0, 8.0, and 10.0) were observed. These results pave the way for developing of photosensitizers-functionalized ETT and photodynamic action to combat hospital-acquired infections like VAP [40].

Overall, the development and application of antimicrobials coatings for ETT have shown great promise and continue to progress. Significant results are being obtained with a wide family of the antimicrobial coating, including photosensitizers. From perspective, these *in vitro* methodologies developed so far could be applied in *ex vivo* and *in vivo* tests to evaluate and optimize these antimicrobial medical devices to be applied in clinical trials. In sum, this approach possesses excellent potential to reduce the number of deaths worldwide and decrease healthcare costs.

3.3 Lower respiratory tract infections and current treatment challenges

Lower respiratory infections are the fourth-largest cause of death worldwide and the main cause of death in low-income countries [14]. The most frequent lower respiratory infections are acute bronchitis and bronchiolitis, influenza, and pneumonia [41]. In Brazil, pneumonia is the number one cause of hospitalization [42]. It is also the main worldwide cause of death of children younger than 5 years old [43]. Although the number of hospitalizations has decreased over the past decades, the in-hospital mortality increased, mainly explained by the aging of the population and the occurrence of pneumonia cases that are more difficult to treat [42].

The European Respiratory Society defines pneumonia as an acute illness of the lower respiratory tract that includes cough and at least one other symptom: new focal chest signs, new lung shadowing shown by radiography, otherwise unexplained fever for more than 4 days, or otherwise unexplained tachypnea/dyspnea [41]. Community Acquired Pneumonia (CAP) is contracted from contact with the infection in day-to-day life [41]. It is predominantly bacterial in origin, being *Streptococcus pneumoniae* its most prevalent pathogen [44]. Other important agents are *Haemophilus influenza*, *Pseudomonas aeruginosa* [44, 45]. Also, about 30% of cases are coinfections with viruses [46]. However, in the vast majority of CAP cases, there is no investigation of the etiological agent [42]. In such situations, the treatment is based on the most prevalent microorganisms of that locality [42].

Hospital Acquired Pneumonia (HAP), also called nosocomial pneumonia, is the one that develops after at least 48 hours after the patients' admission [47]. Its reported mortality rate ranges from 20 to 50%, the highest among nosocomial infections [47]. As mentioned above, ventilator-associated pneumonia (VAP) is the one contracted at least 48–72 hours after endotracheal intubation [41]. The most relevant HAP and VAP agents are also bacteria, like *Staphylococcus aureus, Pseudomonas aeruginosa*, *Escherichia coli*, and *Klebsiella*, *Acinetobacter*, and *Enterobacter* species [48]. Knowledge of the etiological agents is essential in treating these infections since patients who receive the wrong initial therapy have a high risk of mortality and morbidity [47]. However, the delay in starting the treatment also leads to poor prognostic [47]. A significant concern in HAP and VAP cases is the present of methicillin-resistant *Staphylococcus aureus* (MRSA), which is associated with elevated mortality rates and treatment costs [49]. Traditionally, the first-choice drug for MRSA infections is vancomycin, which due to its low penetration in the lungs and high renal toxicity, leads to a failure rate the can reach 70% [49].

Even with new drugs like linezolid, tigecycline and ceftaroline, persists the difficulty in increasing the success rate of treatments and the worry with the development of resistance [49, 50]. Linezolid, for example, was approved for clinical use in 2000, and cases of resistance in patients were reported as early as 2002 [51]. In a study from 2014, the occurrence of non-susceptibility to this antibiotic remained relatively low, but several different resistance mechanisms had already been observed by then [51].

Another approach to hinder the burden of pneumonia is vaccination. Two types of vaccines are currently available for *S. pneumoniae*, the main agent in CAP: the pneumococcal polysaccharide vaccine (PPV) has been recommended for adults since the mid-1980's, but it lacks efficacy in neonates and infants [52]; the pneumococcal conjugate vaccines (PCVs), designed to overcome that, were first approved in 2000 [53]. However, pneumococcal vaccination faces two main challenges: first, each vaccine is only effective against the serotypes contained in it; second, the reduction of the said serotypes increases the colonization of other serotypes that are not covered by the vaccines, and of other pathogen species like *S. aureus* and *H. influenza* [52]. Thus, new vaccines need to be developed continuously, similarly to what happens to antibiotics [52].

In face of so many challenges, PDT using indocyanine green (ICG) and infrared light has been studied in the treatment of bacterial pneumonia. ICG is a water-soluble dye that emits fluorescence when exposed to infrared light [54]. Its absorption peak in human plasma is 805 nm [55]. It is desirable to have the light excitation at this range because it penetrates deeper into biological tissue, since it is less absorbed by water, melanin and hemoglobin [56].

In an *in vitro* study by Leite *et al.*, the *in vitro* inactivation of *S. pneumoniae* was effective using concentrations of ICG as low as 5 μM when combined with a 780 nm laser device or 10 μM when using an 850 nm LED. In these conditions, the treatment was safe for RAW 264.7 macrophages, and seemed to enhance their ability to fight the bacteria [57]. Other studies have also investigated similar protocols for other relevant pneumonia pathogens. Topaloglu *et al.* found an effective *in vitro* killing of *S. aureus* using 84 J/cm^2 of light (809 nm) with 6 μg/mL of ICG, and of *P. aeruginosa* using 125 μg/mL ICG and 252 J/cm^2 [58]. Kassab *et al.* had similar results for *S. aureus*, and showed that the same protocol, with up to 200 J/cm^2 and 10 μM of ICG, was harmless to multiple mammalian cell lines [59].

The first *in vivo* investigation of the proposed protocol, performed by Geralde *et al.*, found a reduction in the bacterial burden and an increase in the survival rate of SKH-1 hairless mice infected with *S. pneumoniae* after a single PDI session using ICG 100 μM and 120 J/cm^2 of light at 780 nm, with a waiting interval of 3 minutes [60]. In this study, the light exposure did not seem to be harmful to the animals. Additionally, the ICG alone was no different form the control, suggesting that the activation with light was essential to the observed effects. It was then demonstrated that nebulization would be a viable delivery method for ICG to reach the lungs. ICG is compatible with air-jet nebulization in multiple concentrations, and it reaches and distributes in the lungs similarly as intranasal instillation [59, 61]. Additionally, mice exposed to pulmonary PDT using ICG and 216 J/cm^2 of light at 808 nm showed no clinical signs of toxicity or histological damage to the lungs, liver or stomach 7 days after the treatment [59]. Replicating such results in larger models and patients might be challenging due to the layers of biological tissue the light needs to go through to reach the target. Nonetheless, aPDT using ICG and infrared light shows good efficacy and safety in pre-clinical studies, and has great potential to become a treatment for lower respiratory infections.

4. Nanotechnology and future perspectives for aPDT

Antimicrobial Photodynamic Therapy is one of the main option that have been investigated against resistant bacteria. However, even with the use of some photosensitizers in the clinic, especially for tumor treatment and already approved by the FDA, some restrictions of these molecules, such as low solubility, little tissue penetration, low specificity and little accumulation in the target cells are some of the characteristics that hinders the greater use of this technique as the gold standard in various diseases [62] Nanotechnologies is one possibility to increase the efficacy of molecules with poor pharmacokinetics and pharmacodynamics properties, including PS [63].

Drug delivery is, therefore, one of the most challenges for aPDT [64]. For this reason, nanotechnology has been used in PDT as a possibility to increase its effect. Nano-systems can be stable (even under light), present good optical properties and high penetration in the tissue, as the skin (for topical application), have more specificity (with surface functionalization) and be more efficient in ROS production [62]. Nanomaterials can be used as PS itself or to load the PS (as carrier), opening several possibilities to conjugate nanotechnology with aPDT.

The nanoparticles used as drug carrier present some advantages in relation to traditional molecules, such as the transport in the blood circulation of hydrophobic substances, the incorporation of some antigen given them desired properties, the facility to enter in the target and yet, it is possible to control drug delivery [64]. Thus, several types of nanoparticles, with different sizes, shapes and functions, have been synthetized in the last years, including for aPDT [65]. They are classified according to their material: inorganic (as metal nanoparticles), organic (as liposomes) and nanocomposites, organic or inorganic [66].

Some nanomaterials have been explored under irradiation, showing photodynamic effect and have been applied in different tests. Gold and Silver nanoparticles, nanomaterials based in silica and silicon, quantum-dots, carbon-based materials and nanoparticles from organic molecules are examples of the materials already used in photodynamic therapy and its multimodal conjugation treatments in several application [62].

The nanosystems also enable the delivery of PS with desirable optical characteristics, such as the use of absorption by two photons or upconversion nanoparticles and can result in high penetration into the tissue. Thus, they can be activated from X-ray to infrared, reaching regions of the body that previously were not possible with traditional PDT. This prospect of applying nano PDT can make this technique extremely useful in the context of respiratory diseases, especially due to the current concern about infections caused by resistant bacteria, the pandemic of the coronavirus, or the next outbreaks that are yet to come [64].

However, it is still necessary to overcome the barrier between *in vitro* and *in vivo* studies to reach nanotechnology's clinical applications. Viral, fungal and bacterial infections characterize a global public health problem and, with the coronavirus pandemic, humanity saw the urgency to invest in new therapeutic possibilities, especially because new pandemics have been predicted. The advent of nanotechnology has helped to provide quick answers to urgent problems [63]. The scientific and clinical community's joint efforts and their integration into industry are needed to respond quickly to respiratory diseases [67].

APDT is increasingly becoming a viable option for upper and lower airway infections and nanosystems can help to break traditional PDT barriers. The search for highly efficient PS has been one of the main research lines when it comes to improving PDT. Many molecules synthesis methods have been explored, as well as the synthesis of nanoparticles, but they are usually complicated and, especially with nanoparticles, are difficult to apply for large-scale production. Thus, simpler synthesis methods with functionalization of these nanometric systems have been gaining relevance in the scientific community, since it is one of the challenges for the clinical implementation of nano-PDT [68]. It is also necessary to understand the parameters beyond the laboratory, such as dose, irradiation and clinical efficacy [69].

5. Conclusions

Increased resistance to antibiotics has a direct impact on humanity and is one of the most important public health problems worldwide. Especially in the respiratory tract (lower and upper), which involves pharyngotonsillitis, pneumonia and infections by endotracheal tube, new therapeutic possibilities are needed. APDT has been shown to be highly effective against the microorganisms that cause these diseases and several protocols with different photosensitizers and illumination devices have been developed to make aPDT a great therapeutic option. New molecules and nanotechnology have been developed to improve aPDT and break down barriers to clinical applications.

Acknowledgements

The authors would like to thank CEPOF, the Brazilian National Council for Scientific and Technological Development (CNPq), the Coordination for the Improvement of Higher Education Personnel (CAPES), and the São Paulo Research Foundation (FAPESP, grants 2013/07276-1, 2018/18188-0, 2016/14033-6, 2019/13569-8).

Conflict of interest

The authors declare no conflict of interest.

Author details

Natalia M. Inada*, Lucas D. Dias, Kate C. Blanco, Giulia Kassab, Hilde H. Buzzá and Vanderlei S. Bagnato
São Carlos Institute of Physics, University of São Paulo, São Carlos, São Paulo, Brazil

*Address all correspondence to: nataliainada@ifsc.usp.br

References

[1] Singer AC, Shaw H, Rhodes V, et al. Review of antimicrobial resistance in the environment and its relevance to environmental regulators. Front Microbiol 2016; 7: 1-22.

[2] Ventola CL. The antibiotic resistance crisis: part 1: causes and threats. P T 2015; 40: 277-283.

[3] Wright GD. Molecular mechanisms of antibiotic resistance. Chem Commun 2011; 47: 4055-4061.

[4] Weidenmaier C, Peschel A. Teichoic acids and related cell-wall glycopolymers in Gram-positive physiology and host interactions. *Nature Reviews Microbiology*. Epub ahead of print 2008. DOI: 10.1038/nrmicro1861.

[5] Winstel V, Xia G, Peschel A. Pathways and roles of wall teichoic acid glycosylation in Staphylococcus aureus. Int J Med Microbiol 2014; 304: 215-221.

[6] Peterson E, Kaur P. Antibiotic resistance mechanisms in bacteria: Relationships between resistance determinants of antibiotic producers, environmental bacteria, and clinical pathogens. *Front Microbiol*. Epub ahead of print 2018. DOI: 10.3389/fmicb.2018.02928.

[7] Bengtsson-Palme J, Kristiansson E, Larsson DGJ. Environmental factors influencing the development and spread of antibiotic resistance. *FEMS Microbiology Reviews*. Epub ahead of print 2018. DOI: 10.1093/femsre/fux053.

[8] Molster CM, Bowman FL, Bilkey GA, et al. The evolution of public health genomics: Exploring its past, present, and future. *Frontiers in Public Health*. Epub ahead of print 2018. DOI: 10.3389/fpubh.2018.00247.

[9] Beceiro A, Tomás M, Bou G. Antimicrobial resistance and virulence: A successful or deleterious association in the bacterial world? *Clinical Microbiology Reviews*. Epub ahead of print 2013. DOI: 10.1128/CMR.00059-12.

[10] Coculescu BI. Antimicrobial resistance induced by genetic changes. *Journal of medicine and life*.

[11] Russotto V, Cortegiani A, Raineri SM, et al. Bacterial contamination of inanimate surfaces and equipment in the intensive care unit. *Journal of Intensive Care*. Epub ahead of print 2015. DOI: 10.1186/s40560-015-0120-5.

[12] Chambers HF, Deleo FR. Waves of resistance: Staphylococcus aureus in the antibiotic era. Nat Rev Microbiol 2009; 7: 629-641.

[13] Bose J, Kloesener MH, Schulte RD. Multiple-genotype infections and their complex effect on virulence. *Zoology*. Epub ahead of print 2016. DOI: 10.1016/j.zool.2016.06.003.

[14] World Health Organization (WHO). The top ten causes of death. *The top 10 causes of death*.

[15] Bush K, Courvalin P, Dantas G, et al. Tackling antibiotic resistance. *Nature Reviews Microbiology*. Epub ahead of print 2011. DOI: 10.1038/nrmicro2693.

[16] Antibiotic resistance threats in the United States. Antibiotic resistance threats. *https://www.cdc.gov/drugresistance/pdf/ar-threats-2013-508.pdf* 2013; 22-50.

[17] Walsh CT, Wencewicz TA. Prospects for new antibiotics: A molecule-centered perspective. *Journal of Antibiotics*. Epub ahead of print 2014. DOI: 10.1038/ja.2013.49.

[18] Jablonski A. Efficiency of Anti-Stokes Fluorescence in Dyes. Nature 1933; 131: 839-840.

[19] Harris F, Chatfield L, Phoenix D. Phenothiazinium Based Photosensitisers - Photodynamic Agents with a Multiplicity of Cellular Targets and Clinical Applications. *Curr Drug Targets*. Epub ahead of print 2005. DOI: 10.2174/1389450054545962.

[20] Ferretti JJ, Stevens DL, Fischetti V a. *Streptococcus pyogenes*: Basic Biology to Clinical Manifestations. *Streptococcus pyogenes Basic Biol to Clin Manifestations*.

[21] Bisno AL, Gerber MA, Gwaltney, Jr. JM, et al. Practice Guidelines for the Diagnosis and Management of Group A Streptococcal Pharyngitis. *Clin Infect Dis*. Epub ahead of print 2002. DOI: 10.1086/340949.

[22] Gerber MA, Baltimore RS, Eaton CB, et al. Prevention of rheumatic fever and diagnosis and treatment of acute streptococcal pharyngitis: A scientific statement from the American Heart Association Rheumatic Fever, Endocarditis, and Kawasaki Disease Committee of the Council on Cardiovascular Disease i. *Circulation*. Epub ahead of print 2009. DOI: 10.1161/CIRCULATIONAHA.109.191959.

[23] Lin MH, Fong WK, Chang PF, et al. Predictive value of clinical features in differentiating group A beta-hemolytic streptococcal pharyngitis in children. J Microbiol Immunol Infect 2003; 36: 21-25.

[24] Gunnarsson RK, Holm SE, Söderström M. The prevalence of beta-haemolytic streptococci in throat specimens from healthy children and adults: Implications for the clinical value of throat cultures. Scand J Prim Health Care 1997; 15: 149-155.

[25] Carapetis JR, Steer AC, Mulholland EK, et al. Review The global burden of group A streptococcal diseases. 2005; 5: 685-694.

[26] Chiappini E, Regoli M, Bonsignori F, et al. Analysis of Different Recommendations From International Guidelines for the Management of Acute Pharyngitis in Adults and Children. Clin Ther 2011; 33: 48-58.

[27] Spinks A, Glasziou PP, Del Mar CB. Antibiotics for sore throat (Review). Cochrane database Syst Rev 2013; 11: CD000023.

[28] Kate Cristina Blanco, Sigrid dos Santos Souza VSB. *Turmeric and LED in the treatment of sore throat*. Londres, 2019. Epub ahead of print 2019. DOI: https://doi.org/10.1186/ISRCTN14862781.

[29] Hijazi MH, Macintyre NR. Advances in infection control: Ventilator-associated pneumonia. Semin Respir Crit Care Med 2000; 21: 245-262.

[30] Kollef MH, Sharpless L, Vlasnik J, et al. The impact of nosocomial infections on patient outcomes following cardiac surgery. Chest 1997; 112: 666-675.

[31] Timsit JF, Esaied W, Neuville M, et al. Update on ventilator-associated pneumonia. F1000Research 2017; 6: 1-13.

[32] Shorr AF, Zilberberg MD, Kollef M. Cost-Effectiveness Analysis of a Silver-Coated Endotracheal Tube to Reduce the Incidence of Ventilator-Associated Pneumonia. Infect Control Hosp Epidemiol 2009; 30: 759-763.

[33] Hashemi MM, Rovig J, Bateman J, et al. Preclinical testing of a broad-spectrum antimicrobial endotracheal tube coated with an innate immune synthetic mimic. J Antimicrob Chemother 2018; 73: 143-150.

[34] Micek ST, Skrupky LP. Current concepts in the prevention and

treatment of ventilator-associated pneumonia. J Pharm Pract 2010; 23: 25-32.

[35] Fernandez JF, Levine SM, Restrepo MI. Technologic advances in endotracheal tubes for prevention of ventilator-associated pneumonia. Chest 2012; 142: 231-238.

[36] Stewart PS, Costerton JW. Antibiotic resistance of bacteria in biofilms. Lancet 2001; 358: 135-138.

[37] Inglis TJJ, Millar MR, Jones JG, et al. Tracheal Tube Biofilm as a Source of Bacterial Colonization of the Lung. 2018; 27: 2014-2018.

[38] Barnes M, Feit C, Grant T, et al. Acta Biomaterialia Antimicrobial polymer modifications to reduce microbial bioburden on endotracheal tubes and ventilator associated pneumonia. Acta Biomater 2019; 91: 220-234.

[39] Polívková M, Hubáˇ T. Antimicrobial Treatment of Polymeric Medical Devices by Silver Nanomaterials and Related Technology. Epub ahead of print 2017. DOI: 10.3390/ijms18020419.

[40] Zangirolami AC, Dias LD, Blanco KC, et al. Avoiding ventilator-associated pneumonia : Curcumin-functionalized endotracheal tube and photodynamic action. 2020; 1-7.

[41] Gibson GJ, Loddenkemper R, Sibille Y, et al. (eds). Acute Lower Respiratory Infections. In: *European Lung White Book*. European Respiratory Society, 2013, pp. 210-223.

[42] Corrêa RDA, Lundgren FLC, Pereira-Silva JL, et al. Brazilian guidelines for community-acquired pneumonia in immunocompetent adults - 2009. J Bras Pneumol 2009; 35: 574-601.

[43] Wallihan R, Ramilo O. Community-acquired pneumonia in children: Current challenges and future directions. J Infect 2014; 69: S87–S90.

[44] Cillóniz C, Ewig S, Polverino E, et al. Microbial aetiology of community-acquired pneumonia and its relation to severity. Thorax 2011; 66: 340-346.

[45] Isturiz RE, Luna CM, Ramirez J. Clinical and economic burden of pneumonia among adults in Latin America. Int J Infect Dis 2010; 14: e852–e856.

[46] Gupta RK, George R, Nguyen-Van-Tam JS. Bacterial pneumonia and pandemic influenza planning. Emerg Infect Dis 2008; 14: 1187-1192.

[47] Nair GB, Niederman MS. Nosocomial Pneumonia. Lessons Learned. *Crit Care Clin* 2013; 29: 521-546.

[48] Jones RN. Microbial Etiologies of Hospital-Acquired Bacterial Pneumonia and Ventilator-Associated Bacterial Pneumonia. Clin Infect Dis 2010; 51: S81–S87.

[49] Torres A. Antibiotic treatment against methicillin-resistant Staphylococcus aureus hospital- and ventilator-acquired pneumonia: a step forward but the battle continues. Clin Infect Dis 2012; 54: 630-632.

[50] Gould IM, David MZ, Esposito S, et al. New insights into meticillin-resistant Staphylococcus aureus (MRSA) pathogenesis, treatment and resistance. Int J Antimicrob Agents 2012; 39: 96-104.

[51] Mendes RE, Deshpande LM, Jones RN. Linezolid update: Stable in vitro activity following more than a decade of clinical use and summary of associated resistance mechanisms. Drug Resist Updat 2014; 17: 1-12.

[52] Feldman C, Anderson R. Review: Current and new generation pneumococcal vaccines. J Infect 2014; 69: 309-325.

[53] Gibson GJ, Loddenkemper R, Sibille Y, et al. (eds). Immunisation against respiratory diseases. In: *European Lung White Book*. European Cystic Fibrosis Society., 2013, pp. 306-315.

[54] Lim C, Vibert E, Azoulay D, et al. Indocyanine green fluorescence imaging in the surgical management of liver cancers: Current facts and future implications. J Visc Surg 2014; 151: 117-124.

[55] Fickweiler S, Szeimies R-M, Bäumler W, et al. Indocyanine green: intracellular uptake and phototherapeutic effects in vitro. J Photochem Photobiol B Biol 1997; 38: 178-183.

[56] Huang Y, Chen A, Hamblin M. Low-level laser therapy: an emerging clinical paradigm. SPIE Newsroom 2009; 1-3.

[57] Leite IS, Geralde MC, Salina ACG, et al. Near-infrared photodynamic inactivation of *S. pneumoniae* and its interaction with RAW 264.7 macrophages. *J Biophotonics*. Epub ahead of print 2017. DOI: 10.1002/jbio.201600283.

[58] Topaloglu N, Gulsoy M, Yuksel S. Antimicrobial Photodynamic Therapy of Resistant Bacterial Strains by Indocyanine Green and 809-nm Diode Laser. Photomed Laser Surg 2013; 31: 155-162.

[59] Kassab G, Cheburkanov V, Willis J, et al. Safety and delivery efficiency of a photodynamic treatment of the lungs using indocyanine green and extracorporeal near infra-red illumination. *J Biophotonics* 2020; 50: jbio.202000176.

[60] Geralde MC, Leite IS, Inada NM, et al. Pneumonia treatment by photodynamic therapy with extracorporeal illumination - an experimental model. *Physiol Rep*. Epub ahead of print 2017. DOI: 10.14814/phy2.13190.

[61] Kassab G, Geralde MC, Inada NM, et al. Nebulization as a tool for photosensitizer delivery to the respiratory tract. J Biophotonics 2019; 12: e201800189.

[62] Chen J, Fan T, Xie Z, et al. Advances in nanomaterials for photodynamic therapy applications: Status and challenges. Biomaterials 2020; 237: 119827.

[63] Uskoković V. Why have nanotechnologies been underutilized in the global uprising against the coronavirus pandemic? Nanomedicine (Lond) 2020; 15: 1719-1734.

[64] Chatterjee DK, Fong LS, Zhang Y. Nanoparticles in photodynamic therapy: An emerging paradigm. Adv Drug Deliv Rev 2008; 60: 1627-1637.

[65] Sztandera K, Gorzkiewicz M, Klajnert-Maculewicz B. Nanocarriers in photodynamic therapy—in vitro and in vivo studies. Wiley Interdiscip Rev Nanomedicine Nanobiotechnology 2020; 12: 1-24.

[66] Baranwal A, Srivastava A, Kumar P, et al. Prospects of Nanostructure Materials and Their Composites as Antimicrobial Agents. 9. Epub ahead of print 2018. DOI: 10.3389/fmicb.2018.00422.

[67] Navarro-Torné A, Vidal M, Trzaska DK, et al. Chronic respiratory diseases and lung cancer research: A perspective from the European Union. Eur Respir J 2015; 46: 1270-1280.

[68] Yan K, Zhang Y, Mu C, et al. Versatile nanoplatforms with enhanced

photodynamic therapy: Designs and applications. Theranostics 2020; 10: 7287-7318.

[69] Dharmaratne P, Sapugahawatte DN, Wang B, et al. Contemporary approaches and future perspectives of antibacterial photodynamic therapy (aPDT) against methicillin-resistant Staphylococcus aureus (MRSA): A systematic review. Eur J Med Chem 2020; 200: 112341.

Chapter 12

Nanomaterials for Enhanced Photodynamic Therapy

Lucas F. de Freitas

Abstract

Photodynamic therapy is a non-invasive option for eliminating superficial tumors and to control infections. However, despite some protocols are already approved for the clinic, PDT applications could be much broader if some of its main hindrances were overcome. For instance, the most efficient photosensitizers are hydrophobic, so if one injects them intravenously they tend to aggregate and to be internalized by phagocytes in the blood, impairing the delivery to the target site. In addition, visible light has a limited penetration in tissues, therefore the main applications of PDT are limited to superficial tumors unless an invasive procedure is used for the light to reach deeper sites. Another setback is the hypoxia that commonly happens in tumors, hindering the full potential of PDT as it depends on a constant oxygen supply. In this chapter the reader will find some strategies based on Nanotechnology to overcome these and other obstacles for PDT to reach its full clinical potential, i.e. hypoxia-reverting protocols, X-ray-driven PDT, Cherenkov radiation-driven PDT, and active tumor-targeting.

Keywords: photodynamic therapy, nanotechnology, active targeting, X-PDT, CR-PDT

1. Introduction

Nanotechnology consists on the development of materials with dimensions usually between 1 and 100 nm, where the properties of matter are significantly different than their bulk counterparts, and can be tuned to the desired application. These novel chemical and physical properties are usually derived from quantum effects and from the drastically increased surface-to-volume ratio. Furthermore, since many biological structures, i.e. proteins, organelles, viruses, etc., can be found within the nanometric scale, synthetic nanostructures have easy access to biological systems.

Although Nanotechnology started purely as a physical and materials science, soon the medical properties of nanomaterials became evident, and the new era of nanomedicine and nanopharmacy started. Nanomaterials are now recognized as excellent therapeutic and diagnostic tools, and thousands of novel compounds and nanostructures are developed every year, for the most diverse applications.

As you will see in this chapter, Nanotechnology can help practitioners to overcome several hindrances of photodynamic therapy that have so far prevented this approach from reaching a broader clinical success. Over the last decade, nanostructures have been applied as drug delivery platforms for PDT, and as strategies to enhance the efficiency of photosensitizers in generating ROS upon irradiation.

The nanoparticles can be organic or inorganic, can assume a multitude of shapes and sizes within the nanoscale, can act as photosensitizers themselves or as energy transducers. Even further, nanocarriers prevent the complications that arise from the poor solubility of photosensitizers in aqueous media, and increase the tumor accumulation in order to preserve healthy tissues. We are going to discuss in details the most relevant data regarding the enhancement of PDT by the use of nanomaterials.

2. Nanotechnology in combination with PDT

2.1 Main hindrances of PDT

There is a plethora of photosensitizing compounds available, but the majority of them did not present the requirements for clinical trials, i.e. good solubility, target selectivity, sufficient light absorption on the desired wavelength, and low accumulation in distant sites, especially the skin [1]. One of the biggest hindrances of photosensitizers is their hydrophobicity and consequent tendency to aggregate in aqueous environments, making the intravenous administration difficult unless some kind of delivery system is used [2, 3]. Besides, it is desirable that the photosensitizers accumulate preferentially in the target tissue rather than in healthy sites in order to avoid toxicity, therefore strategies of targeted delivery are often necessary to increase the therapeutic efficiency, and nanoparticle systems offer great advantages in this regard [1].

Besides the tendency to aggregate when photosensitizers are injected intravenously, they tend to be distributed to the whole body in a non-specific way, and to be taken up by plasma proteins or phagocytes, decreasing significantly the efficiency of PDT. To increase the specific delivery and avoid side effects, several carriers have been developed to take advantage of the enhanced permeation and retention (EPR) effect or to actively target tumors and enhance specific accumulation, such as polymer and metal nanoparticles, micelles and liposomes, and magnetic nanoparticles. The EPR effect is caused by the leaky vasculature common to tumor tissues, due to the sinusoid capillaries and the fenestrated endothelial cells, plus the inefficient lymphatic drainage from tumor sites. The active targeting, on the other hand, is actually a plethora of strategies to increase specific tumor accumulation of a drug or therapeutic compound [3].

Another obstacle for photodynamic therapy is the limited penetration of light, so it is used mostly for superficial tumors, or with the help of optic fibers introduced in the patient. Recently, researchers have been developing strategies to produce light inside of the body with the help of nanoparticle scintillators. These materials are able to convert external X-ray photons, which can reach deeper sites in the organism, into visible light photons that could excite a photosensitizer in a process called X-PDT. Another approach to excite photosensitizers with endogenous light is with Cherenkov radiation in a process referred as CR-PDT. Cherenkov radiation is generated when a particle exceeds the speed of light in a defined medium, and is common with the decay of several medical radioactive isotopes [4].

Photosensitizers that absorb in the NIR region, such as indocyanine green (absorption around 800 nm) and aluminum sulfophthalocyanine (absorption around 790 nm), although being able to be used in deeper regions due to the deeper penetration of NIR light, tend to be less efficient in generating singlet oxygen than other photosensitizers that absorb in lower wavelengths. Upconversion nanoparticles (UCNs) can overcome these limitations. The process where the absorption of multiple photons – usually two or three – from a given wavelength leads to the emission of photons from a shorter wavelength is referred as photon upconversion. This can be used as a strategy to reach deeper tissues with longer wavelengths and excite photosensitizers that absorb in shorter wavelengths and would not be reachable by light otherwise [5].

UCNs usually consist in inorganic luminescent materials, usually made with lanthanide elements that absorb NIR light and emit UV-visible light that can be used to excite more efficient photosensitizers. Other than the possibility of exciting photosensitizers in deeper regions and prevent photobleaching, enhancing PDT efficacy, they can carry a plethora of hydrophobic photosensitizers, either loaded physically or chemically [6, 7].

2.2 Nanomaterials used for PDT enhancement

Nanostructured delivery systems for photosensitizers can provide some major advantages in PDT. The first one is regarding the increased quantity of dyes that can be delivered to the target cell due to the large surface-to-volume ratio, while the second one refers to the prevention of the premature release of the dyes before reaching the target, enhancing the specific accumulation in the target tissue and diminishing the side effects. The third is somehow related to the second, since the loaded dyes find few obstacles in the blood stream and acquire an amphiphilic character once conjugated with nanostructures, enhancing the tumor accumulation as well. Another advantage is the privileged accumulation of nanosized materials in tumor tissues due to the enhanced permeability and retention (EPR) effect. Finally, their surface can be functionalized with a plethora of groups, so that their biodistribution, pharmacokinetics, cell uptake and surface chemistry can be tuned according to the desired application [8]. **Figure 1** summarizes the main advantages of nanotechnology combined with PDT.

Both biodegradable and non-biodegradable nanoparticles can be used to potentiate photodynamic therapy (PDT). In the case of biodegradable nanoparticles

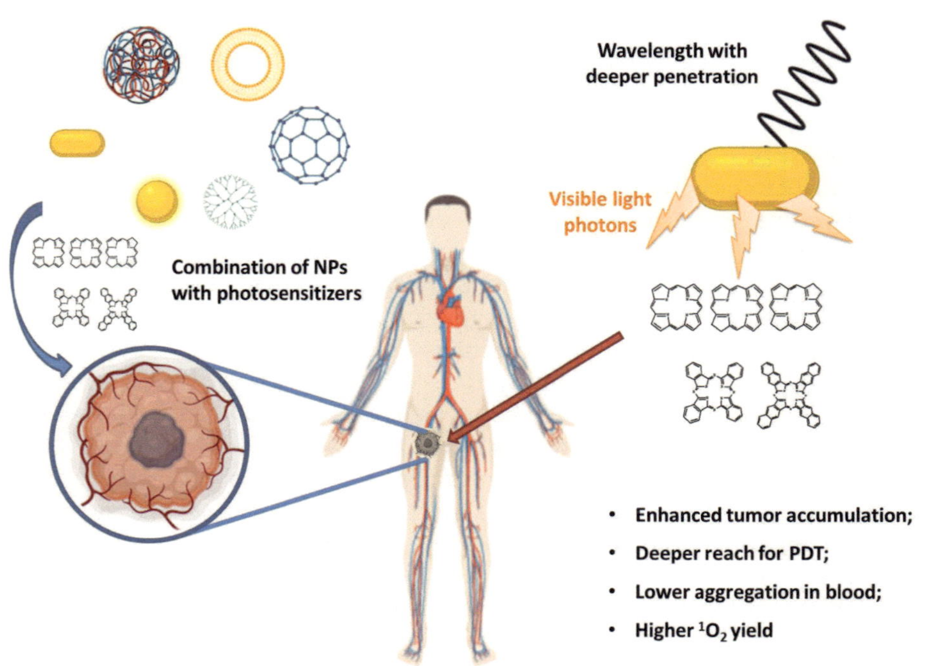

Figure 1.
The combination of nanoparticles with photosensitizers and its main advantages for tumor ablation.

(generally polymers and lipid-based structures), the photosensitizers are trapped inside them and are released in a controlled manner, so that singlet oxygen can be generated due to the exposition to light. On the other hand, when non-biodegradable nanoparticles are used, usually the photosensitizers are adsorbed on their surface (either external or internal, in case of porous structures), and they do not need to be released completely to generate singlet oxygen [1].

Regarding biodegradable nanoparticles, many photosensitizers have been encapsulated with water-soluble polymers, such as meso-tetra(hydroxyphenyl) porphyrin, bacteriochlorophyll, verteporfin, various phthalocyanines, methylene blue, and hypericin. Their singlet oxygen efficiency depends much on the polymer. Poly lactic glycolic acid (PLGA), for instance, has demonstrated good results compared to other polymers, along with poly lactic acid (PLA) and poly ethylene glycol (PEG). The pharmacodynamics of different polymer nanoparticles may differ from one another, and so do their bioavailability, thus the PDT efficiency may be different according to the nature of the polymer [1].

Non-biodegradable nanoparticles are mostly metallic or ceramic-based (especially silica), but polyacrylamide was also reported as a photosensitizer nanocarrier. Nevertheless, solid silica nanoparticles present higher singlet oxygen yield than polyacrylamide nanoparticles, i.e. 2 to 3-fold more singlet oxygen production by silica nanoparticles loaded with methylene blue compared to their polyacrylamide counterparts [1].

Plasmonic materials, a very important class of non-biodegradable nanomaterials, have proven to act as photosensitizers in the right conditions, and if they have photosensitizers attached to their surface, they can enhance the photodynamic efficiency of the dye. It was observed that semiconductor nanoparticles that present the suitable energy gap can be used as photosensitizers and can also be conjugated with other organic dyes. In these conjugated materials, energy can be transferred from the excited nanoparticles to the photosensitizers through a FRET mechanism [5].

Gold and silver nanoparticles are more stable and present higher extinction coefficients than organic dyes, but if one desires to use them to generate singlet oxygen, O_2 molecules must be adsorbed on their surface in order to provide a rapid energy transfer between the two. Furthermore, the energy transfer from the nanoparticles to the adsorbed oxygen molecules is more efficient in low-energy surface states of metal nanoparticles rather than the high-energy states. When these conditions are fulfilled, it is believed that the PDT antitumor efficiency can be up to 10 times that of chemotherapeutics like doxorubicin [5].

Gold nanorods have been developed by different authors in order to carry phthalocyanines via adsorption onto the nanoparticle surface, either chemically with a thiol group or via electrostatic interaction. The formation of a phthalocyanine layer covering the nanoparticle prevents the aggregation of the hydrophobic photosensitizer and enhances the photodynamic activity [2, 9].

Camerin and collaborators compared the efficacy of a phthalocyanine in its free form and conjugated with gold nanoparticles in ablating B78H1 amelanotic melanoma tumors in mice. The results showed that the accumulation of photosensitizer in the tumor is enhanced when they are bound to the nanoparticles, and as a consequence, the damage was significantly more intense and the tumor growth was significantly slower than the tumors treated with the free phthalocyanines [2].

Several cases of enhancement of the photosensitizer efficiency by plasmonic nanoparticles (due to a strong energy transfer and the prevention of photobleaching) have been reported in the literature, with various photosensitizers and nanoparticle morphologies and materials [9–13]. One interesting example was demonstrated by [14], because the PDT efficiency of the photosensitizer conjugated with gold nanoparticles was comparable to the free photosensitizer, but the hyperthermal effect contributed to a more intense cytotoxicity against the tumor cells.

The material and the morphology of the plasmonic nanoparticles influence on the extinction coefficients and, consequently, on the energy transfer efficiency. Gold nanourchins, for instance, present an intense extinction coefficient at 940 nm, which is within the therapeutic window, and the singlet oxygen production was intense and sufficed to eliminate cancer HeLa cells while preserving normal NIH-3 T3 fibroblasts. Gold bipyramids can be efficient singlet oxygen generators if the wavelength used overlaps with the surface plasmon resonance peak, even more efficient than methylene blue. Silver and gold nanocubes are unable to generate singlet oxygen, while in the form of nanoprisms the opposite occurs [5].

This dependence on the morphology can be explained by theoretical calculations showing that O2 can be adsorbed on Au(111), Ag(111), Au(110), Ag(110), Au(100), and Ag(100) surfaces, but on Au(111), Au(100), and Ag(111) surfaces oxygen can remain in molecular form and be excited to its singlet state, whereas on the other surfaces it dissociates into its atomic form. This can only be altered when some defects are present in the crystalline structure [5].

Quantum dots are other promising materials for photodynamic therapy. Graphene quantum dots, for example, reduced tumor cell viability to 20% in a 1.8 μM concentration, compared to 35% cell viability when the same concentration of PpIX was used. Similar results were obtained for ZnO quantum dots irradiated with blue light [5].

Silica is also widely used as a nanomaterial because it is non-toxic and optically transparent, and their surface chemical functionalization is easily achieved due to the presence of several hydroxyl groups on its surface. When it comes to PDT, silica can act as a carrier of photosensitizers, protecting them from enzymatic degradation and enhancing their permeation in tumors [5]. **Figure 2** shows some of the most important nanomaterials used in combination with PDT.

2.3 Recent advances in X-PDT

X-ray driven PDT makes use of scintillating materials and/or radiosensitizers (**Figure 3**). High-Z elements, for instance, have inner shell electrons which are very efficient in capturing X-ray photons and converting them into relaxed electrons and visible light photons. Thus, the most common scintillators are nanoparticles of high-Z elements doped with rare earth elements, and present

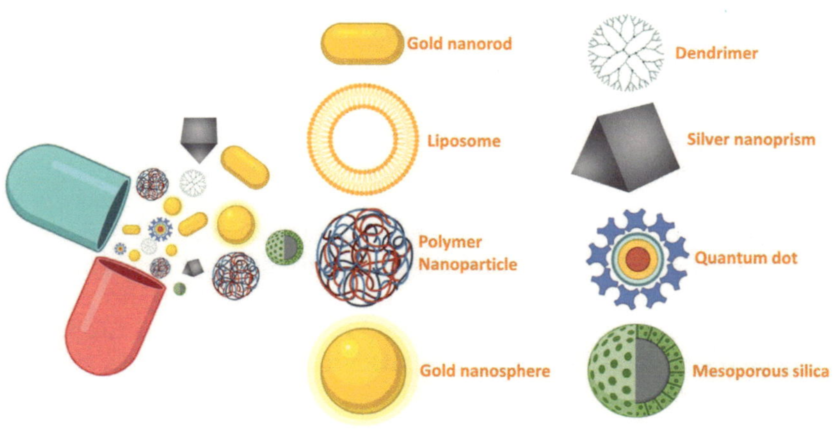

Figure 2.
Some of the various morphologies and types of nanoparticles used in combination with PDT.

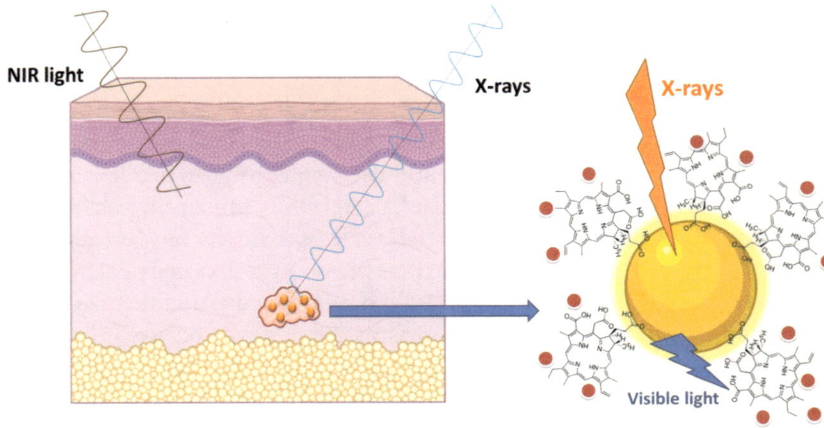

Figure 3.
Deeper penetration of X-rays and it use for X-PDT. The red circles symbolize singlet oxygen generated by the interaction of the excited photosensitizer and molecular oxygen.

useful properties for medical imaging and high-energy physics. The materials can be designed as films, coordination compounds, vitroceramics, metal-organic frameworks (MOFs), and hybrid organic-inorganic materials, and characteristics such as nanometric size, defects, coatings and media interaction influence on their scintillation properties [4].

Nanoscintillators can be basically divided in doped and semi-conductors scintillators. Lantanides are the most explored as doped scintillators due to their high density, high-Z, and significant intensity of luminescence, while semiconductor scintillators are mostly composed of porous Si, Si nanocrystals, ZnO, CdSe, CdS, PbS, and CuBr [4].

The efficiency of X-PDT is largely affected by the intensity of X-Ray luminescence, the singlet oxygen yield of the photosensitizer, and the way the photosensitizer is bound to the nanomaterial (either by covalent bonding, electrostatic interactions, or by pore loading). Furthermore, part of the tumor ablation might be due to the generation of UV photons during the scintillation process, apart from the photodynamic effect. The radiosensitization effect must also be considered, since high-Z materials generate ROS whenever their electrons are excited by X-rays into states above the conduction band edge, consequently producing electron hole pairs that interact with water producing hydroxyl radicals, and the electrons generate superoxide and peroxide radicals when they react with O_2. Those ROS increase the cytotoxicity of the materials under X-ray irradiation [4].

Nanoscale metal-organic frameworks (nMOFs) consist of the self-assembly of metal ions or clusters and bridging ligands, usually organic polydentate. These materials are used as a means to put scintillators and photosensitizers closer to each other, enhancing the singlet oxygen generation efficiency [4].

Nanosized MOFs are usually biodegradable, offering a significant advantage over other nanomaterials, depending on the desired application. They encompass a virtually infinite possibility of structures due to the large availability amount of organic linkers and metallic parts; however, it is of utmost importance to select the components in accordance with the desired application in order to optimize the results. In the medical field, the use of MOFs is still in the prelude, since more pharmacokinetic, pharmacodynamics and biological characterization studies must be performed so that these materials reach clinical trials [15].

Regarding the use of lanthanides as scintillators, Dou et al. synthesized UCNs (NaYF4:Yb,Tm) covalently conjugated with chlorin e6 to prevent the premature release of the photosensitizer and tested them *in vitro*. The nanoparticles were more efficient than the free photosensitizer even at low concentrations, and the efficacy can be fine-tuned by adjusting the dose of Ce6-UCNs and the laser power [7]. On the other hand, non-lanthanide materials such as SiC/SiOx core/shell nanowires functionalized with azide groups and porphyrin derivatives were tested for X-PDT and demonstrated significant efficacy. This material showed to be non-cytotoxic in the dark, and emits fluorescence at 545 nm when irradiated with X-rays, exciting the porphyrin derivative in the process [4].

Another example of experimental X-PDT was performed by Sivasubramanian et al. using BaFBr:Eu^{2+} nanoparticles loaded with porphyrins. When irradiated with 3 Gy of X-rays, the nanoparticles generated luminescence that matched the excitation wavelengths of the photosensitizer, leading to photodynamic effect that damaged the DNA, the mitochondria, and generated intense oxidative stress, significantly killing prostate cancer cells *in vitro* [16].

One of the main concerns about X-PDT is the radiation dose that needs to be applied to the patients. In order to diminish the amount of radiation that the patient must be exposed to, some scintillators that present persistent luminescence upon irradiation, rather than fluorescence, are the option. Fluorescence is a phenomenon that lasts for a few nanoseconds, while persistent luminescence can persist for minutes to hours after the excitation, therefore the required dose of radiation for excitation can be significantly decreased. There are evidences that persistent luminescence decreases the rate of oxygen consumption during PDT and may avoid the undesired hypoxia that hinders the photodynamic efficacy [4].

2.4 Recent advances in CR-PDT

Cherenkov radiation-driven PDT, symbolized in **Figure 4**, takes advantage of the fact that most radiopharmaceuticals accumulate in tumors in a selective manner, therefore the photodynamic ablation may occur in a more localized way. However, the generation of Cherenkov radiation occurs in low fluence rates, usually not enough to enable a good photodynamic efficiency [4].

There is a significant advantage, though, of CR-PDT over X-PDT, which is the possibility of targeting multiple metastases easier than with external X-rays.

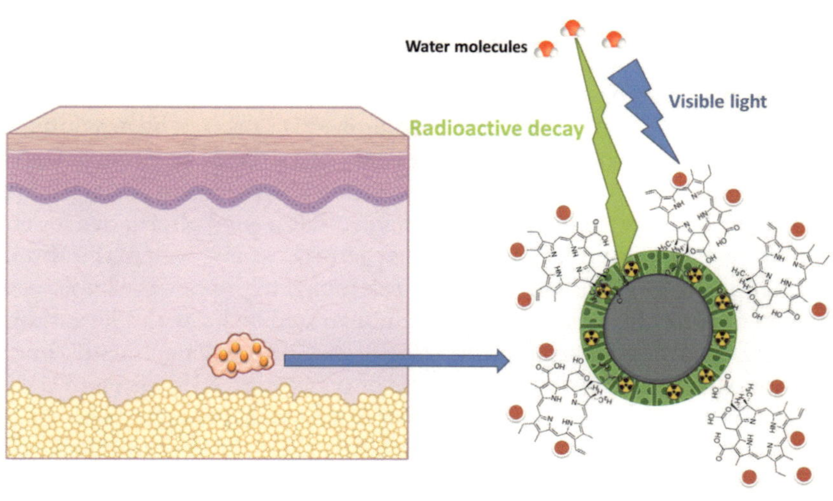

Figure 4.
Cherenkov radiation being generated after radionuclide decay, and its ability to excite photosensitizers in order to perform PDT. The red circles symbolize singlet oxygen.

Furthermore, even if the photons generated by the radionuclides are in much lower number than external irradiation (and possibly insufficient to exert significant phototoxicity), it is likely that the damage induced directly by the radionuclides contribute synergistically for the success of tumor ablation with CR-PDT [17].

An example of experimental CR-PDT was performed by Kamkaew et al. The authors encapsulated the radionuclide ^{89}Zr with chlorin e6 into a mesoporous silica nanoparticle. The zirconium Cherenkov radiation emission is mostly in the UV region, but there is a significant emission in the blue region around 400 nm, corresponding to one of the absorption peaks of chlorin e6. The results *in vitro* showed high levels of DNA damage when the photosensitizer is present compared to the radionuclide alone, while in vivo results showed complete tumor remission after 14 days, even with a sublethal radiation dose of 15 MBq. However, a significant amount of radioactive nanoparticles were found in the liver after 14 days, so strategies to avoid toxicity to health tissues must be applied [18].

Nevertheless, much progress is yet to be made before X-PDT and CR-PDT become official clinic protocols, despite all the successful results that have been obtained so far. The mechanisms of cell death by the combination of radiotherapy and PDT must be fully understood, and the materials used as scintillators must be fully characterized and optimized [4].

2.5 Hypoxia-reverting strategies

PDT efficacy in tumors is limited by the oxygen supply to the tumors, which tends to be reduced due to deteriorated microcirculation, especially in the tumor center. Since PDT consumes oxygen, it increases even further the local hypoxia, preventing the technique to reach its full potential. Therefore, some strategies to increase the availability of oxygen to the tumors while PDT is occurring have been developed in order to increase the tumor ablation [3]. Cheng and co-workers, for instance, loaded photosensitizers that are activated at 780 nm into perfluorocarbon nanodroplets enriched with oxygen with average size of 200 nm. The use of the nanodroplets also increases the half-life of singlet oxygen, so the PDT efficiency is enhanced both *in vitro* and *in vivo*. With intravenous administration, the tumors were significantly ablated, but with intratumor administration the tumors were eliminated completely [19].

It was observed by Kim et al. that O_2 can be efficiently produced via Fenton reaction in cancer tissues due to the abundancy of H_2O_2 derived from the tumor metabolism, especially when mesoporous silica nanoparticles are conjugated to manganese ferrite nanoparticles, which are classical Fenton catalysts, and loaded with chlorin e6. This system enabled a continuous PDT process by providing the tissue with the necessary amount of O_2 via Fenton reaction, and could act as a contrast agent for magnetic resonance imaging, acting as a theranostic material [20].

In this regard, cerium oxide nanoparticles provide a good alternative for converting hydrogen peroxide into molecular oxygen and water, even in the absence of light irradiation. They are, therefore, a smart strategy to provide the hypoxic tissues with oxygen to enhance PDT efficacy, as demonstrated by Jia et al. The authors used a mesoporous core-shell structure consisting of $NaGdF_4$:Yb,Tm@$NaGdF_4$ upconversion nanoparticles coated with CeO_x capable of converting NIR light into UV light, which activates cerium oxide to produce ROS. Since the nanoparticles have a hollow interior, they can also be used as a drug carrier for a combined chemotherapy, besides being very efficient in tumor ablation by PDT [21].

Although most of the oxygen-generating strategies make use of the excess of hydrogen peroxide caused by the intense metabolism of tumors, which can react with iron cations generating O_2 and hydroxyl radicals. There is a class of materials, however, that uses water as the source of oxygen, the so-called water-splitting materials, commonly used for solving energy and environmental problems. Since water is the major component of the organism, there is a virtually endless supply of oxygen to be used for PDT enhancement. Metal-free C_3N_4 decorated with carbon dots (in order to enhance the water-splitting upon irradiation with red light) was used by Zheng et al. as a water-splitting material. The nanocomposite was conjugated with the compound PpIx-PEG-RGD, consisting of the photosensitizer protoporphyrin IX with polyethylene glycol and the peptide sequence RGD (arginine, glycine, and asparagine) for active tumor targeting and photodynamic therapy. Under 630 nm irradiation, there was an increased O_2 concentration and singlet oxygen production, enabling a significant cell killing without the occurrence of hypoxia [22].

Red blood cells (RBCs) can be used as photosensitizer and oxygen carriers at the same time in order to increase the efficacy of PDT in hypoxic situations. Wang et al., for example, coupled the photosensitizer Rose Bengal and a hypoxic probe on the surface of RBCs. Upon low levels of oxygen, the hypoxic probe can switch to an active state and undergo an orthogonal near-infrared upconversion, resulting in the release of O_2 from the oxygenated hemoglobin when 980 nm light is applied. The photodynamic process is, thus, kept for longer and results in a better tumor ablation [3].

Oh the opposite side of the previous strategies, a protocol has been developed in order not to avoid the hypoxia in the tumors, but to use it to potentiate chemotherapy after PDT has been performed. This is possible with the use of hypoxia-activated prodrugs such as triapazamine or apaziquone. He and collaborators used nanoscale metal-organic frameworks (NMOFs) as porous nanocarriers of photosensitizers and hypoxia-activated chemotherapeutics. Both *in vitro* and in vivo results indicate an on-demand release behavior of the nanoparticles and an intense tumor ablation, therefore it consists on a promising antitumor strategy [23].

2.6 Tumor-targeting and specific delivery strategies for PDT using nanomaterials

One of the most common strategies of actively targeting specific organs or tissues is by the use of antibodies. Stuchinskaya and collaborators combined the versatility of gold nanoparticles with a hydrophobic photosensitizer (zinc phthalocyanine derivative), preventing its aggregation before reaching the target, and decorated the nanoparticle with tumor-specific antibodies (anti-HER2 for breast cancer) by covalent bonds formed with the coating layer of polyethylene glycol. There was a high efficiency in singlet oxygen generation in cancer cells after a selective targeting [24].

Active targeting can also make use of membrane proteins that are overexpressed in tumor cells, i.e. some integrins and neuropilin-1. By coupling ligands like RGD (a tripeptide composed of arginine, glycine, and aspartate), biotin, and folic acid to nanocarriers, the tumor accumulation is significantly enhanced [3]. Organelle targeting is also an option, especially when it comes to mitochondria. Several lines of evidence show that targeting the mitochondria for PDT avoids drug-resistance by tumor cells via a decreased level of intracellular ATP (the drug resistance phenotype in tumor cells is often associated with overexpressed ATP-driven transmembrane efflux pumps), besides the fact that damage to the mitochondria often leads to cell death [25]. Targeting the lysosomes can be additionally useful because the leakage of protons and hydrolases into the cytoplasm can damage inner structures and lead to cell death [3].

Another reason that makes organelle-targeting important is the short action range of singlet oxygen (no more than 20 nm), so a localized photosensitizer excitation is required. Hou et al. developed a Fe_3O_4@Dex-TPP nanoparticles that enhance the oxygen concentration in tumor cells via Fenton reaction, target the mitochondria (via the triphenylphosphine group, TPP), and are able to be imaged by magnetic resonance imaging due to the magnetic behavior of Fe_3O_4. This system was loaded with the photosensitizer protoporphyrin IX and grafted with a reduced glutathione-responsive moiety. Upon internalization, Fe^{2+} and Fe^{3+} ions are liberated from the Fe_3O_4 core and diffuse into the cytoplasm, then oxygen is produced by Fenton reaction (Fe^{2+} reacting with the excess of H_2O_2 producing O_2 and hydroxyl radical (•OH). This allows the PDT process to keep occurring, enhancing the therapeutic efficacy [25].

One of the strategies for specific delivery is the development of pH-sensitive materials that make use of the mild acidity environment found in tumors (around 6.5 to 7.2). Ai and co-workers developed upconversion nanoparticles with a low-pH insertion peptide that in acidic environments allow the insertion of the nanoparticles into the plasma membrane. They observed a large accumulation in the tumor tissue compared to healthy tissues [26].

Calcium phosphate is a biocompatible and biodegradable material, as it is the main component of hard tissues such as bones and teeth. It is sensitive to pH, maintaining its stable structure in physiological pH and dissolves in acidic environments, therefore it can be useful for controlled delivery to tumors. Another advantage relies on the fact that, once inside the cells, calcium phosphate nanoparticles dissolve and liberate calcium ions across lysosomal membranes, impairing the osmotic pressure of the cell and leading it to necrosis [27].

Liu et al. fabricated calcium phosphate-encapsulated core-shell structured nanoparticles (UCNPs-Ce6@SiO2@Calcium phosphate-Doxorubicin), characteristic for being biodegradable, biocompatible, pH-sensitive (which enables the liberation of the chemotherapeutic in the tissue), and provides therapeutic efficiency by PDT upon irradiation with 808 nm due to the presence of Chlorin e6 in its structure. Finally, due to the presence of rare earth elements, it can be used as an imaging tool for diagnostic purposes [27].

Another strategy is the development of nanomaterials that can be degraded by enzymes that are overexpressed in tumors, such as matrix metalloproteinases (MMPs) and hyaluronidase. One good example is the nanomaterial developed by Li et al. [28], which consisted of hyaluronic acid nanoparticles conjugated with chlorin e6 that disassemble in the presence of hyalurinodase and liberate the photosensitizer. This way, they can act as theranostic materials, meaning they can use as diagnostic tools and therapeutic agents. Another example was the MMP2-responsive chimeric peptide nanoparticles coupled with protoporphyrin-IX, which turn from a sphere into large fibers when MMP-2 is present, and this sphere-to-fiber transition contributes to the augmented tumor retention of the nanoparticles [29].

Dai et al. developed a peptide nanoparticle coupled with protoporphyrin-IX (PpIX-Ahx-K8(DMA)-PLGVR-PEG8) responsive to both pH and enzyme. This nanoparticle assumes a spherical shape while in circulation and avoids nonspecific uptake, and when in tumor environments they undergo a charge reversal and cleavage of the PLGVR sequence by MMP-2. Simultaneously, the DMA group is detached because of the low pH. This logic worked to enhance even more the specific uptake by tumor tissues [23].

A very intricate nanosystem combining tumor-targeted PDT with antiangiogenesis therapy and reduced glutathione (GSH) was developed by Min et al.. It consisted on a porphyrinic zirconium-metal-organic framework nanoparticle that can act simultaneously as a photosensitizer and a carrier of the vascular endothelial growth factor receptor 2 (VEGFR2) inhibitor apatinib. MnO2 covers the nanoparticle core in order to consume the intratumoral GSH, and the whole system is decorated with a camouflage made of a tumor cell membrane. The tumor specificity was much enhanced, and so was the ablative efficiency of the combined treatment provided by this nanomaterial [30].

In addition to the previous strategies, some researchers have developed nanoparticles that are activated by near-infrared light for selective photodynamic therapy, protecting healthy tissues like the skin. The mechanism of action of these systems is based on the blockage of photodynamic action from the photosensitizer by a co-loaded NIR dye via a fluorescence resonance energy transfer (FRET) effect. The photosensitizer action is recovered once the NIR dye is photobleached by NIR light irradiation in the specific site. Dong et al. developed $CaCO_3$-PDA-PEG hollow and porous nanoparticles loaded with chlorin e6 for this purpose, and observed that they are degraded in acidic environments such as tumors, liberating the photosensitizer in a selective manner. The generation of singlet oxygen was enhanced in the acidic environment, and the photosensitizer was taken up more efficiently when administered within the nanoparticles, compared to the free photosensitizer and other formulations. It is worthy to mention that when chlorin e6 is injected in a liposomal formulation, the mice present significant weight loss, probably due to an intrinsic toxicity, and this does not happen in the $CaCO_3$-PDA-PEG formulation [31].

Jeong et al. tested human serum albumin nanoparticles loaded with chlorin e6 in order to develop a more biocompatible system for enhanced PDT efficacy. The nanoparticles, with circa 88 nm in diameter, proved to be non-cytotoxic in the dark, but produced significant amounts of singlet oxygen upon irradiation with the appropriate wavelength. Remarkably, when injected in mice they provided a very specific tumor delivery compared with the free photosensitizer, and simultaneously provided a good imaging property die to the fluorescence of chlorin e6 [32].

PDT can be not only an adjuvant for chemotherapy, but also for immunotherapy, and nanotechnology can potentiate the results and enable the combination of the two therapies in one single approach. That is what was demonstrated by Xu et al. when they developed mesoporous silica nanoparticles made of amorphous silicon dioxide. The nanoparticles were relatively small (around 80 nm in diameter) in order to enhance the cell internalization and avoid side effects, and the pores were large (around 5–10 nm) in order to optimize the drug loading capacity. The nanoparticles were loaded with CpG oligodeoxynucleotide, which is a Toll-like receptor-9 agonist for immunotherapy, and chlorin e6. The authors observed an effective accumulation in tumors in vivo after intravenous injection, and the treatment induced cell damage and the recruitment of dendritic cells. With the immune response elicited, there was a strong cancer vaccination effect, therefore tumors in distant sites can also be affected by the treatment [21].

Finally, a novel phenomenon has been calling the attention of researchers, namely aggregation-induced emission (AIE) of photosensitizers. Some fluorophores are poor light emitters when they are in a single molecule state, but they become strong emitters when aggregated, enabling bioimaging with significant biocompatibility and photostability. Besides, they can generate singlet oxygen in the aggregated state, so they can act as efficient PDT agents. Liu and coworkers synthesized AIEsomes, which are lipid structures conjugated with compounds with AIE property, and tested their efficacy in vivo. Their compounds were biocompatible, provided efficient bioimaging and loading efficiency, ultimately leading to a significant photodynamic effect [33].

3. Conclusion

Photodynamic therapy has long proven to be an efficient way to eliminate tumors and control infections in a non-invasive way. PDT consists on the use of light-absorbent compounds named photosensitizers, which are able to excite O_2 from its ground triplet state to its excited singlet state, or to generate reactive oxygen species whenever they are irradiated with an appropriate wavelength. Much success has been achieved so far, and some PDT protocols are already available for the treatment of tumors, skin infections and for dentistry applications.

Nevertheless, the full clinic potential of PDT is yet to be achieved, mainly due to some limitations of the technique, i.e. the lack solubility of photosensitizers and limited stability in aqueous media such as the blood and the biological tissues (which makes the administration to patients somewhat difficult), the limited penetration of light, especially in the visible spectrum (limiting most of the applications to superficial sites), and the hypoxia that is usually present in tumor tissues, especially the center, and is increased during photodynamic action (since PDT is intrinsically dependent on oxygen, hypoxia hinders the full therapeutic potential of PDT).

Nanotechnology offers potential solutions to these limitations due to the intrinsic properties of nanomaterials, derived mainly from quantum effects that appear in matter in the nanometric scale, and from the surface chemistry that is often optimized in nanomaterials. Nanoparticles can act as photosensitizers given the necessary conditions, or can potentiate the photodynamic properties of attached photosensitizers. Additionally, nanocarriers can be loaded with hydrophobic photosensitizers, avoiding their aggregation and enhancing their specific accumulation in the target site. Finally, upconversion, scintillating and/or radiosensitizing nanomaterials enable the application of PDT in deep-seated tumors because they absorb wavelengths that reach deeper into the organism and emit visible light that can excite photosensitizers in the vicinity.

Nevertheless, some more studies must be performed in order to develop nanoplatforms that join the advantages of both Nanotechnology and Photodynamic Therapy, with good biocompatibility and with optimized clinical results. The potential, though, is strong for Nano-PDT to become various protocols for the most diverse medical applications.

Acknowledgements

The author would like to thank Fundação de Amparo à Pesquisa do Estado de São Paulo – FAPESP for all the financial support. Fapesp grant number 2018/15598-2.

Conflict of interest

The authors declare no conflict of interest.

Author details

Lucas F. de Freitas
Nuclear and Energy Research Institute – IPEN/CNEN, São Paulo – SP, Brazil

*Address all correspondence to: luk_freitas@yahoo.com.br

References

[1] Bechet D, Couleaud P, Frochot C, Viriot ML, Guillemin F, Barberi-Heyob M. Nanoparticles as vehicles for delivery of photodynamic therapy agents. Trends Biotechnol. 2008;26(11): 612-21.

[2] Camerin M, Magaraggia M, Soncin M, Jori G, Moreno M, Chambrier I, et al. The in vivo efficacy of phthalocyanine-nanoparticle conjugates for the photodynamic therapy of amelanotic melanoma. Eur J Cancer [Internet]. 2010;46(10):1910-8. Available from: http://dx.doi.org/10.1016/j.ejca.2010.02.037

[3] Dai X, Du T, Han K. Engineering Nanoparticles for Optimized Photodynamic Therapy. ACS Biomater Sci Eng. 2019;5(12):6342-54.

[4] Cline B, Delahunty I, Xie J. Nanoparticles to mediate X-ray-induced photodynamic therapy and Cherenkov radiation photodynamic therapy. Wiley Interdiscip Rev Nanomedicine Nanobiotechnology. 2019;11(2):1-18.

[5] Krajczewski J, Rucińska K, Townley HE, Kudelski A. Role of various nanoparticles in photodynamic therapy and detection methods of singlet oxygen. Photodiagnosis Photodyn Ther [Internet]. 2019;26(December 2018):162-78. Available from: https://doi.org/10.1016/j.pdpdt.2019.03.016

[6] Idris NM, Gnanasammandhan MK, Zhang J, Ho PC, Mahendran R, Zhang Y. In vivo photodynamic therapy using upconversion nanoparticles as remote-controlled nanotransducers. Nat Med. 2012;18(10):1580-5.

[7] Dou QQ, Teng CP, Ye E, Loh XJ. Effective near-infrared photodynamic therapy assisted by upconversion nanoparticles conjugated with photosensitizers. Int J Nanomedicine. 2015;10:419-32.

[8] Lucky SS, Soo KC, Zhang Y. Nanoparticles in photodynamic therapy. Chem Rev. 2015;115(4):1990-2042.

[9] Freitas LF, Hamblin MR, Anzengruber F, Perussi JR, Ribeiro AO, Martins VCA, et al. Zinc phthalocyanines attached to gold nanorods for simultaneous hyperthermic and photodynamic therapies against melanoma in vitro. J Photochem Photobiol B Biol [Internet]. 2017 Aug;173:181-6. Available from: https://linkinghub.elsevier.com/retrieve/pii/S101113441730283X

[10] Vankayala R, Kuo C-L, Sagadevan A, Chen P-H, Chiang C-S, Hwang KC. Morphology dependent photosensitization and formation of singlet oxygen (1Δg) by gold and silver nanoparticles and its application in cancer treatment. J Mater Chem B [Internet]. 2013;1(35):4379. Available from: http://xlink.rsc.org/?DOI=c3tb20806k

[11] Fales AM, Yuan H, Vo-Dinh T. Silica-Coated Gold Nanostars for Combined Surface-Enhanced Raman Scattering (SERS) Detection and Singlet-Oxygen Generation: A Potential Nanoplatform for Theranostics. Langmuir [Internet]. 2011 Oct 4;27(19):12186-90. Available from: https://pubs.acs.org/doi/10.1021/la202602q

[12] Yang Y, Hu Y, Du H, Ren L, Wang H. Colloidal plasmonic gold nanoparticles and gold nanorings: shape-dependent generation of singlet oxygen and their performance in enhanced photodynamic cancer therapy. Int J Nanomedicine [Internet]. 2018 Apr;Volume 13:2065-78. Available from: https://www.dovepress.com/colloidal-plasmonic-gold-nanoparticles-

and-gold-nanorings-shape-depend-peer-reviewed-article-IJN

[13] Ke X, Wang D, Chen C, Yang A, Han Y, Ren L, et al. Co-enhancement of fluorescence and singlet oxygen generation by silica-coated gold nanorods core-shell nanoparticle. Nanoscale Res Lett. 2014;9(1):1-8.

[14] Nagy-Simon T, Potara M, Craciun A-M, Licarete E, Astilean S. IR780-dye loaded gold nanoparticles as new near infrared activatable nanotheranostic agents for simultaneous photodynamic and photothermal therapy and intracellular tracking by surface enhanced resonant Raman scattering imaging. J Colloid Interface Sci [Internet]. 2018 May;517:239-50. Available from: https://linkinghub.elsevier.com/retrieve/pii/S0021979718301474

[15] Lismont M, Dreesen L, Wuttke S. Metal-Organic Framework Nanoparticles in Photodynamic Therapy: Current Status and Perspectives. Adv Funct Mater. 2017;27(14):1-16.

[16] Sivasubramanian M, Chuang YC, Lo LW. Evolution of nanoparticle-mediated photodynamic therapy: From superficial to deep-seated cancers. Molecules. 2019;24(3).

[17] Glaser AK, Zhang R, Andreozzi JM, Gladstone DJ, Pogue BW. Cherenkov radiation fluence estimates in tissue for molecular imaging and therapy applications. Phys Med Biol [Internet]. 2015 Sep 7;60(17):6701-18. Available from: https://iopscience.iop.org/article/10.1088/0031-9155/60/17/6701

[18] Kamkaew A, Cheng L, Goel S, Valdovinos HF, Barnhart TE, Liu Z, et al. Cerenkov Radiation Induced Photodynamic Therapy Using Chlorin e6-Loaded Hollow Mesoporous Silica Nanoparticles. ACS Appl Mater Interfaces [Internet]. 2016 Oct 12;8(40):26630-7. Available from: https://pubs.acs.org/doi/10.1021/acsami.6b10255

[19] Cheng Y, Cheng H, Jiang C, Qiu X, Wang K, Huan W, et al. Perfluorocarbon nanoparticles enhance reactive oxygen levels and tumour growth inhibition in photodynamic therapy. Nat Commun. 2015;6:6-13.

[20] Kim J, Cho HR, Jeon H, Kim D, Song C, Lee N, et al. Continuous O2-Evolving MnFe2O4 Nanoparticle-Anchored Mesoporous Silica Nanoparticles for Efficient Photodynamic Therapy in Hypoxic Cancer. J Am Chem Soc. 2017;139(32):10992-5.

[21] Jia T, Xu J, Dong S, He F, Zhong C, Yang G, et al. Mesoporous cerium oxide-coated upconversion nanoparticles for tumor-responsive chemo-photodynamic therapy and bioimaging. Chem Sci. 2019;10(37):8618-33.

[22] Zheng DW, Li B, Li CX, Fan JX, Lei Q, Li C, et al. Carbon-Dot-Decorated Carbon Nitride Nanoparticles for Enhanced Photodynamic Therapy against Hypoxic Tumor via Water Splitting. ACS Nano. 2016;10(9):8715-22.

[23] He Z, Dai Y, Li X, Guo D, Liu Y, Huang X, et al. Hybrid Nanomedicine Fabricated from Photosensitizer-Terminated Metal–Organic Framework Nanoparticles for Photodynamic Therapy and Hypoxia-Activated Cascade Chemotherapy. Small. 2019;15(4):1-11.

[24] Stuchinskaya T, Moreno M, Cook MJ, Edwards DR, Russell DA. Targeted photodynamic therapy of breast cancer cells using antibody-phthalocyanine-gold nanoparticle conjugates. Photochem Photobiol Sci. 2011;10(5):822-31.

[25] Hou H, Huang X, Wei G, Xu F, Wang Y, Zhou S. Fenton Reaction-Assisted Photodynamic Therapy for Cancer with Multifunctional Magnetic Nanoparticles. ACS Appl Mater Interfaces. 2019;11(33):29579-92.

[26] Ai F, Wang N, Zhang X, Sun T, Zhu Q, Kong W, et al. An upconversion nanoplatform with extracellular pH-driven tumor-targeting ability for improved photodynamic therapy. Nanoscale [Internet]. 2018;10(9):4432-41. Available from: http://xlink.rsc.org/?DOI=C7NR06874C

[27] Liu S, Li W, Dong S, Gai S, Dong Y, Yang D, et al. Degradable Calcium Phosphate-Coated Upconversion Nanoparticles for Highly Efficient Chemo-Photodynamic Therapy. ACS Appl Mater Interfaces. 2019;11(51):47659-70.

[28] Li F, Du Y, Liu J, Sun H, Wang J, Li R, et al. Responsive Assembly of Upconversion Nanoparticles for pH-Activated and Near-Infrared-Triggered Photodynamic Therapy of Deep Tumors. Adv Mater. 2018;30(35):1-7.

[29] Zhang Y, Vecchio D. Potentiation of antimicrobial photodynamic inactivation mediated by a cationic fullerene by added iodide: in vitro and in vivo studies. Nanomedicine. 2015;10:603-14.

[30] Min H, Wang J, Qi Y, Zhang Y, Han X, Xu Y, et al. Biomimetic Metal–Organic Framework Nanoparticles for Cooperative Combination of Antiangiogenesis and Photodynamic Therapy for Enhanced Efficacy. Adv Mater. 2019;31(15):1-11.

[31] Dong Z, Feng L, Hao Y, Chen M, Gao M, Chao Y, et al. Synthesis of Hollow Biomineralized CaCO3-Polydopamine Nanoparticles for Multimodal Imaging-Guided Cancer Photodynamic Therapy with Reduced Skin Photosensitivity. J Am Chem Soc. 2018;140(6):2165-78.

[32] Jeong H, Huh M, Lee SJ, Koo H, Kwon IC, Jeong SY, et al. Photosensitizer-Conjugated Human Serum Albumin Nanoparticles for Effective Photodynamic Therapy. Theranostics. 2012;1:230-9.

[33] Li Y, Wu Q, Kang M, Song N, Wang D, Tang BZ. Boosting the photodynamic therapy efficiency by using stimuli-responsive and AIE-featured nanoparticles. Biomaterials [Internet]. 2020;232(October 2019):119749. Available from: https://doi.org/10.1016/j.biomaterials.2019.119749

Chapter 13

Synergic Influence of Parameters Involved in the Polymeric Nanoparticle Preparation on the Efficacy of Photodynamic Therapy

Barbara Silva Figueiredo, Julyana Noval de Souza Ferreira, Vannyla Viktória Viana Vasconcelos, Priscila Ponate de Souza, Rafaela Vergna De Angeli and André Romero da Silva

Abstract

The challenge was always great for lipophilic photosensitizer use in the photodynamic therapy (PDT) for treatment of internal body diseases. Photosensitizer metabolism in liver, incompatibility of the molecules in the gastric acid, aggregation in the bloodstream, opsonization of molecules and phagocyting process hamper the application of the free lipophilic photosensitizer in disease treatment using PDT. This problem has been partially resolved using the drug delivery system to encapsulate the photosensitizer. Many studies have been reported using polymeric nanoparticles to encapsulate the lipophilic photosensitizer showing excellent results for PDT, but few nanoparticulate formulations are available at the pharmacies. The absence of deep knowledge about the influence of synergic effect of parameters used in the nanoparticle preparation on its properties, the photobleaching process of encapsulated photosensitizer and the molecule aggregation into the nanoparticle can decrease the photodynamic efficacy for the lipophilic photosensitizer. Our research group has studied the influence of many parameters on the nanoparticulate properties of several encapsulated phthalocyanines and porphyrin using factorial design, evaluating the free and encapsulated compound aggregation, efficacy to reduce the viability of cancer cells, the photooxidation of the biomolecules and the influence of photobleaching. This work shows the most important results to be consider in the optimization of the polymeric nanoparticle.

Keywords: polymeric nanoparticle, factorial design, phthalocyanine, porphyrin, photodynamic therapy, photooxidation, cancer cells, photobleaching

1. Introduction

Photodynamic therapy (PDT) is an important therapeutic modality used in the treatment of cancer and several non-malignant diseases, including infections and dental treatments [1–5]. It is characterized by the administration of a photosensitizer (PS), a light source to activate it and oxygen molecules (**Figure 1**) [6]. After administration of the photosensitizer, the diseased tissue is irradiated with

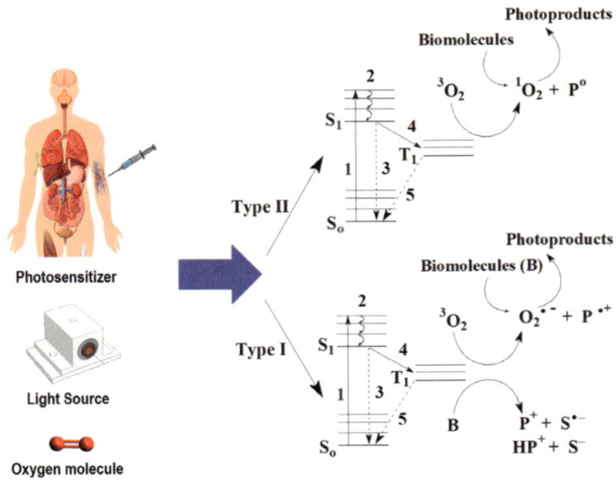

Figure 1.
PDT mechanism involving the combination of a photosensitizer, a light source and oxygen molecules. After excitation to a higher energy state (1), the photosensitizer may suffer rotovibrational decays to the excited state S_1 (2), from which the photosensitizer can suffer energy decay to the fundamental state S_0, via fluorescence (3), intersystem crossing (4) or phosphorescence (5).

visible light, causing the excitation of the PS to a singlet electronic state (S_1), which can be deactivated to the fundamental state (S_0) through radiative processes (fluorescence or phosphorescence) or non-radioactive (internal conversion, intersystem crossing or vibrational relaxation). Among these processes, intersystem crossing is essential for PDT. It consists of a prohibited transition by spin from the excited singlet electronic state (S_1) to the excited triplet state (T_1). In this state, the PS can interact with oxygen molecules or other biomolecules that are present in the irradiated tissue generating reactive oxygen species (ROS) that can cause damage to diseased tissues [7, 8]. These ROS can be generated by two mechanisms, [9] involving energy transfer (type II mechanism) or electron transfer (type I mechanism) (**Figure 1**).

The success of the treatment, fundamentally, depends on the photochemical, photobiological and pharmacokinetic properties of the photosensitizer. New porphyrin and phthalocyanine derivatives have been synthesized and encapsulated because their photochemical properties are suitable for PDT [10–12]. In general, hydrophobic photosensitizers tend to form aggregates in aqueous medium, affecting their bioavailability and their ability to generate reactive oxygen species, [13] and consequently, reducing their efficacy in treatment by PDT. In addition, lipophilic molecules hamper the administration of photosensitizer by parenteral via [14]. The nanocarrier systems has proven to be quite effective to solve this problem since they facilitate the administration of the hydrophobic photosensitizer, protect the photosensitizer from aggressive environments and decreasing its aggregation state [15].

Many studies show prominent results with polymeric nanoparticles as carriers of lipophilic photosensitizers due to the benefits associated with their application in PDT for cancer treatment [16–18] such as effectively increase in the amount of PS in the target tissue due to a greater volume/area ratio; prevent the premature release of the photosensitizer, avoiding its accumulation in healthy tissues; maintaining drug concentration at therapeutically appropriate intervals in blood circulation and tissues; greater ability to penetrate the target tissue due to its size; in addition to protecting drugs from liver inactivation and enzymatic degradation [15].

Another advantage of polymeric nanoparticles is their biocompatibility and biodegradability, once it is degraded by enzymatic processes that generates non-toxic and biocompatible products, being removed from the body by physiological pathways. An example is the nanoparticle of poly(lactide-co-glycolide) (PLGA), a polymer approved by the Food and Drug Administration (FDA) and that we used in our research [15]. However, it also be reported that the use of nanomaterials in contemporary clinical practice need to be monitored because of the unpredicted effects of the cumulative exposes of non-biodegradable nanoparticle in the human body [19].

Few nanoparticulate formulations are on the shelves of pharmacies due to the lack of knowledge of the combinatorial influence of the parameters used in the preparation of the nanoparticles on the fundamental properties for maximum therapeutic potential, [5] a fact that hampers the scale up process for the production of nanoparticulate formulations. Besides, the poor batch-to batch reproducibility to prepare polymeric nanoparticle, the low solubility of some polymers in water that requires the use of organic solvent to synthesize the nanoparticle, the low glass transition temperature of some polymers that limit the use of them to prepare the nanoparticulate formulation and the high cost of biodegradable polymers are drawback that hamper the development of nanoparticulate pharmaceutic formulation for using in PDT. For these reasons, we have studied the influence of the parameters involved in the preparation of polymeric nanoparticle loaded with several porphyrin and phthalocyanine derivatives (**Figures 2-4**) that have different physicochemical properties (**Table 1**).

Given these considerations, we present an overview of the main results obtained by our research group on the influence of several preparation parameters on the final properties of polymeric nanoparticles loaded with photosensitizers for

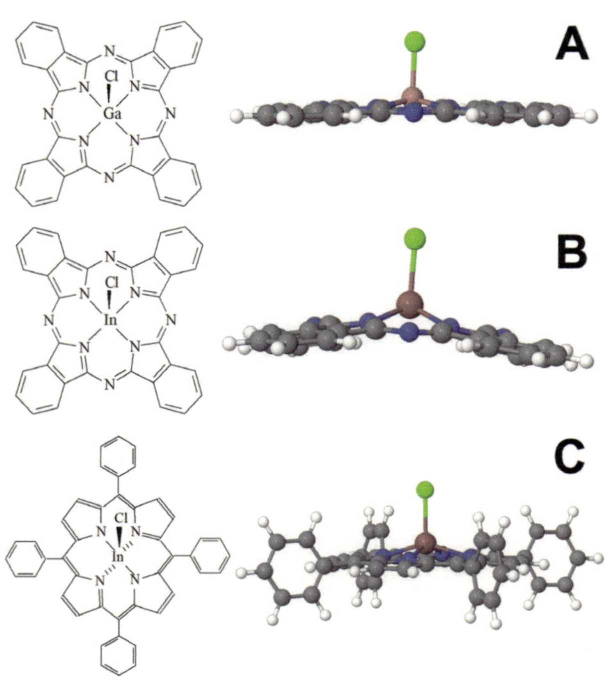

Figure 2.
Molecular structures optimized by Avogadro and MOPAC software for (A) gallium phthalocyanine chlorine (GaPc), (B) indium phthalocyanine chlorine (InPc) and (C) chloro(5,10,15,20-tetraphenylporphyrinato) indium (III) (InTPP).

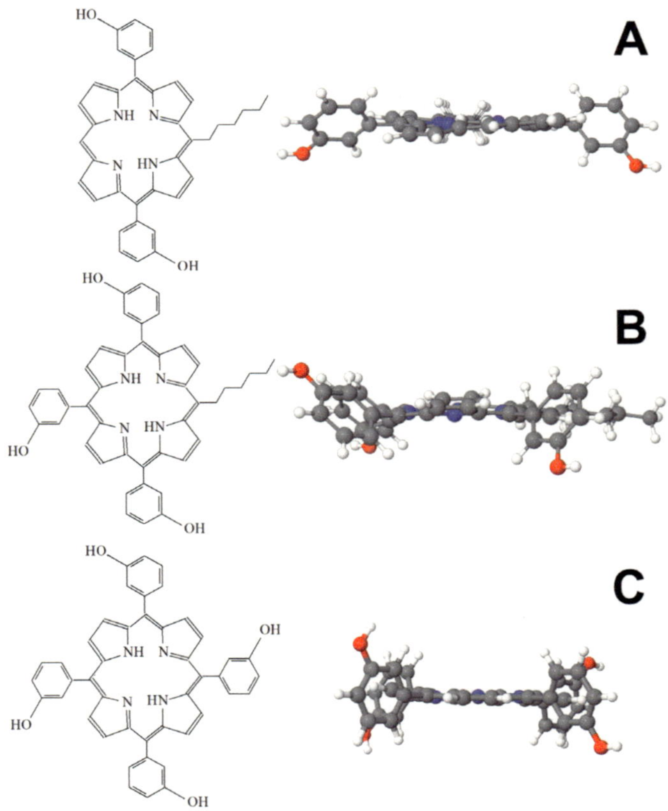

Figure 3.
Molecular structures optimized by Avogadro and MOPAC software for (A) 5-hexyl-10,20-bi(3-hydroxyphenyl) porphyrin (hex-m-bisHPP), (B) 5-hexyl-10,15,20-tri(3-hydroxyphenyl)porphyrin (hex-m-trisHPP) and (C) 5,10,15,20-tetra(3-hydroxyphenyl)porphyrin (m-THPP).

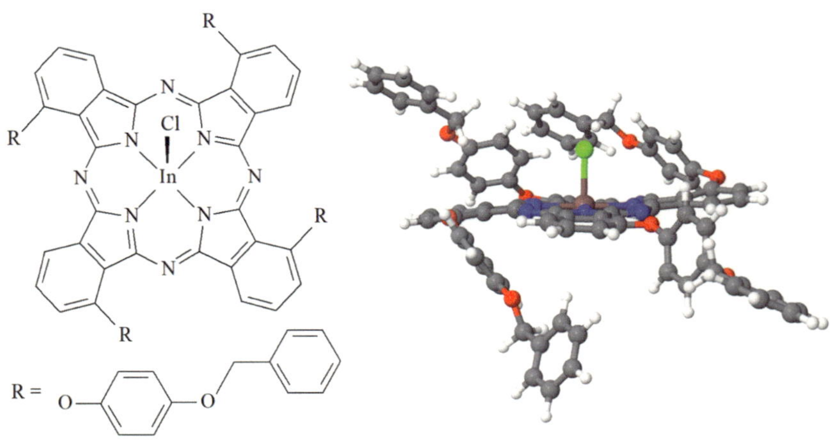

Figure 4.
Molecular structures optimized by Avogadro and MOPAC software for 1,4-(tetrakis[4-(benzyloxy)phenoxy] phthalocyaninato) indium(III) chloride (InTBPPc).

application in PDT, besides regarding the effect of encapsulation in reducing the photobleaching process of photosensitizer and on the efficiency of nanoparticles containing photosensitive compounds in reducing the viability of cancer cells or in biomolecules photooxidation.

Compound	GaPc	InPc	InTPP	m-THPP	Hex-m-BisHPP	Hex-m-TrisHPP	InTBPPc
Heat of Formation / kj/mol [$]	867.59016	866.26780	912.86350	418.11873	569.44802	412.25908	545.82102
Volume / Å^{3} [$]	596.57	606.78	782.35	781.06	691.12	799.51	1555.32
Ionization Potential / EV [$]	7.304876	7.272500	7.860061	8.012104	7.779898	7.811042	7.160890
Energy Difference HOMO-LUMO / EV [$]	4.862	4.903	5.965	6.185	5.969	6.106	4.922
Dipole Moment / D [$]	7.00151	7.40825	4.43138	3.91867	2.74405	1.76290	8.27066
Log P*	4.52	1.67	2.33	6.82	6.78	7.57	9.17
Log S*	−4.04	−4.59	−6.12	−5.23	−5.10	−5.33	−6.52
Polarizability**	66.75	67.90	90.90	87.68	75.43	87.05	157.27
HLB**	4.20	4.50	3.40	3.22	3.20	3.05	7.63

Values were calculated from ALOGPS 2.1 Program http://www.vcclab.org/lab/alogps/
**Values were calculated from MarvinSketch 20.16 Program.*
$ *Values were calculated from MOPAC 2016 Program.*

Table 1.
Physicochemical properties of the studied photosensitizers.

2. Influence of nanoparticles preparation parameters on their final properties

The development of carrier systems involves a lot of study of the variables used in the formulations preparation and their influences on the nanoparticulate properties that reflect on the cellular uptake of nanoparticles, its bioavailability and, consequently, the photodynamic efficiency. The approach to analyze the individual effect and the combinatorial effect (synergistic or antagonistic) of the parameters is usually done by factorial design of experiments, which all levels (experimental domains) of a factor are combined with all levels of the other factors of the experiment [16].

The influence of factors on the characteristics of nanoparticles is intrinsically linked to the production process [16, 20, 21]. Many works have shown the individual effects of some parameters involved in the nanoparticles preparation stage on their properties. However, the influence of a parameter used in a polymeric nanoparticles formulation will not always produce the same response for similar formulations [5].

There are significant challenges to consolidate polymeric nanoformulations in the pharmaceutical market since small changes in the composition of the formulation, for example, the encapsulated drug, can influence the nanoparticles properties, such as the particle size, the surface charge, the residual amount of emulsifier on the surface of the particles, and encapsulation and recovery efficiencies of the nanoparticles [5].

2.1 Size

The particle size used for the treatment of oncological and non-oncological diseases depends on the administration route and/or the type of diseased tissue. For example, in intravenous administration, the particles must be smaller than 5 μm in order to circulate through the capillaries, however, smaller sizes are necessary for nanoparticles reach the tumor vessels and remain longer in the blood stream [5, 8, 22].

Researches have shown that nanoparticles with sizes smaller than 200 nm have a longer circulation time in the bloodstream due to the reduction of the recognition of the nanoparticle by plasma proteins (opsonin) that signal the reticuloendothelial system to act in the phagocytosis process of the nanoparticles. Remaining longer in the circulatory system, smaller diameter particles could interact more effectively with cell membranes, presenting greater capacity of cellular internalization due to the overexpression of porous in tumor cells membranes, a fact that would result in greater efficiency of nanoparticulate photosensitizers in reducing cell viability through PDT [5, 8, 22].

A highly significant parameter in causing changes in the nanoparticles size was the stirring rate used in the preparation process. The increase of stirring rate leads to smaller sized nanoparticles due to the better dispersion of the organic phase in the aqueous phase, reducing the droplet size of the organic phase and, consequently, the nanoparticle size [20].

Although the stirring rate is considered the main factor responsible for the size reduction of the nanoparticle, in some formulations this parameter is not significant [23]. In the preparation of PLGA-PEG nanoparticles loaded with chloro(5,10,15,20-tetraphenylporphyranato) indium(III) (InTPP – **Figure 2C**), the ethanol percentage in the aqueous phase was the main parameter responsible for size decrease, not the stirring rate [20].

Our group demonstrated that the individual increasing in the ethanol percentage in the aqueous and organic phases contribute to reduce the nanoparticles size. The ethanol present in the aqueous phase causes an increase in viscosity while the addition of ethanol in the organic phase accelerates the separation of phases from the PLGA during the dispersion of the organic phase in the aqueous phase. These effects hinder the coalescence of organic droplets dispersed in the aqueous phase, preventing an increase in the nanoparticles size [16, 20].

Analyzing two preparation methods, the PLGA-PEG nanoparticles loaded with gallium phthalocyanine (GaPc - **Figure 2A**) prepared by the Emulsification-Diffusion Method (EDM) were smaller in size than the nanoparticles prepared by the Emulsification-Evaporation Method (EEM). In the EDM method, the organic solvent is dispersed in the aqueous phase generating droplets that are stabilized by colloidal stabilizing agents, however, the rapid efflux of solvent can cause the formation of aggregates and a population with varying sizes [5].

The aqueous phase temperature is another factor that can positively or negatively influence the nanoparticles size. The increase in temperature reduces the viscosity of the mixture between the organic phase and the aqueous phase, favoring the coalescence of organic solvent drops and consequently increasing the particles size, but the increase in temperature also favors the diffusion of the organic solvent into the aqueous phase, favoring the reduction of particle size. In the EDM method the effect of coalescence is more pronounced, causing the size increase, while in the EEM method the diffusion of the organic solvent to the aqueous phase is more pronounced, decreasing the nanoparticle size [5].

Combinatory effects of two parameters can also be significant for nanoparticle size. The binary effect between changing the method from EEM to EDM and increasing the aqueous phase temperature tends to increase the nanoparticles size [5]. Univariate methods do not allow to identify the combinatory effect that could be important for a determinate nanoparticulate property being necessary the use of factorial design.

The ratio between the photosensitizer mass and the polymer mass is also a parameter that can influence the nanoparticle size. In the study of the preparation of PLGA nanoparticles loaded with three porphyrins (Hex-m-bis-HPP, Hex-m-tris-HPP and m-THPP - **Figure 3A-C**, respectively) with different amphiphilicities, [16] the effect of the porphyrin/polymer mass ratio on the nanoparticle size was only significant in m-THPP nanoparticles, which the increase in the mass ratio caused a reduction in size. The low polymer concentration reduces the organic phase viscous resistance against the shear force during the emulsification process, favoring the reduction of the organic phase droplets size dispersed in the aqueous phase and, consequently, reducing the nanoparticles size [16].

Different results have also been reported in the literature, not observing any effect of the photosensitizer mass/polymer mass ratio on the PLGA nanoparticles size loaded with bupivacaine [24], while others have reported that an increase in the proportion decreased the nanoparticles size [25, 26].

Another parameter that can also influence the nanoparticles size is the polyvinyl alcohol (PVA) concentration, which is the most used emulsifier in formulations preparation stage. In some cases, the effect of increasing the PVA concentration on the particle size may be very similar to the effect of the stirring rate. It is known that PVA molecules anchor in the aqueous/organic interface formed during emulsification, causing a decrease in interfacial tension and favoring the mechanical and spatial stabilizations of the organic droplets dispersed in the aqueous phase [27]. In addition, polymeric PVA chains not anchored to the nanosphere surface can increase the aqueous phase viscosity. The reduction in interfacial tension and the increase in viscosity caused by PVA favor a decrease in the nanosphere size [20].

Emulsification time is a factor that may or may not be significant on size. In the preparation of PLGA-PEG nanoparticles containing gallium phthalocyanine, this parameter did not significantly influence the nanoparticles size [5], however some studies have already shown that it can increase or decrease the size [28]. As stated earlier, each parameter behaves in a particular way according to the parameters used in the preparation of nanoparticles. All these influences on size were summarized in **Figure 5**.

Besides the preparation parameters, the physicochemical properties of photosensitizers can also influence nanoparticles size. The polymeric PLGA-PEG nanoparticles loaded with GaPc or InTBPPc had different results for size distribution. The average diameter of the InTBPPc nanoparticles was 1.3 times greater than for nanoparticles with GaPc. According to the optimized structures designed by the molecular modeling program (**Figure 2A** and **4**), it was shown that InTBPPc has a volume of 1555.32 $Å^3$ (**Table 1**), that is 2.6 times greater than GaPc. This result suggests that the molecular size of the encapsulated phthalocyanine may influence the increase in the size distribution and the nanoparticles diameter [29].

The storage of lyophilized samples at certain temperatures is another factor that can influence the particles size. Studies were conducted with the PLGA-PEG nanoparticles loaded with GaPc (**Figure 6**) to evaluate the influence of the formulation storage at different temperatures on the nanoparticles size. The experiments were carried out with a formulation characterized by presenting 88.9% of the nanoparticles with a diameter smaller than 199.9 nm, an important outcome since particles smaller than 200 nm remain longer in the circulatory system [5]. The experiments suggest that the temperature of 20°C is more suitable for storage purposes of the formulations for 4 weeks, due to the results of less variation in the average diameter of the particles. Even considering the statistical variation of the measurements, there are changes in the PLGA-PEG nanoparticles size that may be associated with the aggregation of the particles during the storage period and the difficulty of disintegrating them during the process of redispersion in water. Such average size variations were greater for lower or higher temperatures than 20°C.

Similar analysis was performed with lyophilized formulations of PLGA-PEG nanoparticulate loaded with InTBPPc (**Figure 7**) for only 12 days at temperatures of 5°C and 35°C. Before the storage process, the formulation was characterized with a population of 98.9% of the particles with an average diameter smaller than 199.9 nm. In the short storage period, the generation of small and large aggregates

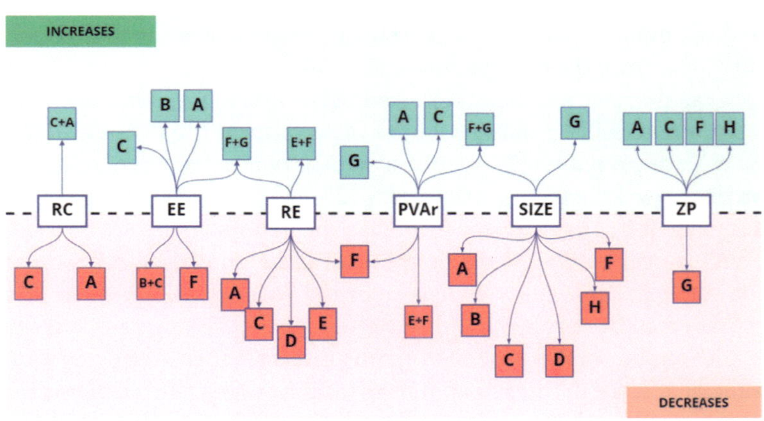

Figure 5.
Effects of some parameters involved in the nanoparticles preparation stage [(A) stirring rate, (B) PVA concentration, (C) ethanol concentration in the aqueous phase, (D) ethanol concentration in the organic phase, (E) emulsification time, (F) changing the preparation method from EEM to EDM, (G) aqueous phase temperature, (H) photosensitizer mass/polymer mass ratio] over different nanoparticulate properties [(RC) residual chloroform, (EE) entrapment efficiency, (RE) recovery efficiency, (PVAr) residual PVA, size, (ZP) zeta potential].

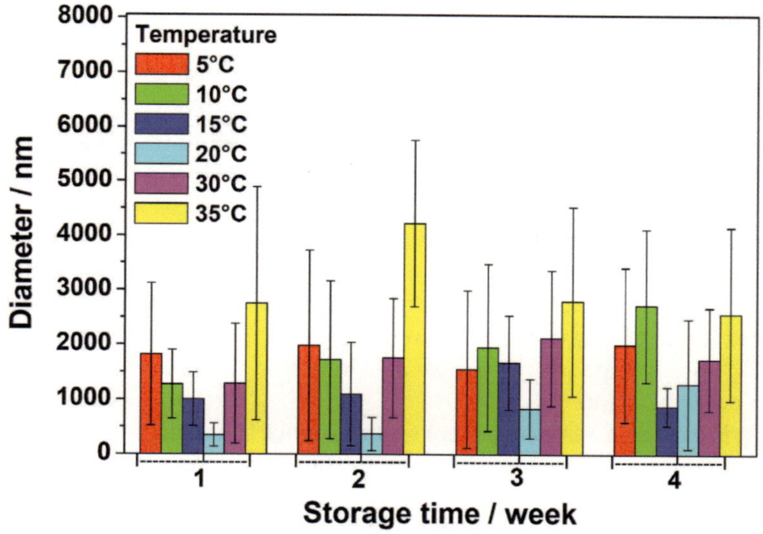

Figure 6.
Average diameter of the PLGA-PEG nanoparticle loaded with GaPc after storage for 1–4 weeks in different temperatures.

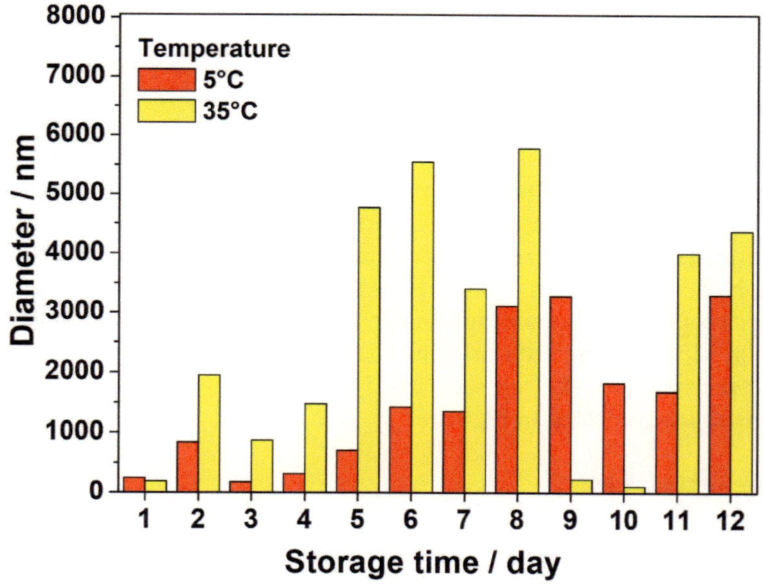

Figure 7.
Average diameter of the PLGA-PEG nanoparticle loaded with InTBPPc after storage for 12 days in different temperatures.

was observed at temperatures of 5°C and 35°C, with the size variation being greater for the temperature of 35°C in the first 8 days. This temperature is above the PLGA-PEG glass transition temperature (Tg at 30°C), [30] a fact that favors particle aggregation. Therefore, it can be concluded that storage temperatures, whether low or high, can influence the formation of aggregates, a fact that could reduce the photosensitizer efficiency during PDT.

2.2 Zeta potential

The zeta potential is a property related to the particles physical stability that can be used to measure the magnitude of the repulsion or attraction. The maximization of the repulsive forces between the nanoparticles, minimizes the interactions responsible for colloidal instability, consequently interfering in the photodynamic efficacy of an encapsulated photosensitizer [5, 20].

Nanoparticles coated with amphiphilic polymers, such as PEG, usually have a higher zeta potential due to the increase in the contact surface and, consequently, to the shielding of the nanoparticle surface charge [31–34]. Therefore, the greater surface area (ratio of surface area/volume) of the nanoparticle, the greater is the residual PVA percentage at the nanoparticle interface and, consequently, the greater is the zeta potential value [5].

Thus, it is expected the parameters that influence the nanoparticles size will also be significant on the zeta potential values. As the stirring rate is one of the main factors in causing the decrease of the nanoparticles size, it will also be expected that this factor is able to affect the zeta potential, increasing its value [20].

GaPc-loaded PLGA-PEG nanoparticles presented higher zeta potential values when prepared by EDM than those prepared by the EEM. This fact corroborates with the results obtained from the nanoparticle prepared by the EEM, which presented greater sizes and smaller values of zeta potential, suggesting that they are more stable from an electrostatic point of view [5].

The increase in the aqueous phase temperature also caused a significant decrease in the absolute value of the zeta potential, because this factor induced an increase in the nanoparticles size which have less residual PVA adsorbed on their surfaces, resulting in a smaller zeta potential [5].

In the preparation of PLGA nanoparticles containing three porphyrins (m-THPP, Hex-m-bisHPP and Hex-m-trisHPP) with different amphiphilicities, each formulation presented a different response of the preparation parameters related to the zeta potential, with results intrinsically linked to particle size. For Hex-m-bisHPP-loaded nanoparticles, the increase in the ethanol percentage in the aqueous phase caused an increase in the zeta potential due to the decrease of the nanoparticle size. While for nanoparticles containing m-THPP, the porphyrin/polymer mass ratio was the only significant factor that caused an increase in the zeta potential value since this factor decreased the particle size [16]. The summary of all influences on the zeta potential was indicated in **Figure 5**.

2.3 Entrapment efficiency

The entrapment efficiency relates the amount of drug that was effectively encapsulated/adsorbed on the nanoparticle. This property depends on the physicochemical properties and the interaction between the photosensitizer, the carrier matrix and the surrounding environment. Studies have shown that higher entrapment efficiency is associated with better photodynamic efficiencies for a short period of light activation [19, 35].

The diffusion process of the photosensitizer from the organic phase to the aqueous phase has significantly influenced the substance entrapment efficiency during the nanoparticle preparation process. Results have shown that the individual increase in the PVA concentration and the ethanol concentration in the aqueous phase tend to increase the photosensitizer encapsulation. The aqueous phase viscosity increases with the PVA and ethanol concentrations, which favors the formation of smaller sizes nanoparticles, having a specific surface area (area/volume) that allows a greater number of PVA molecules at the interface of the organic/aqueous phase. This hinders the diffusion of photosensitizers from the organic phase to the aqueous phase, favoring an increase in nanoparticle encapsulation. On the other hand, the combinatory effect caused by the simultaneous increase in the concentration of PVA and ethanol in the aqueous phase decreases the entrapment efficiency of InTPP in PLGA nanoparticles, as experiments showed that PVA and ethanol favor the solubilization of InTPP in aqueous medium [20].

When the method is changed from EEM to EDM, the entrapment efficiency decreases since the EDM method favors the formation of smaller diameter nanoparticles, facilitating the organic solvent diffusion into the aqueous phase and decreasing the entrapment efficiency of the photosensitizer in nanoparticles [5].

The increase of the aqueous phase temperature combine with the change in the preparation method also influences the photosensitizer entrapment efficiency. In the EEM method, the increase in the aqueous phase temperature causes the more effectively evaporation of the organic solvent, leading to fast polymer coacervation and, consequently, the organic/aqueous interface solidification. This increases the photosensitizer entrapment efficiency in the PLGA-PEG nanoparticles prepared by EEM. In the EDM method, the same increase in the aqueous phase temperature favors the solvent diffusion from the organic phase to the aqueous phase that carries the photosensitizer out of the nanoparticle, decreasing the entrapment efficiency [5]. All effects of parameters on entrapment efficiency were registered in **Figure 5**.

In addition to the parameters used in the nanoparticle preparation, the physicochemical properties of the photosensitizer may interfere on the entrapment efficiency. As an example, molecules of greater polarity tend to diffuse more easily from the organic phase to the aqueous phase, decreasing the entrapment efficiency [16]. The theoretical calculations compared to experimental results have suggested that photosensitizers with higher volume tend to be less efficiently encapsulated by nanoparticles. This was observed for InTBPPc molecules and also for Hex-m-TrisHPP molecules (**Table 1**). Molecules that have close volume values have shown similar entrapment efficiency as GaPc and InPc (**Figure 2A**, **B**, respectively).

2.4 Recovery efficiency

The recovery efficiency calculates the percentage of nanoparticle that has been produced and recovered. It is a property that has economic importance and has great value for the pharmaceutical industries, since they aim to reduce the production costs of the nanoparticulate formulation.

The nanoparticles size influences directly the recovery efficiency. Smaller nanoparticles are expected to be less recovered during the washing step than larger nanoparticles since the sedimentation rate of the particles in a centrifugal field is proportional to the square particle diameter. Thus, the parameters that influence the nanoparticles size tend to influence the recovery efficiency [20].

Parameters that cause a reduction in size, such as stirring rate, the EDM preparation method, the ethanol concentration in the aqueous or organic phase, as well as the emulsification time can favor the decrease of the recovery efficiency [5, 20].

Synergistic effects can be significant for recovery efficiency. For example, increasing the aqueous phase temperature together with the change in the preparation method, or increasing the emulsification time together with the change from the EEM method to EDM, can increase the recovery efficiency [5]. All effects of the parameters used to prepare of nanoparticles on the recovery efficiency are shown in **Figure 5**.

2.5 Residual polyvinyl alcohol (PVA)

PVA is the emulsifier most commonly used in the polymeric nanoparticles preparation. Even with the washing steps during the process, aiming to reduce the excess of PVA, an amount of these molecules remains adsorbed to the nanoparticle polymeric matrix due to the orientation of the PVA hydrophobic part in the organic phase, keeping molecules attach on the surface of the particle after the coacervation process [31]. This residual PVA on the particles surface can interfere on the nanoparticles physicochemical and biological properties, such as the size, release profiles of encapsulated drugs and intracellular uptake of the nanoparticles.

PVA tends to be adsorbed on the nanoparticle surface through the hydrophobic part of vinyl acetate, which tends to anchor the polymer in the aqueous/organic interface formed during the emulsification process. Smaller sized particles have a greater specific surface area, so it requires a greater amount of PVA to stabilize the emulsion droplets. Thus, these nanoparticles retain a greater amount of PVA adsorbed on its surface. Therefore, parameters that influenced the particle size, tend to affect the percentage of residual PVA [5, 16, 20, 22].

As the ethanol in the aqueous phase and the stirring rate favor the preparation of smaller nanoparticles, it is expected a higher amount of residual PVA on the small nanoparticle surface. However, the relation between the nanoparticles size and residual PVA is not immutable. An example is the PLGA-PEG nanoparticles containing gallium phthalocyanine [20]. It was reported that the aqueous phase temperature increased the nanoparticles size and the residual PVA while the change in the preparation method from EEM to EDM decreased the nanoparticles size and the residual PVA. Therefore, a different situation that it was expected. Probably, the presence of PEG linked to PLGA hindered the interactions of PVA molecules with the organic/aqueous interface [20].

Residual PVA can also be influenced by synergistic effects. For example, changing the preparation method from EEM to EDM, associated with an increase in the aqueous phase temperature can cause an increase in the residual PVA. However, the increase of the emulsification time together with the change of the preparation method can reduce the residual PVA [5]. All influences of the parameters used in the preparation of polymeric nanoparticle were summarized in the **Figure 5**.

It should be noted that the residual PVA values can still vary according to the number of washing steps and the method used to wash the nanoparticle suspension [5, 22].

2.6 Residual chloroform

The organic solvent can be retained by nanoparticles during the preparation of the nanoparticulate formulation, becoming a residual organic impurity. Therefore, the quantification of solvent residual is necessary to eliminate toxicological risks for patients. According to the American Pharmacopeia, the residual chloroform limit is 60 ppm for pharmaceutical formulations. Thus, it is very important to evaluate the influence of the factors involved in the nanoparticle preparation on the residual chloroform concentration [20].

The percentage of residual chloroform, as described for other properties, is also related to the nanoparticle size. Thus, there is a tendency to reduce residual chloroform linked to the reduction in the nanoparticles size.

In the preparation of PLGA-PEG nanoparticles containing chloro(5,10,15,20-tetraphenylporphyranato) indium(III) (InTPP - **Figure 2C**), the influence of four parameters on the residual chloroform percentage was studied: PVA concentration, stirring rate, ethanol percentage in the aqueous phase and in the organic phase [20].

The stirring rate and the ethanol percentage in the aqueous phase were the factors that significantly influenced the residual solvent, favoring the decrease of residual chloroform. The increase in the stirring rate favors the organic phase dispersion into the aqueous phase, generating small organic droplets that favor the fast solvent diffusion into the aqueous phase. On the other hand, ethanol in the aqueous phase hinders the coalescence of organic droplets dispersed in the aqueous phase, favoring the formation of smaller diameter particles [20].

Although the individual effects of ethanol in the aqueous phase and the increase in stirring rate cause a decrease in residual chloroform, the synergistic effect of the simultaneous increase of these factors caused an increase in residual chloroform. Both factors favored the decrease in the nanoparticles size. Small size nanoparticles tend to present a higher residual PVA percentage on the particles surface, which makes difficult the solvent diffusion from organic droplets into the aqueous phase. This diffusion becomes even more difficult after the solidification of the polymeric matrix surface layer during the process of evaporation of the organic solvent, favoring the residual increase of chloroform in the nanoparticles [20]. All influences on residual chloroform have been reported in **Figure 5**.

3. Photobleaching

Experimental results have shown that the photobleaching process can hinder the photodynamic efficiency of photosensitive compounds [36, 37]. Photodegradation of photosensitizers can reduce the concentration of these photoactive compounds in diseased tissue, decreasing the efficacy of PDT to reduce cell viability, leading to an incomplete treatment. On the other hand, photobleaching can reduce the photosensitivity of healthy tissues after irradiation due to the lower amount of reactive oxygen species generated in the photodynamic process motivated by the destruction of photosensitizer molecules. Considering that phthalocyanines are photosensitizers that tend to suffer photobleaching, [37] as well as to aggregate in aqueous medium, our group evaluated the ability of polymeric nanoparticles to reduce the aggregation of these lipophilic molecules and also the effect of photobleaching [29].

The laser power and the concentration of free phthalocyanine significantly influenced the photobleaching for concentrations in which the molecule is in the monomeric state since the photosensitizer aggregation state tends to decrease the photobleaching process due to the difficulty to produce reactive oxygen species [29].

Works have shown that the encapsulation of photosensitizers decrease the effect of photobleaching in phthalocyanines when compared to free molecules due to the scattering of light caused by the polymeric matrix [5, 7, 8, 29]. More soluble photosensitizers tend to be more susceptible to suffer photobleaching and even encapsulated can be photodegraded according to the laser power and irradiation dose used, limiting its ability to be used as a good photosensitizer in photodynamic therapy [29]. The short storage period at several temperatures did not cause significant influence in the photobleaching behave of the encapsulated phthalocyanines, probably due to the aggregation process of the particles (**Figures 6**, 7) (results not showed).

4. Photooxidation

Phthalocyanines are a class of compounds used as photosensitizers due to their chemical, electronic and spectroscopic properties, [38, 39] in particular, due to the intense absorption of these compounds in the therapeutic window and their ability to generate singlet oxygen in the presence of a light source.

Researchers have shown that the presence of heavy atom in the phthalocyanine structure favors the generation of singlet oxygen due to the increase in spin-orbital coupling and, consequently, the transition of the photosensitizer from an excited singlet state to a triplet state (intersystem crossing) [40–42]. In addition, the literature suggests that photooxidative mechanisms for singlet oxygen are usually more efficient due to their greater diffusibility and higher reaction rate constants with substrates [43, 44]. However, the metallophthalocyanines present limited solubility in certain solvents due to the symmetry of molecular structure, hamper their application in PDT [29].

The chemical structure of phthalocyanines has been modified by introducing substitutes in the peripheral or non-peripheral positions of the phthalocyanine nucleus to reduce the molecule symmetry and consequently increase the polarity and solubility of the phthalocyanines [41, 42]. Besides, studies show that encapsulation improves the photodynamic efficiency of the photosensitizer, as well as decreases side effects such as photosensitivity of the skin after photodynamic treatment, and reduces molecular aggregation compared to phthalocyanines dissolved in aqueous medium [5, 7, 8, 29, 45].

We have studied the photodynamic efficiency of different porphyrins and phthalocyanines encapsulated in polymeric nanoparticles (**Figures 2-4**). As an example, gallium phthalocyanine (GaPc - **Figure 2A**) and 1,4-(tetrakis[4-(benzyloxy) phenoxy] phthalocyaninato) indium(III) chloride (InTBPPc - **Figure 4**) are convenient photosensitizers for PDT. These compounds have high singlet oxygen (0.41 and 0.94, respectively) and triplet (0.69 and 0.97, respectively) quantum yield. However, InTBPPc has more interesting features for use in PDT [29].

The photooxidation of simple molecules (as dimethylanthracene (DMA) and tryptophan (Trp)) was used to evaluate the photodynamic efficiency of each free and encapsulated phthalocyanines. It is notable that the asymmetry caused by (benzyloxy)phenoxy group in phthalocyanine seems to increase the photodegradation of InTBPPc, due to the greater solubility of the photosensitizer which favors the reduction of its aggregation state. The decrease in the aggregation state favors the generation of singlet oxygen and consequently, the efficacy of the free photosensitizer in photooxidizing simple molecules such as DMA and Trp, as well as the phthalocyanine photobleaching [29]. Therefore, free InTBPPc was more efficient than free GaPc in photooxidate DMA and Trp molecules, due to its lower aggregation state and the higher capacity of free InTBPPc to generate singlet oxygen. However, the encapsulated GaPc proved to be more efficient than the encapsulated InTBPPc in photooxidate the Trp molecules, corroborating that the encapsulation can enhance the photosensitizer photocytotoxicity and reduce the aggregation state of the free photosensitizer [29].

We have demonstrated that the photocytotoxicity of encapsulated photosensitizers depends on the incubation time, the photosensitizer concentration and the laser power [5, 7, 8, 16, 29]. However, these observations cannot be considered a fact for all free or encapsulated photosensitizers due to their solubility characteristics, their states of aggregation and the influences of the parameters used in the nanoparticles preparation on the nanoparticulate properties. For example, the aggregation state of free InPc decreases the photodynamic efficiency of this photosensitizer, so that the viability of tumor cells is not altered by increasing the concentration and laser power [7].

We have observed that each nanoparticulate formulation should be treated in a particular way, taking care to do generalizations about certain conclusions as susceptible to be applied to all formations. An example was the result observed with InTBPPc, the encapsulation process did not increase its efficiency in the photooxidation process of Trp due to the photobleaching process suffered by the photosensitizer [29]. In general, the encapsulation process of photosensitizers has not created barriers for the singlet oxygen generation, and has increased the uptake of photosensitizer into the cancer cells, improving the efficiency of the phthalocyanines and porphyrins to reduce the viability of cancer cells [7, 8, 16].

It was also shown that the photocytotoxic activity of nanoparticles loaded with porphyrins did not depend on the different amphiphilic characteristics of the compounds, probably due to the encapsulation process [16]. Even the similarities in photodynamic efficacy are related to the degree of similarity in the internalization of each encapsulated photosensitizer inside tumor cells [16].

5. Future perspectives and challenges

The greatest challenge when it comes to oncology is prepared drugs with high specificity to promote the death of malignant cells without harming healthy ones. PDT has been used with successful to treat several cases of cancer with a lesser side effects than those treated by conventional chemotherapy. New photosensitizers have been synthesized to increase the photodynamic efficiency on the disease tissues and to facilitate the photosensitizer administration during the treatment. However, the hydrophobicity of new compounds should not limit their use in PDT. The use of nanoparticles as carrier has motivated the research in PDT since results had showed very promising advances in reducing the viability of the cancer cells due to the specificity achieved by the targeted or magnetic drug delivery system and due to the increase of the bioavailability of the nanoparticle. But the synthetic control is a very challenger for preparing a targeted polymeric nanoparticle in order to maintain the reproducibility of the nanoparticulate properties and its efficiency in the cancer treatment. Thus, there is much to be studied about the synthetic particularities of the polymeric nanoparticulate formulation for greater clinical application in the cancer treatment by PDT. In this sense, the development of nanoparticulate systems consistently involves a lot of work to study the several variables and its synergistic or antagonistic combinations that influence the properties of nanoparticulate formulations. Besides, the decrease of the entrapment efficiency of the photosensitizer associated to decrease of the nanoparticle size, the influence of combinatory effect of the photobleaching of encapsulated photosensitizer and the aggregation state of the compound into the nanoparticle, the establishment of adequate loading of photosensitizer into the nanoparticle and the uptake of the polymeric nanoparticle into the disease cells should be considered to development nanoparticulate formulation with high photodynamic efficiency to reduce the viability of the cancer cells.

6. Conclusions

In this chapter we demonstrate the most significant parameters in decreasing the nanoparticles size were the increase in stirring rate and PVA concentration. Other factors that also reduced the particles size were the increase in the ethanol percentage in the aqueous phase and in the organic phase, and the increase in the photosensitizer mass/polymer mass ratio. Nanoparticles prepared by the EDM showed smaller sizes than the nanoparticles prepared by the EEM but are less stable. The aqueous phase temperature showed double behavior in relation to the nanoparticles size, increasing or decreasing the size depending on the method used to prepare the nanoparticle. The other properties evaluated, such as zeta potential, entrapment and recovery efficiencies, residual PVA and residual chloroform, are dependent on the size of the nanoparticle. Therefore, parameters that are significant in relation to size will also influence these properties. Properties as zeta potential, residual PVA and entrapment efficiency presented an inversely proportional relation with nanoparticle size while the recovery efficiency and residual chloroform were directly proportional. In most of the properties some significant binary effects were observed, but their influence was not predominant in the results.

Besides the parameters used in the nanoparticle preparation, the physicochemical properties of the photosensitizer can interfere on the entrapment efficiency, as well as the washing step of the nanoparticulate formulation can influence the residual PVA and the recovery efficiency. The short storage period of the nanoparticulate formulation can affect the characteristics of the particle, favoring the nanoparticle aggregation in different temperature.

We have shown that the encapsulation of photosensitizers reduces the photobleaching effect due to light scattering caused by the polymeric matrix, however more soluble photosensitizers even encapsulated can suffer photobleaching according to the laser power and irradiation dose used in the experiment, limiting their ability to be used in PDT. The aggregation of the photosensitizer also causes a reduction in its photodynamic efficiency because it reduces the singlet oxygen generation, but the encapsulation improves the photosensitizer efficiency since the entrapment can reduce the aggregation of the lipophilic compounds in aqueous medium.

The photocytotoxicity of encapsulated photosensitizers depends on the incubation time, the photosensitizer concentration and the laser power, as well as the uptake of photosensitizer into the cancer cells. Drug delivery systems have improving the efficiency of the phthalocyanines and porphyrins to reduce the cell viability. However, the generalization of the conclusions about preparation of nanoparticulate formulations and photooxidation conditions should be done carefully, each nanoparticulate formulation behaves in a characteristic way and should be treated singularly.

Acknowledgements

We thank the Conselho Nacional de Desenvolvimento Científico e Tecnológico (CNPq) (800,304/2012-8, 800,470/2013-3, 800,708/2014-8), the Foundation for Research and Innovation Support of Espírito Santo (FAPES) (54,623,804/11, 0945/2015, 0388/2016) and the Federal Institute of Espírito Santo for financial support of the scientific initiation grants. We also thank the access to equipment and assistance provided by the National Institute of Science and Technology on Photonics Applied to Cell Biology (INFABIC) at the State University of Campinas for the confocal microscopy analysis. INFABIC is co-funded by Fundação de Amparo a Pesquisa do Estado de São Paulo (FAPESP) (2014/50938-8) and Conselho Nacional de Desenvolvimento Científico e Tecnológico (CNPq) (465,699/2014-6).

We also thank the Prof. Tebello Nyokong from Rhodes University (South Africa), the Prof. Mahmut Durmus from Gebze Technical University (Turkey) and Prof. Mathias O. Senge from Trinity College Dublin (Ireland) for providing samples of the new synthesized photosensitizers so that our group could carry out some of the works cited in the text.

Author details

Barbara Silva Figueiredo[1], Julyana Noval de Souza Ferreira[1], Vannyla Viktória Viana Vasconcelos[1], Priscila Ponate de Souza[2], Rafaela Vergna De Angeli[2] and André Romero da Silva[2]*

1 Federal University of Espírito Santo, Health Sciences Center, PostGraduate Program in Biochemistry and Pharmacology, Vitória-ES, Brazil

2 Federal Institute of Espírito Santo, Department of Chemistry, Aracruz-ES, Brazil

*Address all correspondence to: aromero@ifes.edu.br

References

[1] Zhang C, Chen W, Zhang T, Jiang X, Hu Y. Hybrid nanoparticle composite applied to photodynamic therapy: strategies and applications. J Mater Chem B. 2020;8:4726-4737. DOI: 10.1039/d0tb00093k

[2] Cheng G, Li B. Nanoparticle-based photodynamic therapy: news trends in wound healing applications. Materials Today Advances 2020;6:100049. DOI: 10.1016/j.mtadv.2019.100049

[3] De Freitas LM, Calixto GMF, Chorilli M, Giusti JSM, Bagnato VS, Soukos NS, Amiji MM, Fontana CR. Polymeric nanoparticle-based photodynamic therapy for chronic periodontitis in vivo. Int J Mol Sci. 2016;17. DOI: 10.3390/ijms17050769

[4] Xu C, Akakuru OU, Ma XH, Zheng JP, Zheng JJ, Wu AG. Nanoparticle-based wound dressing: recent progress in the detection and therapy of bacterial infections. Bioconjugate Chem. 2020;31(7):1708-1723. DOI: 10.1021/acs.bioconjchem.0c00297

[5] Lorenzoni D, Souto CAZ, Araujo MB, Berger CS, Da Silva LCD, Baratti MO, Ribeiro JN, Endringer DC, Guimarães MCC, Da Silva AR. PLGA-PEG nanoparticles containing gallium phthalocyanine: Preparation, optimization and analysis of its photodynamic efficiency on red blood cell and Hepa-1C1C7. J Photochem Photobiol B Biol. 2019;198. DOI: 10.1016/j.jphotobiol.2019.111582

[6] Abrahamse H, Hamblin MR. New photosensitizers for photodynamic therapy. Biochem J. 2016;473(4):347-64. DOI: 10.1042/BJ20150942

[7] Souto CAZ, Madeira KP, Rettori D, Baratti MO, Rangel LBA, Razzo D, Da Silva AR. Improved photodynamic action of nanoparticles loaded with indium (III) phthalocyanine on MCF-7 breast cancer cells. J Nanoparticle Res. 2013;15(9). DOI: 10.1007/s11051-013-1879-8

[8] Da Silva AR, Inada NM, Rettori D, Baratti MO, Vercesi AE, Jorge RA. In vitro photodynamicactivityofchloro(5,10,15,20-tetraphenylporphyrinato)indium(III) loaded-poly(lactide-co-glycolide) nanoparticles in LNCaP prostate tumour cells. J Photochem Photobiol B Biol. 2009;94(2):101-12. DOI: 10.1016/j.jphotobiol.2008.10.010

[9] Da Silva AR, Ribeiro JN, Rettori D, Jorge RA. Type II photooxidation mechanism of biomolecules using chloro(5,10,15,20-tetraphenylporphyrinato)indium(III) as a photosensitizer. J Braz Chem Soc. 2008;19(7):1311-20. DOI: 10.1590/s0103-50532008000700013

[10] Zheng YL, Li ZY, Chen HJ, Gao Y. Nanoparticle-based drug delivery systems for controllable photodynamic cancer therapy. Eur J Pharm Sci. 2020;144. DOI: 10.1016/j.ejps.2020.105213

[11] Syuleyman M, Angelov I, Mitrev Y, Durmus M, Mantareva V. Cationic amino acids linked to Zn(II) phthalocyanines for photodynamic therapy: synthesis and effects on physicochemical properties. J Photochem Photobiol A Chem. 2020;396. DOI: 10.1016/j.jphotochem.2020.112555

[12] Zhdanova KA, Savelyeva IO, Ignatova AA, Gradova MA, Gradov OV, Lobanov AV, Feofanov AV, Mironov AF, Bragina NA. Synthesis and photodynamic antimicrobial activity of amphiphilic meso-arylporphyrins with pyridyl moieties. Dyes and Pigments. 2020;181. DOI: 10.1016/j.dyepig.2020.108561

[13] Vara J, Gualdesi MS, Bertolotti SG, Ortiz CS. Two phenothiazine dyes as photosensitizers for the production of singlet oxygen. Photophysics,

photochemistry and effects of aggregation. J Mol Struct. 2019;1181:1-7. DOI: https://doi.org/10.1016/j.molstruc.2018.12.078.

[14] Koberlik M, Madiyalakan R, Woo T, Haddadi A. Antitumor efficacy of photodynamic therapy using novel nanoformulations of hypocrellin photosensitizer SL052. Photochem. Photobiol. 2012;88:188-193. DOI: 10.1111/j.1751-1097.2011.01035.x

[15] Lucky SS, Soo KC, Zhang Y. Nanoparticles in photodynamic therapy. Chem Rev. 2015;115(4):1990-2042. DOI: 10.1021/cr5004198

[16] Da Silva AR, Da Silveira JM, Senge MO, Jorge RA. Effects of preparation conditions of poly(lactide-co-glycolide) nanoparticles loaded with amphiphilic porphyrins and their photoactivities. J Nanosci Nanotechnol. 2014;14(8):6274-6286. DOI: 10.1166/jnn.2014.8855

[17] Xiao SH, Chen XQ, Ye QH, Chen KZ, Xiao WL, Guan XQ, Huang BC, Liu GW, Wei H, Peng YR. Prop-2-ynyloxybenzyloxy substituted phthalocyanine-based polymeric nanoparticles: synthesis, photophysical properties andin vitroPDT efficacy. J Coord Chem. 2020;73(8):1232-1244. DOI: 10.1080/00958972.2020.1766683

[18] Kim D, Byun J, Park J, Lee Y, Shim G, Oh YK. Biomimetic polymeric nanoparticle-based photodynamic immunotherapy and protection against tumor rechallenge. Biomater Sci 2020;8:1106-1116. DOI: 10.1039/c9bm01704f

[19] Kendall M, Lynch I. Long-term monitoring for nanomedicine implants and drugs. Nature Nanotechnol. 2016;11(3):206-10. DOI: 10.1038/nnano.2015.341

[20] Da Silva AR, De Oliveira AM, Augusto F, Jorge RA. Effects of preparation conditions on the characteristics of poly(lactide-co-glycolide) nanospheres loaded with chloro(5,10,15,20- tetraphenyl-porphyrinato)indium(III). J Nanosci Nanotechnol. 2011;11(6):5234-46. DOI: 10.1166/jnn.2011.4136

[21] Sah E, Sah H. Recent trends in preparation of poly(lactide-co-glycolide) nanoparticles by mixing polymeric organic solution with antisolvent. J Nanomater. 2015;2015: 1-22. DOI: 10.1155/2015/794601

[22] Da Silva AR, Zaniquelli MED, Baratti MO, Jorge RA. Drug release from microspheres and nanospheres of poly(lactide-co- glycolide) without sphere separation from the release medium. J Braz Chem Soc. 2010;21(2):214-25. DOI: 10.1590/S0103-50532010000200005

[23] Saraf S. Process optimization for the production of nanoparticles for drug delivery applications. Expert Opin Drug Deliv. 2009;6(2):187-96. DOI: 10.1517/17425240902735806

[24] Zhang H, Lu Y, Zhang G, Gao S, Sun D, Zhong Y. Bupivacaine-loaded biodegradable poly(lactic-co-glycolic) acid microspheres. I. Optimization of the drug incorporation into the polymer matrix and modelling of drug release. Int J Pharm. 2008;351(1-2):244-9. DOI: 10.1016/j.ijpharm.2007.10.004

[25] Javadzadeh Y, Ahadi F, Davaran S, Mohammadi G, Sabzevari A, Adibkia K. Preparation and physicochemical characterization of naproxen-PLGA nanoparticles. Colloids Surfaces B Biointerfaces [Internet]. 2010;81(2): 498-502. DOI:10.1016/j.colsurfb.2010.07.047

[26] Sashmal S, Mukherjee S, Ray S, Thakur R, Ghosh L, Gupta B. Design and optimization of NSAID loaded nanoparticles. Pak J Pharm Sci. 2007;20(2):157-62. PMDI: 17416573

[27] Galindo-Rodriguez S, Allemann E, Fessi H, Doelker E. Physicochemical parameters associated with nanoparticle formation in the salting out, emulsification-diffusion, and nanoprecipitation methods. Pharm Res. 2004;21(8):1428-1439. DOI: 10.1023/B:PHAM.0000036917.75634.be

[28] Ganea GM, Sabliov CM, Ishola AO, Fakayode SO, Wagner IM. Experimental design and multivariate analysis for optimizing poly(D,L-lactide-co-glycolide) (PLGA) nanoparticles synthesis using molecular micelles. J Nanosci Nanotechnol. 2008;8(1):280-292. DOI: 10.1166/jnn.2008.011

[29] Fanchiotti BG, Machado MPZ, de Paula LC, Durmuş M, Nyokong T, Gonçalves A da S, et al. The photobleaching of the free and encapsulated metallic phthalocyanine and its effect on the photooxidation of simple molecules. J Photochem Photobiol B Biol. 2016;165:10-23. DOI: 10.1016/j.jphotobiol.2016.10.007

[30] Lochmann A, Nitzsche H, von Einem S, Schwarz E, Mader K. The influence of covalently linked and free polyethylene glycol on the structured and release properties of rhBMP-2 loaded microspheres. J Control Release. 2010;147(1):92-100. DOI: 10.1016/j.jconrel.2010.06.021

[31] Sahoo SK, Panyam J, Prabha S, Labhasetwar V. Residual polyvinyl alcohol associated with poly (D,L-lactide-co-glycolide) nanoparticles affects their physical properties and cellular uptake. J Control Release. 2002;82:105-114. DOI: 10.1016/S0168-3659(02)00127-X

[32] Riley T, Govender T, Stolnik S, Xiong CD, Garnett MC, Illum L, Davis SS. Colloidal stability and drug incorporation aspects of micellar-like PLA-PEG nanoparticles. Colloids Surf B-Biointerfaces. 1999;16(1-4):147-159. DOI: 10.1016/S0927-7765(99)00066-1

[33] Hawley AE, Illum L, Davis SS. Preparation of biodegradable, surface engineered PLGA nanospheres with enhanced lymphatic drainage and lymph node uptake. Pharm Res. 1997;14:657-661. DOI: 10.1023/A:1012117531448

[34] Tobio M, Gref R, Sanchez A, Langer R, Alonso MJ. Stealth PLA- PEG nanoparticles as protein carriers for nasal administration. Pharm Res. 1998;15:270-275. DOI: 10.1023/A:1011922819926

[35] Hamoudeh M, Salim H, Barbos D, Paunoiu C, Fessi H. Preparation and characterization of radioactive dirhenium decacarbonyl-loaded PLLA nanoparticles for radionuclide intra-tumoral therapy. Eur J Pharm Biopharm. 2007;67(3):597-611. DOI: 10.1016/j.ejpb.2007.04.003

[36] James NS, Cheruku RR, Missert JR, Sunar U, Pandey RK. Measurement of cyanine dye photobleaching in photosensitizer cyanine dye conjugates could help in optimizing light dosimetry for improved photodynamic therapy of cancer. Molecules. 2018;23(8):1-11. DOI: 10.3390/molecules23081842

[37] Bonnett R, Martinez G. Photobleaching of sensitisers used in photodynamic therapy. Tetrahedron. 2001;57(47):9513-47. DOI: 10.1016/S0040-4020(01)00952-8

[38] Garcia AM, Alarcon E, Munoz M, Scaiano JC, Edwards AM, Lissi E. Photophysical behavior and photodynamic activity of zinc phthalocyanines associated to liposomes. Photochem Photobiol Sci. 2011;10:507-514. DOI: 10.1039/c0pp00289e

[39] Ishii K. Functional singlet oxygen generators based on phthalocyanines. Coord Chem Rev. 2012;256:1556-1568. DOI: 10.1016/j.ccr.2012.03.022

[40] Koziar JC, Cowan DO. Photo-chemical heavy-atom effects. Acc Chem

Res. 1978;11:334-341. DOI: 10.1021/ar50129a003

[41] Durmuş M, Erdoğmuş A, Ogunsipe A, Nyokong T. The synthesis and photophysicochemical behaviour of novel water-soluble cationic indium(III) phthalocyanine. Dyes Pigments. 2009;82:244-250. DOI: 10.1016/j.dyepig.2009.01.008

[42] Nyokong T. Effects of substituients on the photochemical and photophysical properties of main group metal phthalocyanines. Coord Chem Rev. 2007;251:1707-1722. DOI: 10.1016/j.ccr.2006.11.011

[43] Jori G. The molecular biology of photodynamic action. In: Pratesi R., Sacchi CA., editors. Lasers in Photomedicine and Photobiology. Springer Series in Optical Sciences, vol 22. Springer: Berlin; 1980. p. 58-66. DOI: 10.1007/978-3-540-38270-6_6

[44] Wilkinson F, Brummer JG. Rate constants for the decay and reactions of the lowest electronically excited singlet state of molecular oxygen in solution. J Phys Chem Ref Data. 1981;10:809. DOI: 10.1063/1.555655

[45] Durmuş M, Nyokong T. Synthesis, photophysical and photochemical properties of aryloxy tetra-substituted gallium and indium phthalocyanine derivatives. Tetrahedron. 2007;63(6): 1385-94. DOI: 10.1016/j.tet.2006.11.089